ENGENDERING MIGRANT HEALTH: CANADIAN PERSPECTIVES

Edited by Denise L. Spitzer

A number of studies have shown that on arrival newcomers to Canada are, on average, generally healthier than native-born Canadians. However, research also indicates that after ten years in the country they experience poorer health, including higher rates of chronic disease, than those born in Canada. Migrant women – particularly those from non-European countries – experience the most precipitous decline in health. What contributes to this deterioration, and how can it be mitigated?

Engendering Migrant Health brings together researchers from across Canada to address these and other issues at the intersections of gender, immigration, and health in the lives of new Canadians. Situating their work within the context of Canadian policy and society, the contributors illuminate migrants' testimonies of struggle, resistance, and solidarity as they negotiate a place for themselves in a new country. Topics range from the difficulties of francophone refugees and the changing roles of fathers, to the experiences of undocumented migrants and queer newcomers. Throughout the volume the contributors stress the importance of social solidarity to community and individual health.

DENISE L. SPITZER is the Canada Research Chair in Gender, Migration, and Health and an associate professor at the Institute of Women's Studies, University of Ottawa.

EDITED BY DENISE L. SPITZER

Engendering Migrant Health

Canadian Perspectives

UNIVERSITY OF TORONTO PRESS
Toronto Buffalo London

© University of Toronto Press 2011
Toronto Buffalo London
www.utppublishing.com
Printed in Canada

ISBN 978-0-8020-9836-8 (cloth)
ISBN 978-0-8020-9562-6 (paper)

Printed on acid-free, 100% post-consumer recycled paper with
vegetable-based inks.

Library and Archives Canada Cataloguing in Publication

Engendering migrant health : Canadian perspectives / edited by
Denise L. Spitzer.

Includes bibliographical references and index.
ISBN 978-0-8020-9836-8 (bound).   ISBN 978-0-8020-9562-6 (pbk.)

1. Immigrants – Health and hygiene – Canada.   2. Women immigrants –
Health and hygiene – Canada.   3. Women refugees – Health and hygiene
– Canada.   4. Immigrants – Canada – Social conditions.   5. Refugees –
Canada – Social conditions.   I. Spitzer, Denise L.

RA450.3.E54 2011   362.1086'9120971   C2011-905346-2

This book has been published with the help of a grant from the Canadian
Federation for the Humanities and Social Sciences, through the Aid to
Scholarly Publications Program, using funds provided by the Social
Sciences and Humanities Research Council of Canada.

University of Toronto Press acknowledges the financial assistance to its
publishing program of the Canada Council for the Arts and the Ontario
Arts Council.

 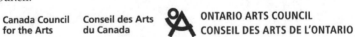

University of Toronto Press acknowledges the financial support of the
Government of Canada through the Canada Book Fund for its publishing
activities.

This book is dedicated
in memory of
Michèle Kérisit
colleague, feminist, and friend

Contents

Part 2: The Sequelae of Suffering

Part 3: Communities, Social Capital, Empowerment, and Resilience

Part 4: Conclusion

Acknowledgments

A collected work such as this one requires the respect, trust, and patience of multiple authors and editors. I am grateful to the talented and compassionate individuals who have shared their work in this volume. We are all indebted to our informants, the women and men who shared their stories with us, and hope that our analyses and perspectives have done justice to their experiences.

I wish to offer special thanks to Michèle Kérisit for her insights and support, to Virgil Duff for his patience, expertise, and enthusiasm for the project, and to the three anonymous reviewers for their insightful and constructive comments. Thanks as well to Joanna Laskey, Luisa Wang, and Kaoutar Kaddouri for their editorial assistance.

Lastly, I would like to thank Michel Arpin, my first reader and best friend: *Merci beaucoup,* tender comrade.

ENGENDERING MIGRANT HEALTH:
CANADIAN PERSPECTIVES

1 Introduction

DENISE L. SPITZER

Is migrating to Canada bad for your health? Perhaps the surprising answer for some is ...'Yes.' While popular wisdom may presume that immigrants from poorer nations come to enjoy a better health care system, more advanced control of infectious diseases, a high standard of sanitation, safer working environments, better quality housing and water in Canada, all of which should contribute to better health standards than in their countries of origin, newcomers who reside in this country for longer than a decade often report a decline in health status. Although this trend is repeated in a variety of immigrant-receiving countries, disaggregating the epidemiological data that gave rise to these observations creates a more complex picture of this phenomenon (Llácer et al. 2007; see also Hyman, this volume). The healthy immigrant effect – so-called, as persons who choose to make migratory journeys tend to be in better health than the native-born populace (Hyman 2007; Newbold 2005b; Ng et al. 2005) – appears to be short-lived, with some immigrants reporting a deterioration of health status the longer they reside in their new homeland (Hyman 2007a; Newbold 2005b; Ng et al. 2005). Notably, non-European immigrants are twice as likely to report declining health status as their counterparts from European countries (Ng et al. 2005).

Within a biomedical context, poor health status is often attributable to deleterious health behaviours such as smoking and excessive alcohol consumption; however, non-European migrants are less likely than the Canadian-born populace to take up these activities (Dunn and Dyck 2000; Ng et al. 2005). Moreover, while newcomers are slightly less active than native-born Canadians, European immigrants who are less vulnerable to experiencing a decline in health status are the group that reports the lowest levels of physical activity (Ng et al. 2005). In addition to their global region of origin, other factors including education, socio-economic class, marital status, official language skills, time of migration, and access to social support contribute to disparate health trajectories. Higher education and income, the ability to communicate in English or French, a spousal relationship, and the presence of a support network appear to militate against this decline of health status (Dunn and Dyck 2000; Newbold 2005b; Ng et al. 2005; Pottie, Ng et al. 2008).

Importantly, gender figures prominently when examining the loss of the healthy immigrant effect. In Canada, women, particularly those from non-European source countries, are most likely to report the steepest decline in self-rated health status compared to other foreign and native-born women and men (Vissandjée et al. 2004; Ng et al. 2005). Further analysis is needed to unpack the healthy immigrant effect – and its apparent loss – that attends to and accounts for both the heterogeneity of gendered, classed, and racialized disparities, and dynamism of this trend.

This book brings together researchers working across Canada to illuminate the complex, gendered dimensions of immigrant, migrant, and refugee health – included here under the rubric of migrant health. Importantly, we situate our work within the context of Canadian policies and society, that is to say, the historical specificities that impact current political and social relations and policy making, and have helped produce the unique profile of Canadian society that newcomers encounter upon arrival. Immigration, social protection, and health care policies help contour the social landscape by forging boundaries of inclusion and exclusion that new Canadians are required to navigate. The voices of immigrants and refugees in Canada are woven throughout the subsequent chapters, offering testimonies of struggle, resistance, and solidarity as individuals and communities negotiate a place for themselves on Canadian territory. Moreover, this collection offers insights into an array of gender issues ranging from changing fatherhood roles and the challenges of gay, lesbian, and bisexual immigrants and refugees to women's trauma narratives and the importance of social solidarity to communal and individual health.

Before offering a brief overview of Canadian immigration and relevant health policies to contextualize the readings in this book, I attempt to critically unpack some of the predominant terms used in discussions of gender, health, and immigration. Thereafter, I summarize some of the dominant issues confronting immigrants, migrants, and refugees in Canada and consider how social location impacts these experiences. Finally, an overview of the book is prefaced by a description of intersectionality and our efforts to continue to operationalize it in our research and analysis.

A Word about Language

Before embarking on our further exploration of migrant health, it is necessary to complicate the meanings of various keywords and concepts that are central to this work. These include the terms *gender, race, visible minority, immigrant,* and *health* (cf. Vissandjée et al. 2007).

Gender

In its perhaps most common and most basic usage, gender is 'regarded as the socially ascribed attributes and roles assigned to the biological categories of, at minimum, the dichotomous pairing of male and female' (Spitzer 2005:80), while sex refers to the biogenetic underpinnings of male and female characteristics in anatomy and physiology (Spitzer 2006). Descriptions such as these invariably freeze-frame dynamic concepts reducing the ability for language to capture not only their complexity, fluidity, and diversity, but also the considerations of hierarchy and power that further inform them (Llácer et al. 2007). Neither sex nor gender is a stable concept nor are they evidence of fixed, 'natural' difference; instead, both are social constructions that may vary across time, socio-economic, geographical, religious, and ethnic boundaries, continuously recreated through performance, and subject to negotiation. The meanings and expectations of gender are expressed through gender ideologies that interact with socio-economic class, ethnicity, sexuality, geography, dis/ability, religion, and age, among other social indicators, to shape social hierarchies and structure access to determinants of health. Moreover, they shore up social disparities through appeals to the fixed and 'natural' nature of sex and gender differences (Mahler and Pessar 2001; Spitzer 2006).

From a population health framework that is meant to inform health and social policies in Canada, health is defined not as the absence of disease, but as the outcome of mutually influential determinants, including socio-economic status, social support, education, employment, both social and economic environments, health behaviours and personal coping skills, health services, gender, and culture (NFH 1997). Importantly, individuals are situated in the dominant social hierarchy as the outcome of the constellation of social indicators of which they are inscribed, resulting in differential exposures to deleterious physical and social effects (Doyal 2002; Spitzer 2005). Neither uniform policies and programs nor a focus solely on health care services provide sufficient theoretical or practical coverage to address health writ large. Efforts to address social and economic inequities, environmental degradation, human rights, and poverty are potentially important interventions to improve the health and well-being of a population (WHO 2006a).

Race

Authors in this text refrain from employing the term *race*, or employing race labels (*Caucasian*, *Oriental*, etc.) without complicating their use of those terms. Race labels are grounded in the presumption that sets of morphological differences among human beings (i.e., hair type, skin pigmentation, stature, etc.) can be collated and categorized under the rubric of four major races. From the time the eighteenth-century Swedish botanist Linaeus (Carl von Linné) introduced the scientific classification of human races, racial differences were imbued with judgments about the moral character and intelligence of each group, with Caucasians described in the most laudable terms (Smedley 1993). Gender figured in the construction of racialized differences producing a disparate range of expectations of roles and behaviour that reinforced stereotypes and which were themselves reinforced by scientific authority (Smedley 1993; Schiebinger 1999). Indeed, disaggregating human beings into disparate and rigid racial categories, a process that was informed by and which helped to further inform colonialism and its aftermaths, has relied on reputed scientific authority to transform race into a scientific 'fact' (Smedley 1993; Graves 2001; Li 2001; Grosfugel 2004).

Although anthropologists such as Franz Boas argued against the scientific validity of race in the early twentieth century, in more recent years geneticists, biologists, and other scientists, including those involved with the Human Genome Project, have likewise concluded that race is a flawed concept and lacking in scientific validity (Graves 2001; Duster 2003; Vissandjée, Hyman et al. 2007). Employing race labels in data collection can only work to reify race and racialized differences. Moreover, the diversity extant within these categories is erased in favour of a more homogeneous image, with little consideration given as to how individuals and groups identify themselves in terms of their origins and affiliation (Plaza 2004; Spitzer 2008). Li (2001) defines the racialization process as one that involves the assignation of social worth and social meaning to each racial category. To foreground the social process that is fundamentally entwined with race discourse, the term *racialized categories* is used throughout this text.

The lack of scientific legitimacy exposes race as a social concept rather than a reflection of biological fact. As a social concept that has relied on scientific authority to discipline racialized populations and provide a rationale for social hierarchy and its various manifestations such as colonialism and slavery, race can also serve as an important identity label and a space for forging solidarity and community (Duster 2003; Spitzer 2008). Notably a reduction or the elimination of the use of the term *race* does not lead to the reduction or elimination of racism. Indeed, systemic racism, embedded in institutions and reflective of dominant values that inform procedures, processes, and expectations (often read as 'common sense') disregards the role of social identifiers (gender, class, etc.) in the creation of social inequalities (Essed 1991; Anderson and Reimer Kirkham 1998; Li 2001). Furthermore, racializing processes help underscore the worthiness and unworthiness of individuals and groups of individuals who can be linked to the nation state through citizenship (Ong 2003).

Visible Minority

A related term, *visible minority*, also requires unpacking. Carty and Brand (1993) situate the uptake of this descriptor in the hands of the Canadian government. Used to speak to the apparently commonly shared experiences of racism, the application of a visible-minority label inevitably denies the unique, historically shaped relations between groups of people that inform experiences of racism and marginalization (Carty and Brand 1993). That said, the critical deployment of visible-minority status can speak to the ways in which individuals are relegated to racialized categories, how they respond to this assignation, and the consequences thereof; however, the contingencies of the term, including the masking of wide diversity of experiences and opportunities, must be made evident (Spitzer 2004).

Refugee/Migrant/Immigrant

The terms *refugee, migrant,* and *immigrant* are generally distinguished by the degree of voluntariness with regards to the decision to emigrate and by the long-term intentions of those attached to these labels to settle in a new country. Citizenship and Immigration Canada (2008a) categorizes newcomers as (1) economic immigrants which includes skilled and business immigrants, live-in caregivers, provincial/territorial nominees and their immediate family members, (2) family class immigrants – spouses/partners, dependent children, parents, and grandparents – and (3) refugees: government or privately-sponsored persons who, fearing persecution, sought asylum in Canada. Refugee claimants, persons who apply for asylum upon or after their arrival in Canada, constitute another subgroup of Canada's foreign-born population (CIC 2008a).

Refugees, who are regarded as the most involuntary of newcomers, are often homogenized into a singular, uneducated, and unskilled mass. For refugees, temporary resettlement in a receiving country may well transform into more permanent residency if the situation in one's home country remains intolerable and/or if their lives built on Canadian soil become more compelling. Migrants refer to those who move temporarily, primarily for work; while the term may refer to movement within the boundaries of a nation state, it is also used to describe those who cross international borders. Temporary foreign workers or labour migrants may well enter the country with the intention of remaining, and, depending upon the temporary worker program in which they entered the country, there could be such opportunities. At times, the term *migrant* is employed to include both voluntary migrants (immigrants) and involuntary migrants (refugees). Importantly, the formal definitions of these terms are often supplanted by more flexible usage of the terms *immigrant* and *migrant* that are often used interchangeably in popular discourse and may further include refugee claimants and undocumented workers. Due to their elasticity and potential disparities between juridical and popular definitions, attention must therefore be paid to these terms to see how these categories are defined and deployed. Indeed, in a collection of this nature, it is difficult to impose a fixed definition given the range of approaches in the use of primary and/or secondary data and differences in foci from lived experience to statistical analyses.

The category under which a migrant enters the country determines not only her or his ability to become a permanent resident, but also structures access to auxiliary health services, education, and settlement services that are meant to assist with their settlement and integration into Canadian society. The assignation of one of these labels, therefore, has important consequences for individuals, their families, and their communities in terms of access to rights, programs, and services. The boundaries, however, between these three categories (immigrant, migrant, and refugee) are fragile and there is considerable slippage between them. For instance, even when political crises compel the out-migration of the population, some may secure employment and enter a safe country as an immigrant rather than refugee. Furthermore, when families emigrate, the decision to do so may not be equally shared; therefore some may be 'involuntary' voluntary migrants.

In essence, the neat divisions among the categories of refugee, migrant, and immigrant belie a much messier reality and much more heterogeneity than had previously been allowed. Lastly, the deployment of ethno-racial terminology may exoticize or 'Other' those cast under these appellations, contributing to the use of 'culture' or 'tradition' as explanations for poor health outcomes wherein cultural groups are collectively and individually held responsible for their own misfortune by clinging in part to their cultural 'eccentricities.' These cultural explanations only serve to mask issues of poverty and socio-economic class (Farmer 1999).

The legacy of migration persists beyond a fixed time period. Newcomers to Canada must reside in the country for three years as permanent residents before they are eligible to apply for citizenship; however, in terms of lived experience, the transition from newcomer to Canadian may proceed at another pace. Statistics Canada, for instance, broadly defines all foreign-born residents as immigrants, distinguishing amongst subgroups by their length of residency in the country; therefore, one can be regarded as an immigrant all one's life. In reality, the immigrant label is more difficult for some to efface, particularly for foreign-born Canadians from non-European countries who are reduced to the most basic of phenotypic characteristics that serve as the basis for their Othering by members of dominant Euro-Canadian society (Spitzer 2004, 2008). Furthermore, studies of second-generation immigrants of colour implicate the role that structural racism plays in constraining social mobility and sustaining social exclusion (Kazemipur and Halli 2001), suggesting that persons of colour are more apt to bear the label of 'immigrant' and henceforth be Othered even if they are Canadian-born.

Situating Canadian Immigration

Returning to the context of this book, concern over Canada's declining population size, the global quest for transnational talent, family reunification, and response to humanitarian concerns are among the visible factors that have informed Canadian immigration policy (Ley and Hiebert 2001; Bannerji 2004; Green and Green 2004). The subtext of immigration policy, however, has at times included a focus on building and maintaining a white, settler society as evidenced most definitively by decidedly racist policies that at various times excluded: Chinese migrants through both the imposition of a head tax that rendered the journey too costly for many and later an outright ban; South Asians in the early twentieth century hoping to enter Canada who were confronted with near-impossible demands that their tickets be purchased in Canada and that they travel non-stop from their homeland; and European Jews who were prohibited from entering the country prior to the outbreak of the Second World War (Abella and Troper 1982; Wickberg 1982; Das Gupta 1994; Jakubowski 1997; Dua 2000). The introduction of a point system in 1967 ostensibly opened up Canada to qualified newcomers based on apparently objective criteria such as profession, work experience, and personal suitability; however, economic interests took precedence and greater efforts were made to attract investors and entrepreneurs to this country to stimulate further economic growth (Green and Green 2004; Jones 2004). As immigration policies became more liberal, citizenship conversely became more restrictive (Sharma 2001). In addition, discourses of diversity and multiculturalism have become increasingly familiar codes for describing – and managing – the presence of 'non-whites' in Canadian society (Li 2001; Castles 2002).

Local, regional, and world contexts have had an impact on immigration policies and realities. Thus while migration has been ongoing for centuries, the intensity, density, and breadth of contemporary global migration is a unique phenomenon (Castles 2002; Tastsoglou and Dobrowolsky 2006). Currently, much of the movement of people around the world is impelled by the forces of global capitalism effected through the neo-liberal principles and policies propagated by institutions such as the International Monetary Fund and the World Bank. Per the demands of these global financial institutions, poorer nations have restructured their economies by devaluing currencies, reducing social spending, and promoting privatization of public resources and shifting production towards export markets (Parreñas 2001; Jaggar 2002; Gunewardena and Kingsolver 2007).

Gendered roles and expectations figure prominently when the movement of peoples across the globe is considered. Approximately half of the world's 191 million migrants are women (Llácer et al. 2007.). As of 2006, Canada receives approximately 129,501 immigrant and refugee women and 122,146 immigrant and refugee men annually (CIC 2007). Approximately 70 per cent of principal applicants to Canada are male (CIC 2005); female members of their households are therefore regarded as dependants.

In recent years, the global demand for household labourers, caregivers, and domestic helpers has grown exponentially. The lure of potential opportunities and/or the pressure from family or peers compels increasing numbers of young women to emigrate. The resultant changes brought to the household and to family networks due to their absence destabilizes gendered notions of men as breadwinners and of women as the centre of home life. As Sassen (2000) indicates, women are increasingly engaged in an epiphenomenon of the institutions that facilitate economic globalization, global survival circuits that involve income-generating activities in the informal economy, that enable the flow of income, goods, and people across borders. Across the globe, women have become increasingly responsible for ensuring the survival of their families (Tastsoglou and Dobrowolsky 2006).

Immigration, Health Care, and Well-being in Canada

Newcomers to Canada are subject to medical surveillance and screening prior to being granted permission to settle in the country. Designated medical practitioners, under contract with Citizenship and Immigration Canada, perform a standardized medical examination and take a chest X-ray to screen for any medical conditions that would eliminate individuals who could potentially pose a public health risk or whose condition would create an excessive burden on the health care system (Gushulak and Williams 2004; CIC 2009a). Notably, all dependents are obliged to undergo medical screening regardless of whether they intend to emigrate with the applicant. Medical practitioners may discuss health issues arising from the examination, but not the outcome of the examination itself (CIC 2009a).

Once in the country, newcomers have access to the Canadian health care system. The Canada Health Act underpins the structure of the Canadian health care system and enshrines its five major pillars: universality, portability, accessibility, comprehensive coverage, and public administration (Wilson 1995). All legal residents are eligible for health care services upon attaining a provincial health care insurance card, although access to those services may differ depending on immigration status, geographic location, and occupational status that may constrain workers' ability to take time off for services or recuperation, among other factors (Spitzer et al. 2003; Varcoe, Hankivsky, and Morrow 2007).

Immigrants and refugees may find themselves with disparate access to health care services depending on their province of residence. While refugees receive immediate access to health services through the Interim Federal Health Program, four provinces – British Columbia, Ontario, New Brunswick, and Québec – impose a three-month waiting period for new arrivals to become eligible for a provincial health care insurance card (CIC 2009b). Newcomers are encouraged to purchase coverage from a private insurer during this period (CIC 2009b). The ability of new arrivals to afford private insurance in addition to the considerable expense of immigration and resettlement is in many cases questionable. Moreover, once eligible for provincial health care insurance, coverage for some services does not extend to permanent residents, nor are all procedures covered in each province, leading to a much more irregular pattern of insurance coverage than might be evident from the claims for universality.

Despite the circulating stereotype to the contrary, immigrants and refugees in Canada tend to underutilize health services (Guruge, Donner, and Morrison 2000). Language barriers and lack of knowledge about health care services are frequently cited as barriers to immigrant and refugee health (Guruge, Donner, and Morrison 2000; Stewart, Anderson et al. 2008); however, broader, more subtle matters are also potent factors in the uptake of health services. Health care institutions are imbued with and are reflective of dominant neo-liberal, capitalist ideology and the prevailing discursive constructions of gender, nation, racialization, and health (Anderson and Reimer Kirkham 1998; Spitzer 2004). As a result, foreign-born individuals and those who are otherwise marginalized in Canadian society may find themselves Othered in the face of standardized policies, procedures, and discourses. In addition, the focus on individual behaviours and risk factors, and notions of personal responsibility for health prevention, maintenance, and recovery, not only operate to brand the Others as receptacles of risk (Ong 2003) and marginalize those unable to afford self-care and supplementary medications and devices, but also contrast with official discourse in Canada that asserts that social determinants of health, in particular gender, poverty, and migration status, are powerfully implicated in health status and outcomes (Anderson and Reimer Kirkham 1998; Thurston and Vissandjée 2005).

Still, research and discussion about immigrant health is often narrowed to considerations of immigrant *health care*. Similarly, the complexity and heterogeneity of persons and experiences that are collected under the rubrics of immigrant, migrant, or refugee, demand a more nuanced and complicated approach to understanding migrant health.

Engendering Migrant Health: An Overview

Social location, the dynamic outcome of intersectionality, shapes the way individuals perceive the world and in turn are perceived by others. I employ the term *engendering* to refer to efforts to make visible the implications of intersectionality (not just gender) and social location on health and well-being. The kinetic instability and heterogeneity of our social landscape creates a complex picture that cannot be adequately addressed given the relative solidity that language can impose. While we must remain cognizant of the slipperiness of labels and social categories – and the diversity contained therein – there are some commonalities shared amongst peoples identified as migrants, immigrants, or refugees that I will summarize here, but which will be elaborated upon in subsequent chapters. These issues include marginalization, livelihood and socio-economic status, identity, and social capital/social support.

Marginalization

A newcomer is not a tabula rasa, a blank slate awaiting the inscription of new life-ways and a new path. Instead, newcomers and Canadian residents alike are embedded in a nexus of long-term, political-economic relations and histories, constituting social hierarchies that haunt current relationships, help construct perspectives of the Other, and contribute to social exclusion. While ethnic affiliation situates newcomers in the social landscape, the association with ethnicity and female gender can be more inflexible than for male counterparts. As the members of society most often charged with the enculturation of subsequent generations and with the maintenance of ethnic boundaries by embodying cultural tradition and mores, women are often under surveillance from themselves and others to ensure they are enacting these appropriately gendered roles (Yuval-Davis 1997a; Spitzer, Neufeld et al. 2003).

While carrying out these roles may be satisfying, in the Canadian context at least, they may have implications for health and well-being. For instance, wearing a hijab may at times be an obstacle to employment for some Muslim women (VanderPlaat 2007). Thus while religious practice and community can provide an important place of communion and support for foreign-born women, marginalization due to one's religious affiliation may still lead to subsequent disappointments and potential barriers to income generation that themselves have potential health impacts (see also Spitzer, chapter 2, this volume). The inability to speak English or French also contributes to marginalization and isolation; notably, refugee women are less likely to be able to communicate in one of our official languages (VanderPlaat 2007). Even when newcomers are eligible for language training, women are most apt to be constrained in their ability to partake due to their household responsibilities, in particular pertaining to caregiving (VanderPlaat 2007). Among foreign-born Canadians, poor French or English language skills are associated with poor self-rated health, and women are most implicated in this trend (Pottie et al. 2008).

The intersections of racialized categorization and gender are also reflected in the marginalization of men – in particular communities including Arabic, Muslim, and African Caribbean – who confront circulating stereotypes as violent patriarchs or as in the case of the latter as laid-back (read 'lazy') Lotharios. Finally, as O'Neill and Sproule (chapter 4, this volume) demonstrate, gay, lesbian, and bisexual immigrants, migrants, and refugees are vulnerable both to homophobia within their own ethnocultural communities, and to the triumvirate of sexism, racism, and homophobia from Canadian society at large.

Livelihood and Socio-economic Status

Immigration has a significant impact on one's livelihood – one's occupation, subsistence, social and socio-economic status, and gender roles that proscribe attitudes towards and aptitudes for work and the organization of the household around work. Lack of recognition of foreign credentials is a widespread and contentious challenge to the value of newcomers' experience and education, precipitating a downward spiral that can lead to poverty and disappointments that have identifiable health impacts (Guruge, Donner, and Morrison 2000; Spitzer, Neufeld, and Bitar 2000; Grant 2005; Schellenberg and Maheux 2007). Professional associations and other regulatory bodies deploy gatekeeping functions that secure the most desirable jobs for the Canadian-educated and Canadian-born (Bauder 2003). Negative assumptions about the value of education and work experience from certain regions are evidence of the discrimination faced by many immigrants of colour (Grant 2005; Teelucksingh and Galabuzi 2005a). As a result, the likelihood of being poor is 50 per cent higher for immigrants to Canada than for the population at large, and is an outcome even more likely for newcomers from non-European source countries (Kazemipur and Halli 2001). Even though skilled workers enter the country because of their education and work experience, the 'devaluation of institutional cultural capital' (Bauder 2003:708) that is effected through state and professional actors often acts as an effective barrier to continuing in previous careers. Deskilling, the loss of mastery and confidence in one's skills over time, is a common occurrence. As a result, Bannerji (2004) suggests, the Canadian working class is over-educated. Dobrowolsky and Tastsoglou (2006) assert that women are particularly susceptible to the condition of brain waste; that is, the loss of employment, remuneration, and challenge commensurate with their education and work experience. Rejection of international credentials and experience leads to disappointment, anger, frustration, bitterness, and stress. For many, these experiences are embedded in 'everyday racism ... the integration of racism into everyday situations ... that activate[s] underlying power relations' (Essed 1991:50) and reinforces social exclusion.

Although men also encounter similar problems with foreign credentials, and although many newcomers simply resign themselves to downward mobility, at least in the short term, if a household is planning to invest in further education for one of its members, the likelihood is that benefit will accrue to a male while women tend to take on and remain in so-called 'survival jobs' (VanderPlaat 2007). Moreover, foreign-born women are less likely to be employed in positions that are commensurate with their occupational and educational background, even though they are as a whole better educated than their Canadian-born counterparts (Chard, Badets, and Howatson-Leo 2000).

Downward social mobility, living in poverty, and disillusionment with one's life can have discernible health effects associated with economic deprivation as well as the impacts of chronic stress (Danso 2001; Krieger, Chen, and Selby 2001; Bauder 2003; see also chapter 2, this volume).

Identity

Identity can be regarded as a resource, a 'strategy for everyday life' (Castles 2002:1158), a process or a space where a network of individuals who share meaning and from which other individuals are rendered abject. Notably 'identity is neither singular nor is it a fixed category, but is instead one that is constantly in the state of creation, maintenance and reconfiguration' (Spitzer 2007:54). Identity can offer ballast against the assaults of a hostile environment or solace in an indifferent one. Even as religious, cultural, sexual, ethnic, or gendered identity can be responded to with discrimination, they are also important sources of strength and support that can mitigate the negative impact of marginalization (Tastsoglou and Dobrowolsky 2006; Spitzer 2007).

Social Capital/Social Support

Social support is critical to health and well-being, and the loss and reconfiguration of social support has important consequences for the health and integration experiences of new Canadians (Simich, Beiser, and Mawani 2003; Stewart, Anderson et al. 2008). Simich, Beiser, and Mawani (2003) reported that the lack of meaningful, supportive relations contributed to ill health among their refugee informants in Ontario. In contrast, newcomers who are able to recreate social networks and provide and receive social support are likely to report better health (Dunn and Dyck 2000; Stewart et al. 2008). Importantly, while immigration may result in the fracturing of social networks, it also provides opportunities for women in particular to transgress gender roles and create new subjectivities for themselves (Dobrowlsky and Tastoglou 2006).

Towards an Intersectional Analysis

Persistent and increasing inequities within the category of 'women' or 'men' are challenging scholars, organizations, policy makers, and advocates to recognize and engage in research that explores multiple axes of difference, recognizing that this approach is not optional, but central to any comprehensive attempt to understand health inequities (Hankivsky 2005, 2007; Krieger et al. 1993; Spitzer 2004; Varcoe, Hankivsky, and Morrow 2007; Whittle and Inhorn 2001; Zoller 2005). The authors in this volume take up the challenge of operationalizing intersectional analysis; that is, attending to the ways in which individuals and communities experience the world from a particular social location forged via the mutually constitutive interactions of various social indicators.

Gender interacts with other social markers such as ethnicity/'race,' socio-economic class, sexuality, religion, and migration status to form hierarchies of inclusion and exclusion that criss-cross our social landscape (Thurston and Vissandjée 2005). Social location offers and constrains access to social and material goods, identities, opportunities, and power.

In recent years, gender-based analysis (GBA) has been promoted and embraced by organizations, including the Government of Canada (see CIC 2005; Spitzer 2006), as a means of assessing the complexities of risks and resiliencies determined by social location as read through the indicators of sex and gender. Instead of presuming that all persons respond uniformly to disease, interventions, and policies, GBA sought to unpack the complex, interlocking components and contexts that contribute to gender hierarchy and demands consideration of these factors in research, policy, and practice (Eichler 2001). GBA is further informed by diversity analysis that includes attention to the social and economic factors that intersect with gender to produce disparate health outcomes, and to health needs of a population characterized by cultural, sexual, geographic, age, and ability diversity (Coleman 2003; Spitzer 2006; Women's Health Bureau 2003). Importantly, these factors are interlinking and fluid, and cannot be treated as discrete variables (Zoller 2005).

For instance, 'the Canadian Research Institute for the Advancement of Women believes that different approaches are needed to make real social and economic change – approaches that offer diverse contributions, and that work from Intersectional Feminist Frameworks (IFF)' (CRIAW 2006:6). A focus on intersectional analysis moves beyond the most basic application of GBA, which privileges gender as an analytical entry point and allows us to 'examine how factors including socio-economic status, race, class, gender, sexualities, ability, geographic location, refugee and immigrant status combine with broader historical and current systems of discrimination such as colonialism and globalization to *simultaneously* determine inequalities among individuals and groups' (Krieger et al. 1993: 5). Emerging from critiques that have highlighted the heterogeneity of women's and men's experiences as well as the problematic nature of the dichotomous pairings of male and female, intersectional analysis attends to the dynamic interactions among gender and other social markers that situates individuals and communities in the social landscape viewed in terms of a matrix of domination where position determines access to power and other resources, rather than ladders representing a fixed hierarchy (Browne, Smye, and Varcoe 2007; Weber and Parra-Medina 2003).

Overview of This Book

This text is divided into four sections. Part 1, Situating Migration, Gender, and Health in Canada, includes four chapters that examine issues that cut across communities. In chapter 2, Spitzer proposes that we give greater attention to the body as the site of our experience and apprehension of the world to enrich the more familiar health determinants framework. She argues that the concept of stress expressed in terms of work, weariness, and worries, carries valence in both perspectives and opens up avenues for collective action, policy development, and program implementation. In chapter 3, Kérisit examines the health and well-being of francophone women of colour. In Canada, language is a highly charged issue, and for minority francophones language can be both a source of discrimination and a potential site of social network formation and solidarity. The complex interactions of gender, ethnicity, and language and their influence on health further underscore the importance of intersectional analysis. In the following chapter, O'Neill and Sproule draw attention to the struggles of sexual minority migrants. Queer newcomers may confront homophobia within their own cultural communities and both racism and homophobia in mainstream Canadian society while contending with potentially disparate cultural constructions and expectations of lesbian, gay, and bisexual individuals (LGB). They argue that settlement services must sensitize themselves to the needs of LGB clientele in order to provide appropriate support services. Rounding off this section, in chapter 5, Este and Tachble offer insights into the impact of immigration on parenting, in particular, fathering roles. Focusing on Sudanese and Russian men, they determine that migrant men's inability to obtain remunerative work erodes their role as family providers. Moreover, as they undertake low-wage labour, they contend with time poverty that limits their interaction with their children and constrains their fathering roles.

In the four chapters that comprise Part 2, The Sequelae of Suffering, authors describe the potentially deleterious impacts of immigration and resettlement. In chapter 6, Hyman focuses attention on the vulnerability of immigrant and refugee women to mental health problems. Focusing on structural issues such as personal and systemic racism, Hyman advocates a more nuanced and socially contextualized approach to mental health issues. Thurston follows in chapter 7 with an overview of the challenges foreign-born women face with regard to intimate partner violence. She argues that the current discourse and array of services have the potential to contribute to foreign-born women's Othering and an increased sense of exclusion. In chapter 8, Simich explores the consequences of liminality, as experienced by undocumented workers, on health and well-being. While insecurity contributes to stress and its aftermath, Simich also indicates that there are opportunities for communion and solidarity as well that can help resolve their liminality. In the final chapter of this section, Dossa exhorts us to witness the embodied narratives of immigrant and refugee women. By grounding suffering within the geopolitical context in which it has emerged and flourished, the telling and active listening/witnessing of those narratives carries even greater significance.

In Part 3, Communities, Social Capital, Empowerment, and Resilience, authors highlight the ways in which newcomers to Canada, collectively and individually, work to mitigate the ill effects of uprooting and resettlement on foreign soil. In chapter 10, Ortiz and the Multicultural Health Brokers Co-op focus on equity, access to health, and the role of cultural brokers to facilitate this process. Highlighting the experiences of cultural brokers who are, generally speaking, much like their foreign-born client base, the authors describe the challenges posed by the multiple demands of gender roles and the importance of gender solidarity and informal social support, as embodied by the community-based cultural brokers, in mitigating their effects. In the subsequent chapter, Torres, Estable, Guerra, and Cermeño examine the impact of activities undertaken by a group of Latin American, community-based health workers in Ottawa on the community and on the workers themselves. These efforts enhance personal and communal empowerment and contribute to increased demands for equality and social justice. In chapter 12, Amaratunga and colleagues describe the activities of the Global Ottawa AIDS Link (GOAL), a collectivity of community members, academics, students, and government representatives that are interested in translating successful programs and approaches used in the global South to address HIV/AIDS among vulnerable populations, most notably foreign-born women in the global North. Due to members' commitment, this innovative 'un-project' has survived despite long periods without financial support and has often used innovative methods to promote HIV/AIDS awareness and prevention in a way that does not contribute to stigmatization. In the final chapter of this section, Vissandjée, Apale, and VanderPlaat provide an overview of social capital and what it means to immigrant and refugee women. They argue that newcomers need space for informal network formation in order to strengthen social capital and empower themselves and their communities.

In the concluding section, Part 4, I offer a reflection on the practical issues, theoretical insights, and policy implications that have emerged from this text.

Conclusion

The authors in this edited collection address the myriad ways in which social location, gender, sexuality, social support, and migration status interact to produce diverse and dynamic health outcomes. Indeed, migrating to Canada may be bad for the health of some foreign-born residents; however, addressing economic deprivation and social marginalization, contributing to the development of social capital, and making room for resilience and resistance, may help enhance the well-being of all new Canadians.

PART 1

Situating Migration, Gender, and Health
in Canada

2 Work, Worries, and Weariness: Towards an Embodied and Engendered Migrant Health

DENISE L. SPITZER

Introduction

What makes foreign-born women in Canada sick? This deceptively simple question underpins each of the selections in this book. In an effort to explore the impact of immigration on women's lived experiences and uncover the factors that contribute to both the maintenance and erosion of health and well-being, I suggest we focus attention on the body as both subject and object. In this chapter, I argue that this focal point can lead us towards an embodied and engendered perspective of immigrant health that can stimulate both theoretical insights and more efficacious interventions that are informed by and that attend to the lived experiences and social realities of targeted populations. To develop this argument, I draw from primary research, epidemiological evidence, and the growing body of literature on immigrant and refugee women and health, to describe how *work*, which includes paid and unpaid labour, *worry*, which I take as a particularly gendered task often pertaining to family and kin, and *weariness*, the response to the erosion of one's hopes and dreams, contribute to the deterioration of the health status of predominantly female migrants in the phenomenon known as the loss of the healthy immigrant effect.

To establish the context for this examination, I begin with brief overviews of immigration and integration in Canada, the population health framework, and notions of embodiment. Then, I introduce the three major categories of activities – work, worry, and weariness – that have an impact on the health and well-being of immigrant and refugee women in Canada and which will catalyse our unpacking of the loss of the healthy immigrant effect. Following, I revisit the two paradigms under consideration, population health and embodiment, in light of our observations of migrant women's lives in Canada. I suggest that these two conceptual frameworks can meet around the notion of stress that is reliant upon the permeability, if not outright erasure, of the boundary between mind and body. Importantly, the conceptual terrain of stress provides a pivot point where population health and embodiment can both engage, providing a potential outlet for bodily meanings to inform policies and programs that are also influenced by the population health framework.

Canadian Context

Canada is one of the most culturally diverse countries in the world, with over 18 per cent of its populace foreign-born (CIC 2005; Ng et al. 2005). Over 50 per cent of the 230,000 immigrants and refugees who enter Canada annually are women (CIC 2005; Ng et al. 2005). Nearly half originate in the Asia/Pacific region, another 20 per cent are from Africa or the Middle East, and 9 per cent were born in South or Central America (C1C 2005). (For further discussion see chapter 1, this volume.)

Newcomers are generally in better health than the average Canadian; however, some immigrants, particularly women from non-European countries, report a deterioration in health status after settling in Canada over the long term[1] (Ng et al. 2005; Vissandjée et al. 2004). This phenomenon, the loss of the healthy immigrant effect, has social, political, and economic implications for host societies, sending countries, and the individuals, households, social networks, polities, and identities that comprise the transnational traffic that characterizes our globalized world (see chapters 1 and 6, this volume, for further discussion).

Examining the Loss of the Healthy Immigrant Effect through Multiple Lenses

To unpack the loss of the healthy immigrant effect, I engage with two theoretical paradigms, embodiment and population health, that bring attention to the body in more or less obvious ways.

Population Health

The population health framework that informs Canadian health policy statements conceptualizes health as the consequence of a complex web of determinants that considers factors beyond individual health behaviours and access to health care to examine the impact of wider societal factors such as socio-economic status, gender, social support, social cohesion, living conditions, childhood development, learning opportunities, and work environment on health status (National Forum on Health 1997; Dunn and Dyck 2000; PHAC 2001; Anderson et al. 2003).

The loss of the healthy immigrant effect, therefore, can be viewed within the context of this framework. For example, Dunn and Dyck's (2000) analysis of the National Population Health Survey revealed that social determinants of health such as social support had a more significant impact on the well-being of foreign-born individuals, populations, and communities, than physical, biological, and material determinants. This association is highly salient as kin groups, familial relationships, and friendships are often fractured during the migratory process, resulting in smaller or non-existent social networks whose presence is vital to good self-reported health status (Stewart et al. 2008). Generally speaking, voluntary migrants experience a decline in socio-economic status upon their arrival in Canada, whereafter they are likely to become relegated to the least affluent echelons of society. The odds of being poor are increased by over 50 per cent for immigrants, and are even greater for those who are non-Europeans, even when controlling for factors such as education, linguistic skills, and age (Kazemipur and Halli 2001). The salience of language to gender and health is reflected in an examination of the Longitudinal Survey of Immigrants to Canada, which found that poor self-reported health status was associated with poor official language skills among female immigrants (Pottie et al. 2008). As communal, familial, or personal prosperity, for instance, enhance access to resources including money, prestige, power, and knowledge, they can mitigate health risks (Anderson et al. 2003); prosperity, however, can often be out of reach for foreign-born Canadian residents, especially women from non-European countries (Chard, Badets, and Howatson-Leo 2000; Kazemipur and Halli 2001).

Indeed, women are most vulnerable to the trend of downward economic and social mobility. Despite the fact that they are generally better educated than their Canadian-born counterparts, immigrant women are less likely to be employed in positions that are commensurate with their skills (Chard, Badets, and Howatson-Leo 2000). Both poverty and the dynamics of downward mobility are associated with poor health outcomes due to a host of factors, including reduced access to good nutrition and auxiliary health care, and the stress of income insecurity (Krieger, Chen, and Selby 2001; National Council of Welfare 2001).

The body makes an appearance in some population health literature – at times regarded in terms of micro-, meso-, and macro-levels. At the micro-level, the body can be conceptualized as both a receptacle of and an exhibit for disease. As the body interacts with social indicators such as gender, socio-economic class, ethnicity, processes of socialization, and sexuality, among others, it can be situated within a matrix, or social hierarchy, that constitutes our complex social landscape. As the macro-level policies and programs direct and discipline collections of bodies in the name of producing healthy and productive workers, the body is transformed as an object of disciplinary regimes.

Embodiment

The population health approach enables us to offer recommendations for interventions, policies, and programs in a manner that is familiar to a host of policy makers and biomedically informed professionals; however, in order to gain a more complete understanding of how individuals respond to and make sense of these changes to their environment, we need to attend to the body as subject.

The body is the site of apprehension of the world; it is through the body that we experience, interpret, reflect, and respond to sensations, sights, and textures; that we experience, order, and share the world, creating intersubjective space where socio-cultural environments influence behaviour and our expectations of others (Spitzer 2009b; Young 2005). For instance, embodiment is the intersubjective ground of experience, an indeterminate field informed by perception and engagement with the world yet suffused through the culturally constructed, material entity of the body (Csordas 1994, 1999; Spitzer 2009b). A focus on embodiment allows us to consider how persons attend to the body, making sense of somatic sensations, and reordering those sensations into a constellation of identifiable symptoms that can be granted a meaningful label, potentially a disease label, that further structures how the person will respond to the condition. In addition, Csordas (1994, 1999) asserts that attention must also be paid to language and the imagery of the body, as it can offer insights into cultural and individual conceptions of life and society (cf. Martin 1990, 1992). Moreover, researchers are urged to examine the perception of the biological and the cultural and the body's interaction with global processes (Csordas

1994, 1999). In summary, bodies incorporate and are understood and experienced through local and global frameworks that imbue sensations, behaviours, and relations with political, economic, biomedical, cultural, and gendered meanings.

These disparate theoretical lenses produce different fields of vision, each focusing on different concepts and issues. While theories of embodiment open up considerations that are flexible, meaning-driven, and often individually focused, population health relies on a priori categories (determinants) that are generally regarded as influencing rather than constituting health and well-being. Population health and embodiment also proffer different explanatory models and interpretive possibilities that enable us to speak with a variety of audiences, from scholars of the body and health professionals, to program makers, front-line community workers, and informants whose lives are highlighted, contributing, one hopes, to further actions, from program planning and policy development to theoretical engagement. In this light, both paths can lead to unearthing the myriad lives of the body – albeit in decidedly different ways.

Work, Worries, and Weariness

Work

Canadian statistics have revealed that gender and country of origin figure prominently in labour market placement and socio-economic mobility of immigrants. For instance, nearly 70 per cent of foreign-born Canadians from Asian and Middle-Eastern countries as compared to 32 to 37 per cent of immigrants from Australia, New Zealand, or the United States were not employed in positions commensurate with those in their home country (Chui 2003:30-2). Forty-three per cent of female immigrants were involved in professional activities prior to migration; however, only 24 per cent maintained professional employment and status after settling in Canada (Chui 2003). Foreign-born women are more likely to have assumed jobs in sales and service sector, where their numbers have tripled, or in the manufacturing sector, where their numbers have quadrupled. Notably, the work is generally not commensurate with the education and skills that immigrant women bring to this country (Chui 2003). While many immigrants take on multiple jobs (Guruge, Donner, and Morrison 2000), immigrant women in particular are likely to avail themselves of so-called 'survival jobs' that fail to make use of their educational backgrounds or skills. These positions are apt to be part-time, offer few or no supplemental benefits, and may be fraught with poor occupational health standards. Best characterized as precarious employment, wages for these positions are often insufficiently remunerative to cover basic expenses, necessitating additional employment. As a result, workers report high rates of work-related stress and exhaustion (Lewchuk et al. 2003) that is further exacerbated by the gendered responsibilities of household and family labour.

Extracting oneself from the expanding realm of precarious employment is decidedly challenging for foreign-born Canadians who face tremendous barriers having their credentials, education, and work experience obtained outside the country accepted by Canadian employers and institutions (Guruge, Donner, and Morrison 2000; Danso 2001; Bauder 2003). As immigrants generally do not have access to adjudication processes before arrival, they cannot anticipate the magnitude of the challenges ahead that often originate in this issue. Importantly, it is country of origin that plays a significant role in determining the credence generally granted foreign credentials, thereby shaping future labour market outcomes (Bauder 2003; Chui 2003). Time poverty and financial demands from both local household members and those anticipating remittances back home, limit the ability for individuals to retrain in another field or study to meet the specificities of Canadian credentials (Bauder 2003; Matsuoka and Sorenson 1999). When decisions are made to invest these limited resources in further education, the recipients are most often male members of the household (Langford, Fantino, and Waijaki 1999). As a result, female immigrants are more likely to undergo downward mobility and the process of deskilling – the erosion of professional abilities, professional status, and self-confidence as a result of a prolonged period of time working outside of a particular occupational arena (Alcuitas et al. 1997). Conducting research with foreign domestic care workers who enter Canada under the auspices of the Live-In Caregiver Program (LCP), we encountered many women and men who although well-educated, have found themselves working in low-status employment to sustain the well-being of and to provide opportunities for their families.[2] As one foreign domestic care worker participating in a focus group reflected:

It's really a privilege serving people, but there is that intimidation, there is that what you call, that pride, it must be pride in me … it came out to the surface that I still look at my job as a nanny as lower than others. So I keep on putting in my mind that, 'No, no, being a nanny is a noble job. Being a housekeeper is a noble job.' But at times that thought slips in ... And although I am trying to accept that I am here doing an equally noble job as I had before, the fact remains that there is still a difference. So the difference I compensate my longingness [sic] to do the past job by doing other things here which is commensurate to the demands of that job.

The structure of the workplace and work relations have an impact on the well-being of employees. The work-lives of foreign-born women in Canada, who disproportionately occupy the lowest ranks of the labour market, are often characterized by their lack of control over the pace and organization of their tasks, coupled with high demands and little latitude over work-related decisions (Brooker and Eakin 2001; Din-Dzietham et al. 2004; Kunz-Ebrecht, Kirschbaum, and Steptoe 2004). Locus of control at work has been demonstrated to be a predictor of symptom-reporting among women (Muhonen and Torkelson 2004), while low decision latitude coupled with high demand and effort-reward imbalance contribute to increases in blood pressure (Din-Dzietham et al. 2004). Additionally, exposure to racism and gender discrimination in the workplace can further exacerbate health problems and contribute to the erosion of perceived health and well-being (Brooker and Eakin 2001; Din-Dzietham et al. 2004).

Home, however, is not necessarily a refuge for women as it often purports to be for men. Lack of control at home and at work can contribute to depression among women (Griffen et al. 2002). One European study found that stress levels among men declined in the evening, whereas women's stress escalated throughout the day and was higher among women with young children in the home, who also reported more mental health problems than men and women without young children in their household (Gjerdingen et al. 2000). The stresses of work and home life may be even further exacerbated as immigrant and refugee women and their families are also in the process of renegotiating gender roles in light of competing gender ideologies, changing familial relations, and potentially unfamiliar forms of labour market participation.

As '[A]n adult woman can expect to spend 17 years of her life caring for children and 18 years helping an aging parent' (Older Women's League in Doress-Worter 1994, cited in Remennick 1999:349), women's caregiving responsibilities further intensify the workload at home. For foreign-born women, care-work in Canada may take on different dimensions than in their home country. Truncated familial support networks, limitations placed by provincial governments on access to auxiliary health services, culturally inappropriate services, and lack of information about what kinds of resources are available to assist family caregivers, all contribute to an intensification of caregiving responsibilities for many immigrant women (Spitzer et al. 2003).

Furthermore, as women assume responsibility for caring for infirm family members, they face increased challenges. The changes wrought by health care reform throughout Canada have included shorter hospital stays. Resultantly, family caregivers are required to perform more complex procedures to help their family member recuperate. Moreover, immigrant family caregivers may not avail themselves of all health and social service programs and resources depending upon their province of residence, their immigration status, and, if applicable, the details of their sponsorship agreement (Armstrong and Armstrong 2001; Elabor-Idenmudia 2000; Spitzer et al. 2003; Steele et al. 2002).

Importantly, although care-work can be regarded as rewarding, it is still emotionally and physically exhausting labour that is often charged with increased significance in the ethnic context. The centrality of care-work to gender and ethnic identities means that women appear reluctant to relinquish these responsibilities regardless of emotional, physical, or financial cost (Neufeld et al. 2002; Spitzer et al. 2003). Even affluent immigrant family caregivers appear unwilling to forgo these responsibilities; although they may be amenable to purchase the services of others to assist with other domestic tasks such as house-cleaning, they are likely to retain intimate care tasks for themselves (Spitzer et al. 2003; Stein et al. 1998).

Worries

In addition to caregiving labour and housework, women are predominantly charged with the tasks pertaining to kin-work that operate to lubricate networks of social relations composed of family and friends (Davis 1997; Di Leonardo 1993). Kin-work responsibilities include tasks ranging from remembering dates of special events, issuing social invitations, and other quotidian activities that facilitate communication and strengthen interpersonal bonds. Among the emotional tasks is worry. Worry enables persons to 'do' something for someone in situations with unknown provenance or potentially ambiguous consequences over which they have little or no control. For instance, wives of fishers have traditionally worried on behalf of their partners who put out to sea under possibly dangerous conditions (Davis 1983). Worry is also a highly gendered activity, with women assuming the primary responsibility for it, in particular with reference to their children, household health, and caregiving responsibilities (Davis 1983; Takeda, Kawachi et al. 2004).

For immigrant and refugee women who may endure separation from family, friends, and relations, gendered worry-work may be both intense and virtually chronic. In Canada, immigration policies are informed by and further entrench the nuclear family by delimiting the types of familial relations that are eligible for sponsorship by permanent residents and citizens – with spouse and children under 22 in one stream – and parents, grandparents, and siblings under 18 years of age in the other (CIC 2008; Côté, Kérisit, and Côté 2001). In either process, sponsors who are permanent residents or citizens must sign an undertaking promising to provide financial assistance to relations for a period of time, up to 10 years, to ensure that they do not avail themselves of financial assistance from the Canadian government (CIC 2008; Côté, Kérisit, and Côté 2001). As foreign-born women are overwhelmingly underemployed, these conditions that require potential sponsors to verify their financial wherewithal before approving the application, can make sponsoring family members particularly difficult, and, as a result, familial reunification can be delayed (Spitzer 2009a).

Furthermore, the regulations that shape the notion of what constitutes a dependent child have significant implications. Using numerical age of either 21 and younger or 18 and younger to determine a parent or sibling's eligibility to sponsor them, may conflict with other cultural constructs of adulthood or childhood that hold social roles as more salient than chronological measurements. As such, unmarried adult offspring may live with their parents and be considered dependent by members of both the household and society, although these children may be an important source of financial and emotional support (Spitzer 2009a). Not being able to sponsor an adult child can have dire consequences for all involved.

For example, while soliciting life stories of Somali, Chinese, and Chilean women negotiating meanings of maturation in Canada,[3] one Chilean informant shared her story about coming to Canada as a refugee following the 1973 coup in that country. While she and her husband were granted refuge in Canada, they were compelled to leave their 19-year-old daughter and elder son while fleeing with their youngest child. After their departure, the siblings took on a perilous journey to

Argentina and successfully appealed to the Canadian government to allow them to join their parents; however, the 'choice' thrust upon the family engendered considerable pain that they each still bore 25 years later (Spitzer 2009b).

Once children do join their family members in Canada, maternal worry-work does not end there. Concerns about integration, balancing their needs for socializing with peers, and fears about the erosion of their ethnic identities can inform parent-child relations (Okeke and Spitzer 2005).

Weariness

Migrating to another country requires considerable stamina, drive, and discipline to see one through the short-term obstacles on the path towards a better life, as personally conceived. Stalled upward mobility, thwarted ambitions, and dashed dreams contribute to worries and compound the costs of poorly waged and poorly regarded work, culminating in weariness – and potentially thoughts of returning to one's home country (cf. Danso 2001). For many newcomers to Canada, especially women from non-European source countries, dreams of a better life for themselves – and their children – may remain unfulfilled as the second generation struggles to ascend the socio-economic hierarchy (Kazemipur and Halli 2000) – although recent evidence clearly demonstrates that not all minority ethnic communities share in the same downward trajectory (Hyman 2007a; Jiménez 2008). As the Canadian-born generation cannot be subject to the same demands for Canadian experience and education as their parents, the failure of second-generation Canadians to fully recover from the downward mobility experienced by their parents' generation is more evidently rooted in racist and anti-immigrant sentiments (cf. Wright 2000; Li 2001; Valverde and Pratt 2002; Jiménez 2008).

Encounters with systemic and personal racism and the disjuncture between their dreams of creating a better life in Canada and their lived experiences can result in chronic stress and the disillusionment I call *weariness*. This weariness can be expressed somatically. At times, bodily pains defy nosological categorization, but are linked by the sufferer to the social and material context of their lives (Spitzer 2007). Complaints are a means through which the body communicates its distress (Scheper-Hughes and Lock 1987; Scheper-Hughes 1991; Lock 1993b; Coker 2004). Marginalized people are also able to resist daily discipline by assuming a sick role that allow sufferers to drop out of obligations, constituting what Scheper-Hughes and Lock (1987) term bodily dissent.

Anthropologists have long noted the potency of metaphors such as nerves, *nerva*, or *nervios* that operate as culturally charged symbols that appear in varied forms throughout the world (Low 1994; Doyal 1995). The deployment of nerves or one of its variants as a diagnostic label enables persons who are generally socially and economically marginalized to articulate distress about their social location through somatic complaints (Doyal 1995), compelling Finkler (1994) to label nerves as the embodiment of adversity. Low (1994:142) states that 'nerves embodies the lived experience of daily life as a metaphor of physical, social, political, and economic distress that has specific meanings within a variety of cultural contexts.' Metaphor, Low goes on, is a means by which we create order out of the chaos of lived experience. For example, female survivors of political violence in El Salvador employed the language of *el calor*, intense heat and a symptom of nervios, as a somatic mode of attention and metaphor, to refer to the unspeakable events that they witnessed or underwent in their homeland (Jenkins and Valiente 1994).

Others may reject what they regard as depoliticized, reductionist diagnostic labels offered by biomedicine, and insist on more holistic explanatory models that are grounded in life experience. In a pilot project that explored both immigrant and health professional perspectives of Type 2 diabetes,[4] Carolina, a refugee from El Salvador, described what exacerbated her diabetes:

> I feel it's because of depression. Being in another country, different clim[ate], different culture, the language, it was too much stress for me ...
> *Interviewer:* What makes your diabetes worse?
> Worse? Not having job! Yeah, that's true; is true. Not having job, having emotional problems, and being unstable in job. For example, you are not sure today if you have job tomorrow; you don't know. Something like that. Coping with many, many things' (Spitzer 2009a:148).

Resisting the Impact of Work, Worries, and Weariness

To portray immigrant women as wholly vulnerable to the deleterious effects of social and material marginalization would be inaccurate. Foreign-born women exhibit myriad ways in which they exert agency and demonstrate resilience (see chapters 10 to 13, this volume). Social and material resources and the power to mobilize those resources constitute a bulwark against the derogating effects of social exclusion that has been termed by anthropologist William Dressler (1991) as 'resistance resources.' Resistance resources refer to the material, social, collective, and personal attributes that help buffer the onslaught of stressors. These may include symbolic resources such as identity, language, and religion that may not only offer the benefits that accrue from a sense of belonging, but also from the material benefits of maintaining and expanding social networks (Fortin 2002; Spitzer 2007b, 2008). Importantly, social networks are essential to enabling immigrant and refugee women to navigate the space of a new country and community by offering instrumental, informational, and emotional support (Elabor-Idenmudia 2000; Remennick 1999; Simich, Beiser, and Mawani 2003).

Health Implications of Work, Worries, and Weariness: A Focus on Stress

A woman's health status is reflective of her location in the social landscape as determined by socio-economic status and social role, but the mechanisms through which these phenomena operate are not clear (McDonough, Walters, and Strohschein 2002). Stress, however, may well provide a key to our understanding of the loss of the healthy immigrant effect, especially as chronic stress can bear particularly potent impact when deeply held convictions are shattered (Helman 1990). Significantly, stress is a concept that potentially carries valence in both population health and embodied perspectives. Within a Western scientific framework, interactions between the material body and socio-cultural environment are often denied except in reference to stress, which can be defined as the response to a perceived threat or situation causing distress that results in both behavioural and neurochemical reactions (Weinstock 1996). Stress is one topic that refutes the mind-body dichotomy, and is grounded in the interaction if not outright unification of mind and body. Advances in psycho-neuro-immunology allow us to employ a more integrated outlook in which psychological distress can be linked to increased risk of morbidity and mortality and to specific disease outcomes (Wales 1995; Dressler, Grell, and Viteri 1995; Lundberg and Parr 2000; Agardh et al. 2003).[5] By identifying the potential mechanisms for these interactions, the relationship between stress and health may inevitably contribute to the dissolution of the boundaries between mind and body.

Wainwright and Calnan (2002:87, in Freund 2006:103) note that: 'Over the life course social experiences become "written" on the body in the form of physiological responses (e.g., as patterns of neuro-hormonal activity), some of which may also be experienced as emotional modes of feeling.' Thus the impact of the interactive phenomena of work, worries, and weariness is borne by the body and expressed somatically in ways that can at times elude the presumed certainty of medical diagnostic categories; however, abundant biomedical evidence lends explanatory power to the relationship between deteriorating and poor health status, migration, gender, and downward social mobility (Lundberg and Parr 2000; Spitzer 2003; Kunz-Ebrecht, Kirschbaum, and Steptoe 2004; VanderPlaat 2007; Weekes, MacLean, and Berger 2005). Stress-related health outcomes can, therefore, be regarded as the result of the embodiment of marginalization. Moreover, low-income women – a disproportionate number of whom, as previously noted, are foreign-born – face challenges engaging in self-care activities that are increasingly expected of patients by health professionals and medical centres as auxiliary supplies and services previously provided by public services are no longer available and offloaded onto patients and their families. Hours of operation of health care services may also be problematic for immigrant, low-income women who may have difficulty taking time off work, finding transportation to the appointment, or finding childcare (Anderson and Reimer Kirkham 1998).

Intersections with ethnicity, exposure to racism, both structural and personal, restricted social and physical mobility, and limited access to power networks have also been linked with poor health and increased stress. Some authors further suggest that the effects are even more deleterious for women, who are often socialized into internalizing their distress (Brooker and Eakin 2001; Karlsen and Nazroo 2002; Din-Dzietham et al. 2004). The structural inequities that constrain the lives of many visible-minority migrant women are composed of multiple exposures to stress, and may have direct health impacts that include the precipitation of Type 2 diabetes (Spitzer 2003).

Understanding the relationship between global processes, social, physical, cultural environments, and individual and community health are best conveyed through attention to the body. Siegrist and Marmot (2004) maintain that individuals experience distress that contributes to health problems such as depression, alcoholism, and cardiovascular disease when they are continually disappointed and frustrated in their efforts, in which they have invested significantly and which have offered little in return.

For Dressler (1991), lifestyle incongruity – the disparity between the ideal life, reflected in mainstream media, and the lived experiences of members of minority communities – lies at the core of long-term stress that contributes to related health outcomes such as hypertension, depression, cardiovascular disease, and Type 2 diabetes (Hyman 2007a; Spitzer 2005). Conversely, successfully adopting a lifestyle that is heralded as ideal in a particular society is associated with lower blood pressure and reduced rates of depression and stress compared to the general population (Dressler, Balieiro, and Santos 1998). Moreover, downward socio-economic mobility appears to have a similar impact (Krieger, Chen, and Selby 2001).

Stress induced by a sense of loss of control or discrepant expectations between ideal lives and lived experiences can result in the launching of a cascade of effects involving the nervous and endocrine systems. The relationship between low socio-economic status and work is particularly relevant for our examination of gender, migration, and health as female members of the working poor employed in high-demand jobs have been shown to have elevated levels of cortisol in comparison to others in the population. Notably, the physiological impact of high-demand work is effectively mitigated by high socio-economic status (Kunz-Ebrecht, Kirschbaum, and Steptoe 2004).

The ability to cope with and adapt to the impact of stress is dependent on access to personal, social, and material resources that are themselves socially distributed (Brooker and Eakin 2001; Freund 2006). A study of Soviet refugees in Israel reinforced the salience of social support to understanding the relationship between stressors and the exhibition of distress (Ritsner, Modai, and Ponizovsky 2000). Importantly, they demonstrated that the variability of and interaction between stressors and social support produce disparate outcomes pertaining to psychological distress. Friends and significant others in particular played a role in mitigating the impact of stressors (Ritsner, Modai, and Ponizovsky 2000). In a multi-site examination of the meanings of social support amongst Chinese immigrants and Somali refugees in Canada,[6] one Chinese Canadian woman shared:

> Friends, they are the best help, because they have the experience, and they can share information with others. You can judge whether things are helpful or not, that will be the best. But the problem is that the people around

you don't have the information either, they're also looking for people who have the information. So you need a bigger circle of friends (Spitzer 2005).

Women especially reported reaching out to individuals outside of their ethnocultural community, such as neighbours and landlords, to provide informational support. Similarly, in a previous study we found that neighbours who were not co-ethnic were called upon to provide support in the form of transportation assistance and childcare as they were not integrated into the individual's web of reciprocity and thus requests were less 'costly' in terms of 'repayments' (Young, Spitzer, and Pang 1998).

Bodily Implications

Apprehension of the world is shaped through the physical, physiological, political, and ultimately cultural processes of perception that enable us to observe, participate in, and interpret the world around us. The body is both subject- and object-inscribed and able to inscribe others (Csordas 1999). Embodied subjects then take in and take up their world, interpreting sensations and perceptions through the discursive constructions of language. Csordas (1999, 2002) refers to the culturally defined ways in which one attends to, and with, one's body to the sensations one apprehends as somatic modes of attention. Categorizing sensations and stirrings into shared discourses enables us to participate in the nexus of intersubjectivity.

Work with foreign domestic care workers in Canada suggests that the expression of somatic complaints such as general aches, pains, and malaise, some of which defy nosological categorization, can be regarded as evidence of the impact of global forces on gendered bodies, and represents the embodiment of inequality (Spitzer 2007). Importantly, when foreign domestic care-workers share this body talk with other care-workers, they are potentially able to deploy their discourses of suffering and sacrifice to enhance social solidarity and mobilize social support (Spitzer 2007). As Dossa (chapter 9, this volume) demonstrates, using the language of the body and sharing testimonies of suffering can bring women together. These interactions can lead to collaborative, critical analysis, to the further mobilization of resources, to the creation of social networks and social capital, and to the potential relief from disburdening themselves. A focus on the body, therefore, has the potential to bring a bottom-up approach to community mobilization grounded in the language and lived experiences of immigrant and refugee women.

Work, Worry, Weariness: Towards an Engendered/Embodied Migrant Health

There are any number of factors that mitigate the negative impact of work, worry, and weariness on the health and well-being of migrant women in Canada. From a population health perspective, work, worry, and weariness may result from and are reinforced by downward social and economic mobility, low-control/high-demand work, loss of social support, and cultural disparities, all of which contribute to the loss of the healthy immigrant effect.

From the perspective of embodiment, we apprehend, understand, and interpret that which we have garnered from our physical and social environments, creating intersubjective spaces to engage with others, deploying body talk that can make reference to somatic modes of attention, metaphors, and the language of the body. The body speaks of its suffering, its alienation, and its strengths through the language of pain and perseverance reflecting the embodiment of inequality and adversity. Talk about the body can mean talk about everything (Davis 1997), and opportunities to share this talk of suffering with others is an important means of reaching out to others with similar experiences to elicit empathy, to recall struggles and the strengths of will to overcome them, and to enhance social solidarity and facilitate social support (see also Coker 2004). The etiologies of the suffering are situated in the social world, where complex webs of relationships from global forces to personal lives are linked and experienced at the level of the body. Deploying the language of stress allows sufferers to negate mind/body dichotomies and the reductionist, decontextualized approach of biomedicine in a manner that is comprehensible if not wholly accepted within the biomedical world view. Notably, both of these perspectives focus on the body and open up a space to forge applied solutions to the challenges faced by immigrant and refugee women.

NOTES

1 Most of the epidemiological information on the health of newcomers to Canada is drawn from analyses of the Longitudinal Survey of Immigrants

to Canada (LSIC). To date, the LSIC includes – but does not distinguish between – voluntary and involuntary migrants (refugees). This conflation not only makes it difficult to determine if the trajectories of immigrants and refugees differ, it also troubles the language used to describe newcomers to the country.

2 From *In the Shadows: Live-in Caregivers in Alberta*, 2000-2002, funded by Canadian Heritage, Status of Women Canada, and Health Canada. Awarded to D.L. Spitzer, S. Bitar, and M. Kalbach.

3 From *Migration and Menopause: The Experiences of Maturation in Three Immigrant Communities*, funded by the Issak Walton Killam Doctoral Scholarship. Awarded to D.L. Spitzer.

4 From *Migrant Experiences of Type 2 Diabetes*, funded by a Humanities, Social Sciences, and Fine Arts grant (University of Alberta). Awarded to D.L. Spitzer.

5 Stressors can activate the sympathetic nervous system and the hypothalamic-pituitary-adrenal (HPA) axis that leads to an increase in glucocorticoids, most notably, cortisol (Freund 2006). Prolonged activation results in insulin resistance and immuno-suppression as cortisol raises blood glucose levels and inhibits glucose uptake in the tissues (Scheder 1988; Lundberg and Parr 2000; Tsigo and Chrousos 2002).

6 From Multicultural Meanings of Social Support. SSHRC grant awarded to M. Stewart, J. Anderson, M. Beiser, D.L. Spitzer, and A. Neufeld.

3 Examining the Health of Immigrant and Refugee Francophone Women Living outside Québec

MICHÈLE KÉRISIT

> I have the feeling that being an immigrant and francophone woman I ask for too much.
>
> Bassolé et al. (2004:88)

Although increasingly present in Canada's provinces outside Québec, immigrants who use French as a first or second language have not been the focus of much research, especially regarding health, and all the more so from a gendered perspective. The primary objective of this chapter is an attempt to fill this gap by giving an overview of the situation of francophone immigrant visible-minority women living outside Québec. I examine the specific barriers they face when they need to access the health care system in general with a focus on issues of mental health. Due both to my research working with immigrant and refugee women coming primarily from Sub-Saharan Africa, and to my desire to disrupt the idea that French-speaking Canadians living outside Québec constitute a homogeneous group, I highlight the experiences of women coming from western and central Africa, who, through colonization, have had to learn French as a second language.

In this chapter, I argue that the situation of francophone immigrant refugee women of colour is embedded in an historical and social juncture between different determinations that make relations of gender, ethnicity, racialization, and language (specific to Canada) a source of both discrimination and emancipation. I adopt a perspective that sees the experience of living as a 'minority' as a dynamic process, differing according to different social locations. The issue is therefore not exclusively to describe the multiple effects of minoritization on the health of French-speaking women of colour who have recently settled in Canada (outside Québec), but also to unravel the process through which this minoritization is constituted.

In order to understand how these processes work, I have divided this chapter into three sections. In the first, I take stock of what is known and not known about the situation of French-speaking immigrant and refugee women living outside Québec. In a second section, I present a review of the literature on health issues affecting all French-speaking persons and communities outside Québec, to help identify the gaps in empirical knowledge and theoretical perspectives that exist in the analysis of health issues for French-speaking newcomers in general, and for women in particular. In this section, I also examine the much broader field of work that has been undertaken on immigrant and refugee women's health in Canada outside of Québec, and conclude that despite its relevance to this situation, this body of work keeps mostly silent on the issue of language. In the next section, I draw from a series of qualitative research projects I have conducted on the situation of francophone immigrant and refugee women of colour living in Ontario to outline a framework for thinking about a gendered approach to the impact of minoritization on the health of francophone women living outside of Québec. The specific issues that I will describe have been taken from the findings of these participatory studies, which mostly revolved around issues of family reunification (Côté, Kérisit, and Côté 2001; Grenon, Kérisit, and Magunira 2008), and the integration of women refugees coming from war-torn countries into Canadian society (Bassolé et al. 2004). A constant thread related to health issues can be read in the interviews my colleagues and I conducted, as most of the women's experiences greatly affected their health and well-being.

A Word about Minoritization

Women are subject to the barriers and inequities that impact all newcomers to Canada through a racialization process specific to Canada at the beginning of the twenty-first century. Due to their inclusion within the French-speaking, officially constituted 'minority,' their specific difficulties are subsumed under attitudes, policies, and practices that affect and constitute francophone minority communities in general. These women, then, have become invisible. Francophone foreign-born women are a minority within Canadian society whose lives are informed by unequal gendered relations that are particularly evident in the health system. As women of colour, attitudes and practices within the women's movement that have made headway in the field of health in the last 30 years can silence the specific combination constituted by their experience as women of colour speaking French and as recent settlers in Canada. Moreover, this 'quadruple burden' of minoritization is to be nuanced by the extremely diverse geographic dispersion of their experiences. It is therefore not surprising that their situation is often understood in terms of a 'minority within a minority,' in a sort of spiralling whirl of minoritization. But rather than portraying women as being crushed under the burden of diverse power relations – thereby denying them agency – belonging to a minority within a minority within a minority, whether because of one's sex or one's ethnicity or one's language, can also become a claim for creating new paths towards empowerment.

French-Speaking Newcomers Who Live Outside Québec

Most researchers recognize the major difficulty in obtaining accurate statistics about francophone newcomers living outside Québec (Forgues and Landry 2006; Citizenship and Immigration Canada 2006a). This is due to three problems that seem to prevent census accuracy: the difficulty in defining who is a francophone within statistical categories employed by Citizenship and Immigration Canada (CIC) and Statistics Canada; the overall mobility of French-speaking newcomers within Canada; and the general lack of Canada-wide empirical studies on the situation of francophone newcomers living outside Québec.

A Question of Definition

Who is a 'francophone'? Each year, CIC reports on the number of new permanent residents who are proficient in English and French, both official languages, and those who are proficient in neither French nor English. For instance, in 2004 Canada accepted as permanent residents 9,435 newcomers who claimed to know French and English or French only; 45 per cent (4,222) of them settled in Toronto and 11 per cent (1,055) in Vancouver (CIC 2006a: 20). These numbers, however, rely on unverified voluntary declaration. In order to have a more accurate picture, CIC undertook a parallel study where language proficiency was systematically accounted for among skilled workers. This study revealed that most people declaring proficiency in both official languages had English as their dominant language, meaning that they used English in most if not all of their everyday conversations and interactions. This drastically reduced the number of newcomers outside Québec using French as their primary language (CIC 2006a:19). Under this definition of 'francophones,' it was estimated that in 2004, 454 settled in Toronto and 116 in Vancouver. 'It would therefore seem that these cities attract French-speaking immigrants far less than originally thought' (CIC 2006a:6). However, we have to keep in mind that these numbers only represent immigrants classified under the 'skilled workers' category and exclude the family reunification class and refugees.

In 2006, although 12,452 newcomers declared that they could speak French and English, 1,865 declared that they had French as a dominant language, which accounted for 0.74 per cent of the number of newcomers for 2006, generally divided equally between men and women. This number has remained constant during the past 10 years; in 2001, for instance, 1,779 persons were in this category (CIC 2007). So if we define newcomers as immigrants that have settled in Canada in the past 10 years, we arrive at a rough estimate of 18,000 new French-speaking immigrants who have settled in provinces other than Québec.

However, these numbers have to be regarded with some scepticism. In fact, although there are no available statistical data, field observations from many agencies report that secondary migration within Canada is frequent among French-speaking newcomers. Many having received their permanent residency status in the province of Québec, then proceeded to move elsewhere in the country, particularly Ontario and the western provinces, namely British Columbia and Alberta (PRA 2004: 101). The number of francophone newcomers living outside Québec is therefore much higher than that implied by the restrictive definition given above, which emphasizes obtaining permanent residence and the first area of settlement, neglecting to take into account secondary mobility. Despite those problems, a relatively recent attempt by the Fédération des communautés Francophones et acadiennes du Canada (PRA 2004) and the Office of the Commissioner for Official Languages (Quell 2002) estimate that 5 per cent of francophones living outside Québec are foreign-born (Forgues and Landry 2006).

Origins and Immigration Status

Approximately 194,000 francophone immigrants have settled outside Québec (CIC 2006a). Most francophone immigrants are recent arrivals, with distinctions to be made between different 'waves,' the older wave having been constituted of European French-speaking people. In recent years, many French-speaking newcomers have arrived under precarious circumstances; indeed, 25 per cent of recent refugees in Canada are francophone (CIC 2006a:19). Conflicts and wars that have developed within North and sub-Saharan Africa explain in great part these numbers. Algeria has been a source of refugees since the turmoil the country has known in the mid-1990s. Recent statistics show Algeria is the second largest source country for immigration to Québec (*Globe and Mail* 2007), and there is no reason to suggest that Algerian newcomers are not also undertaking secondary migration within Canada. The genocide in Rwanda, the conflicts within Burundi, and the insecurity felt by the victims of genocide have displaced a great number of citizens from the Great Lakes regions of Africa. The two wars that took place in the Democratic Republic of the Congo, resulting in 3.9 million deaths between 1998 and 2004 (Coghlan et al. 2006), have also expelled many Congolese citizens from their countries. This is in addition to the 'low-intensity' conflicts taking place in other African francophone countries, such as Côte d'Ivoire and the Congo-Brazzaville, among others, that further contribute to the francophone emigration from the continent.

These newcomers have helped boost the increasing numbers of visible minority francophones living in Canada. Between 1996 and 2001, Ontario saw an increase of 42 per cent (Office des affaires francophones de l'Ontario 2005) of its French-speaking visible-minority population; so have urban centres such as Edmonton and Ottawa (Floch 2003). According to 2001 census data, nearly 75 per cent of visible-minority French-speaking immigrants in Ontario were born outside Canada – compared with 6.8 per cent of other French-speaking Ontarians and 27.9 per cent of the general Ontario population. More than 31 per cent were born in Africa, 30.5 per cent in Asia, and 18 per cent in the Middle East; 56 per cent had arrived within the nine years preceding the 2001 census (OAF 2005).

Our understanding of issues pertaining to women's health has to take these macro-demographic trends into account, for they are embedded in the global population movements of the end of the twentieth century and the beginning of the twenty-first.

Integration and Exclusion from the Labour Market

Francophone newcomers (both men and women) seem to experience severe economic and integration problems. Observation and regionally conducted research show that many of them experience great difficulties entering the labour market (PRA 2004:85-8; CIC 2006a:6). In that regard, the situation of visible minority newcomers is not different from that of many other non-French-speaking recent immigrants. Nevertheless, the specificity of their situation will be highlighted here.

Several explanations have been given for these problems in provinces where English is the dominant language. Besides a problematic command of the English language, the lack of foreign credential recognition can be observed, which is a problem many newcomers face in Canada. This lack of recognition is all the more important because many francophone newcomers have post-secondary degrees, as is also the trend for non-French speakers (OAF 2005). At the other end of the educational spectrum, many of the newcomers originate from countries where formal education has been disrupted by conflicts and wars. A significant number are therefore without the necessary skills to enter a sophisticated labour market where the command of English or French (or English and French) would be a prerequisite. Some of them might also have weak French literacy skills, which further impedes their progress in the overall language acquisition process. Last but not least, many newcomers of colour encounter prejudices over and above the lack of recognition of credentials or Canadian experiences. Studies have shown that many immigrants who have repeated their studies within Canadian institutions still have difficulties finding employment in their fields. Another interesting aspect is the added difficulties facing newcomers who do not come from Commonwealth countries. These newcomers can be left on the margins of social and political integration because they are often not familiar with the operations of government services, decision-making processes, common law, and community governance (CIC 2006a). Finally, the general difficulties of labour market integration is compounded by the lack of access by many francophone newcomers to English-language classes (CIC 2006b: 3).

In conclusion, the dispersion of this population plays itself out differently according to the specific geographical location. Some find themselves in urban settings where 'they may have numbers on their side but do not necessarily have a local weight or visibility' (Floch 2003:61), while others live in urban centres, like Ottawa, which have a sizeable francophone community to somewhat sustain life in French. In addition, issues of socio-economic integration are paramount for francophone immigrants and refugees attempting to settle in Canada. These issues are coloured by the fact that a great number of francophone newcomers come from countries where civil conflicts and wars are or have been recurrent. This induces a measure of further vulnerability in their ability to integrate in Canadian society.

The Health of Francophones and Immigrant and Refugee Women Living outside Québec: What Do We Know?

The focus on health issues among researchers and practitioners interested in the minority French population are relatively recent and have accelerated in the past 15 years. Since the beginning of the 1980s, especially in Ontario and New Brunswick, some pioneers, backed up by legal changes in provincial laws, had started to speak about the right of francophones to receive health services in French (Gilbert et al. 2005). The role of grass-roots women's groups along with the efforts of some leading health practitioners were instrumental in this regard (Coderre 1995). It was not until the beginning of the 1990s, however, that health issues for francophone minority communities came to the foreground.

As a result, we know little concerning the state of health of French-speaking minorities in Canada, let alone that of French-speaking newcomers. An overview of the research production concerning francophone health yields three main foci: first, studies related to the organization, development of, and accessibility to health services in French; second, epidemiological studies focusing on specific provincial situations; and third, monographs on health issues experienced by women.

Research Concerning the Development of French Services

In 1997, following the community protest against the closure of the only French-speaking health institution in Ontario (Montfort Hospital in Ottawa) under the Conservative government of Ontario, the federal government invested important funding into the development of francophone health. This new development has contributed to the formation of such institutions as the Consortiun national de formation en santé and the Société Santé en français; both organizations act as vehicles for 'francophone voices' in matters of health at the federal level, and encourage the development of research on the health of francophone Canadians living outside Québec. However, the restricted jurisdiction of the federal government in the development of services per se makes it difficult to see a uniform strategy in developing access to services that are under provincial jurisdiction. The result of this situation has been an extremely diverse provincial response; therefore, most of the issues concerning the health of francophone minorities can only be understood according to provincial legislation.

Combined with the geographic dispersion of these communities within Canada and within provinces, and the difference in the proportion of French-speaking newcomers within these communities, it becomes extremely difficult to sketch out a portrait of francophone services or the health status of French-speaking Canadians, let alone of the newcomers within this population. As a result, most research on the health of francophone communities focuses on access to services and the governance of the system and has lacked a gender perspective.

Some studies have been conducted under the auspices of major francophone organizations in Canada (FCFA 2001; Beaulieu et al. 2000) or recently established regional networks fostering better access to francophone services under provincial jurisdiction[1] (e.g., Cameron 2005; Réseau francophone de santé du nord de l'Ontario et al. 2006). These studies usually tend to take stock of the existing situation to highlight the gaps in services and to develop strategies to overcome them. Although offering a wealth of knowledge on the development of francophone services, these studies, mostly conducted through partnerships between professional practitioners and community-based researchers, provide relatively little insight into the meanings of health or the everyday experiences of French-speaking Canadians. Furthermore, little attention is given to the necessity of incorporating immigrant and refugee or visible minority issues into the analysis of access to health care services or into the solicitation of foreign-born francophones' participation in the development or governance of francophone health care services.

Other studies have highlighted the role that community-based strategies play in creating services. They have also given some thought to the conditions that are necessary for the emergence of new services or the support and development of existing services (Beaulieu et al. 2000; Cardinal 2001). Cardinal, for instance, adopted a framework based on the role of social movements and social actors to explain the development of services in Ontario in the 1980s and 1990s. For this author, this development has followed the 'structure of political opportunities,' meaning that social actors have been able to make claims for new and better francophone services at some conjuncture in time, when an 'objective' coalition between grass roots claims and political and legislative action could be taken.

The advent of the Harris government in Ontario constituted a closure of such opportunities for the francophones of Ontario at the end of the 1990s and the beginning of the 2000s. Cardinal (2001) notices, however, that these claims are framed according to one dominant question: should the development of services be done within a bilingual system or should one strive for independent French-speaking (potentially multicultural) services? She concludes that this question has overshadowed issues of socio-economic and ethnic or cultural diversity within francophone communities (101). I would argue that this apparent foreclosure is due to the differential power/interplay of actors in the development of francophone services, as health care practitioners and bureaucrats currently have the primary influence on the direction of service development under the scrutiny of institutional and jurisdictional arrangements in the provinces. Community-based, grass-roots claims can still have a voice in the development of services, but this voice is progressively becoming more faint as a more mainstream approach to health defined from an epidemiological perspective of medical intervention becomes popular in French-speaking research and professional communities.

Epidemiological Studies

Epidemiological studies have been undertaken in provinces where the number of French-language speakers could be statistically significant, mostly in Ontario (Picard and Allaire 2005; Boudreau and Farmer 1997). In these relatively rare epidemiological studies, based on the definition of the determinants of health used in major national surveys (Ontario Health Survey 1996-1997 and 1990; Canadian Community Health Survey 2000-2001), some differences in the health status of 'francophones,' 'anglophones,' and people speaking 'another language' are cautiously highlighted. For instance, the 2005 report on the health of francophones in Ontario (Picard and Allaire 2005:139) concluded that compared to English-speaking Ontarians, a smaller number of francophones evaluate their health as being very good or excellent; more francophones are addicted to tobacco; there are more cardiovascular incidences among francophones; more of them tend to be overweight; and lastly, good dental health is less prevalent due to less frequent visits to the dentist. However, as the authors highlight, 'data and results contained in the report are above all observations; the report does not provide explanations ... It establishes that the Franco Ontarian population has specific characteristics and has to face its own challenges but does not determine why' (Picard and Allaire 2005:140). On the positive side, the authors mention that adolescents do not smoke more than their anglophone counterparts and that tobacco addiction is on the decline, that sexual activity among youths is comparable to others, and that mental health consultation has stayed the same compared to other sociolinguistic groups. However, one can say that the overall conclusion that can be drawn from this report is the difference between regions in Ontario, with a specific mention of the population residing in northern Ontario that has a specific socio-demographic profile and specific challenges with regards to health issues.

Authors suggest, with caution, that two main determinants could explain the differences between francophone and anglophone informants: the aging of the francophone population (as compared to others) that is correlated with higher incidence of chronic disease; and lower levels of literacy and income that enhance vulnerability to other ailments and risky lifestyles (Evans, Barrer, and Marmor 1994; Perrin 1998; Raphael 2000).

However, relying on national surveys that until now designated 'francophones' as people whose mother tongue is French, these studies cannot refer to francophones who use French as a dominant language. These limits are highlighted and decried in Picard and Allaire (2005:141), and a major research effort is currently under way to include within the francophone population, people, mostly newcomers, who use French as their official language of choice. To date, no studies, however, have been made public with these new data.

Francophone Women's Health

Francophone minority women have, in fact, been at the forefront of research on the health of French-speaking Canadians and have been pioneers in this field, both through their research and their actions. Since the end of the 1970s, women's groups have been involved in fighting violence against women, and in Ontario, for instance, have established coordinated strategies through a coalition of French services for women. In contrast or complementary to the epidemiological studies cited earlier, most of the studies conducted on women's health are qualitative in nature and strive to understand health or ill health from the perspective of (potential) female patients. Academic and community–based researchers have thus, often in coalition, conducted studies on issues of violence (Brunet and Garceau 2004), poverty (Michaud 2005), and aging (Garceau 1996a; Miron and Ouimette 2007). In 1996 a monograph on the health of Franco-Ontarian women (Andrew et al. 1997) analysed the different factors that allowed the emergence of French health and social services in Ontario from a gendered perspective, and grouped both the meaning women gave to their health and their practice, as well as their capacity for action, as one central factor for the development of services. Many of these works alluded to the importance of including factors pertaining to the health of immigrant women, particularly racialized women, in their analysis. However, since the research agenda is currently mostly undertaken by national organizations defending the rights of francophones to be served in French in health institutions, it would seem that the strong voices of women of the 1980s and 1990s have been subsumed under this general struggle, and there is no evidence of growth in gendered analyses of francophone health needs as was present in the 1990s.

What conclusions can we draw from this brief portrait of research in the field of health for French-speaking minority communities? Three main themes are salient: (a) Apart from very few pockets of thriving French-speaking communities, services are rare or incomplete in most regions and provinces of Canada. There is an effort currently underway to establish some number of services in French through further localized research and collective strategies. These initiatives, however, place a greater emphasis on health needs defined from the perspective of service providers and epidemiological research, and not from the perspective of the patient; (b) Epidemiological studies that are available present their results according to sex, but do not employ a gender lens in their analyses. Even when social determinants of health (social capital, for instance) are taken into account, gender-based analyses are not undertaken; (c) There is a current surge of interest and research by practitioners, and community-based and academic researchers concerning the health of francophone minority individuals, sustained by a major restructuring of francophone minority institutions. Nevertheless, little attention is given to specific women's problems or to gendered analyses of health issues.

A Reading of Linguistic Barriers

Another angle of analysis would be to examine to what degree research conducted in English in Canada on the health of immigrant and refugee women has taken into account the particular issues of the francophone linguistic minority. It seems that the specific case of francophone women is very rarely mentioned, whether recently arrived women or women born in Canada. Even when a gendered and diversity-focused perspective is developed regarding immigrant and refugee women in Canada, very little is done regarding the difficulties that French-speaking women face both in accessing the health system and the problems they face in their everyday experiences of health and disease. In a word, the situation of these women in the social and political Canadian arena becomes invisible, despite the claim of such studies to take into account the intersections of racialization, gender, disability, or sexual orientation.

A complete literature review of all studies that has been conducted on the health of racialized and recent immigrant groups in Canada, especially focused on women, is beyond the scope of this chapter. I will therefore only highlight a few examples drawn from recent reports and work that has attempted to give a general overview of immigrant health in Canada. A literature review conducted by ACCESS Alliance in Toronto (ACCESS Alliance 2005), for instance, highlights the effects of social determinants on the health of racialized groups in Toronto (one of the major Canadian cities with francophone immigrants and refugees). As in many other reports and studies, linguistic barriers are quoted as one of the reasons for the lack of access to services, leading to communication difficulties between health care professionals and patients, with potentially dramatic outcomes. The salient points in this particular report are echoed in other research: 'Linguistic and communication barriers frequently hinder equitable access to health care ... Particularly affected are individuals who do not speak one of Canada's official languages fluently' (11).

A recent publication on women's health in Canada (Morrow, Hankivsky, and Varcoe 2007) focuses on expanding 'the meanings and boundaries of women's health through critical analysis and re-conceptualization of theory, policy and practice within the Canadian context' (4). Yet, despite the pivotal nature of the duality between the two so-called founding nations (French and English) in the makeup of Canadian policies and practice, nowhere can we find a conceptualization or a critical perspective on the place of francophone women within the health care debate, let alone of French-speaking immigrant and refugee women, who are generally assimilated in the broader category of immigrant and refugee women. The two chapters that are closer to these issues (Browne, Smye, and Varcoe 2007; Vissandjée et al. 2007) make no mention of this component of diversity within the immigrant and refugee population and the specific challenges it presents.

The most comprehensive report on language barriers to health care access (Bowen 2001) acknowledges that those individuals who speak an official language are among the constituencies of people facing language barriers to the health care system, depending on their location (13). Nevertheless, the bulk of the report points to the barriers facing those (not necessarily women) who do not speak either official language, or those who use visual language. Bowen, however, raises important points regarding the measurement of proficiency and fluency in either official language. The misunderstandings that can happen in conversations between providers and patients who think they are speaking the same language can lead to many failings in the therapeutic transaction, from misdiagnosis to lack of compliance. Many reports on the health of immigrants and refugees (Mulvihill, Meilloux, and Atkin 2001; Gagnon 2002; Beiser 2005; Oxman-Martinez et al. 2005; Thurston and Vissandjée 2005) also point to the necessity to understand the differences observed between immigrant subgroups, in particular along the lines of Canadian-specific immigration law and regulations, countries of origin, and stages of migration. The significantly greater vulnerability of women refugees to physical and mental problems must be highlighted within this framework.

Bypassing the linguistic divide that exists in most Canadian provinces, the impressive work done on immigrant and refugee women's health still renders the situation of French-speaking women invisible, despite the fact that this has many repercussions on their lives. This body of work, however, points to important issues that can be found among francophone newcomers and among French-speaking, African-born women in particular. The analysis of the issues the latter group faces when they settle in Canada must be understood in the general framework of international migration and the major barriers that all women newcomers face when they arrive in this country. The question raised by the following section will address both the commonality of their situation with other racialized immigrant and refugee women in Canada, and the specificity of the issues these African-born, francophone women face.

French-Speaking Immigrant and Refugee Health: Towards an Analytical Framework

Advocating for the incorporation of women's migration experience as a determinant of their health, Vissandjée and colleagues (2007:221) define four broad areas where this experience affects immigrant and refugee women's health: social exclusion, lack of economic opportunities, the experience of violence, and absence of security and health policy and practices preventing real access to health care services. Acknowledging that these four components are present in all women's health issues, the authors argue that migration patterns the way these social inequities are experienced. My research with French-speaking immigrant and refugee women coming from developing countries certainly confirms their assertions regarding the manner in which migration affects women's health.

The studies on which I base my analysis in this third section of the chapter have examined the impact of legal dispositions existing within the 1978 Law on Immigration and the 2002 Law on Immigration and the Protection of Refugees, concerning the difficulties women met in the course of their integration into Canadian society. The first project (Côté, Kérisit, and Côté 2001) dealt with the effects that spousal sponsorship had on the well-being of women, mostly those coming from the global South. The second study attempted to see how the women's experiences of organized violence in the home country affected their experiences of integration within Canada (Bassolé et al. 2004). This research led us to understand that the vulnerability due to the impact of organized violence (on health and identity) was exacerbated by the difficult conditions these women met in Canada as refugees. The last study (Grenon, Kérisit, and Magunira 2008) examined the process of family reunification and the different strategies that can be brought forward to improve it. Although not directly dealing with the consequences of these difficulties, which have been thoroughly studied by Rousseau (Rousseau, Mekki-Barada, and Morrow 2001; Rousseau et al. 2004), the women we met during group interviews and community workers we interviewed were quite adamant that the length of and obstacles with the family reunification process had a very dramatic effect on the well-being of women. As a matter of fact, many answers were expressed in terms of ill health or mental health issues.

In all three studies, the importance and relevance of a gendered analysis and the impact of racialization within the migration and resettlement phase in Canada were affirmed. Three recurring themes were of particular importance in defining the specific experience of the participants in the three studies: the first- and the second-family upheavals and potential violence within the family during social integration are present in many analyses made in the field of women's health; but the third, which deals with the linguistic issue, has to be unravelled to understand how the minoritization of francophone women impacts their health.

Women, Migration, and Family Upheaval

My research found that women's sense of well-being was linked to their family life and was thus affected by the upheaval caused by immigration. Coming from countries where women are mostly responsible for the well-being of their families and where separation from a spouse is considered a dramatic event for a woman, the gendered nature of the impact of the immigration process, and the obstacles met during resettlement, were very visible.

For instance, spousal sponsorship created a context by which the husband could take control of the woman's life, leaving her little freedom to act as an independent agent in her search for social or economic integration into Canadian society. It seemed obvious that even for those women who had harmonious relationships with their husbands, the very slow and complex procedures that sponsorship introduced into the lives of families impeded the possibility of expedient reunification with other members of their family.

For the women who applied for permanent residency as sponsored spouses within Canada, the waiting period made them very vulnerable to isolation and to the arbitrary authority of their husbands. Moreover, the absence of information on their rights and the emphasis placed on their obligations by immigration personnel meant that sponsored women generally did not have all the necessary information at their disposal that would allow them to assess or even clearly understand their situations. These women found that they were treated as 'minors,' since possibilities for action were limited. The sponsorship regime placed the women de facto in relationships of dependency with regard to their husbands, who could exercise financial and social control. Many women faced blackmail based on a 'sponsorship debt,' in the sense that they owed their life in Canada to their husbands (and sometimes the husbands' family). This debt was seen as the crux of these mechanisms of control. The sponsorship debt made women vulnerable to the position of power their husbands occupied within their marriage – a position reinforced by the integration difficulties these women experienced.

Moreover, by being able to withdraw sponsorship during the waiting period for permanent residency status, and by threatening to do so, the husbands were able to wield a weapon that the sponsorship regime had served to them 'on a silver platter.' During this period, one wife we interviewed felt that she had no choice and most often kept quiet, even if she was abused. When sponsored women became permanent residents and succeeded in understanding the full extent of their rights, they were able to act, develop strategies for autonomy, and make use of some services. This did not, however, mean that they were granted the same rights enjoyed by other permanent residents, as social assistance was denied to them unless they disclosed the abuse to which they were subjected. Francophone immigrant women in Ontario decried the multitude of difficulties that constrained their ability to integrate into Canadian society, including joining the labour market, overcoming language barriers, and facing various forms of racist and sexist discrimination which made the experience of sponsorship very difficult.

Women, bearing the brunt of this dependency, were expressing feelings of psychological distress and depression. Two of the respondents said they tried to commit suicide, while others sought psychological help for depression. One of the participants described the effects of her distress: 'When you don't have anyone, no family to talk to, and you find yourself in this situation, I used to cry night and day. I was depressed ... Now, when I think about it, it was really hard. I started to get pimples all over my face. It was really stressful. I was losing my hair. I just wanted to end it all. No, it was awful.'

In our study on the impact of organized violence and war on the integration of women, as well as in our study of family reunification – which also involved many refugee women from Africa – issues of delayed family reunification with children living in very precarious situations in the home country counted as the most heart-rending narratives from women. Given the length of time it took many of them to obtain permanent residency after claiming refugee status, along with the structural obstacles that existed, particularly in Africa, and the overall poverty experienced by many women making them unable to gather enough money to pay for fees and travel, it took many years before many women could be reunited with their children. This of course affected their well-being and their mental health, all the more so when they were not accompanied by a family member or a spouse. One woman described the effect of being separated from her children: 'Since I came ... I am seriously ill. It happens sometimes that I cannot get up. I do not eat, I do not drink, I just stay like this ... I can die now from thinking of my children.'

Francophone Women and Socio-economic Integration

Many authors have recently documented the impact of some difficult socio-economic integration on the health of immigrants, and immigrant and refugee women in particular. Among these difficulties are the poverty generated by lack of employment opportunities due to the lack of acceptance of foreign credentials and experience, subtle or overt racism, and discrimination, among other challenges. As one refugee woman told us: 'In Canada, you are going to sleep well and hope that you will not be woken up by the sound of bombs and rifles. That you will have ... But you have all the chances to die on social assistance. If you have a car, you will be entitled to do cleaning, small jobs, but if you have a diploma, keep it in your suitcase.'

Isolation and lack of communication also hamper their social integration in the full sense of the word. The women we have met have particularly emphasized the 'coldness' of Canadian social interaction, the anonymous lives they had to live, and of course the absence of family around them, particularly the extended family. One of the women said that the fast and competitive Canadian ways, associated with the loss of extended social ties familiar in Africa, led her, for the first time, to learn the word 'stress.' (See chapter 2, this volume, for further discussion of the concept of stress.) This was particularly moving for the refugees from the Rwandan genocide, where many of our participants had lost their whole families and could not establish relationships with people who had not experienced the traumatic events. Making a parallel between the situation she knew as a persecuted Rwandan during the genocide and her current situation, one woman said: 'Anyway, here also, it is survival at the top.'

Access to Services for Francophone Refugees

As I previously mentioned, most of the francophone immigrant women we met in the second study came from countries where social and civil strife were endemic (Bassolé et al. 2004). Many women had lost their entire families, or had endured torture, sexual exploitation, and extreme violence.

As a result of such suffering their health status was not always stable, and many, as far as we could determine, were still under severe strain and experiencing bouts of depression. At the same time, with the obstacles placed in front of them, not so much because of their immigration status (most, though not all, had obtained refugee status and permanent residency status relatively quickly), but because of poverty and single motherhood, loss of social status, isolation, and family reunification delays, they had the pressures to overcome their own mental, physical, and social vulnerability in order to survive. The strain on them in such circumstances was great, and one can easily imagine the need for help in finding their bearings in a new society. The absence of 'somebody to speak to' was one of the recurring themes in the interviews. (For further examination of social support see contributions by Spitzer, Simich, and Vissandjée and colleagues, this volume).

Women reacted to their trauma in different ways. Some were reluctant to recount what had happened to them, and their voices sounded 'strangled' when they spoke. These were likely the women who needed help the most; yet, they had never been able to seek aid for their plight. There are literally no specialized services in Ontario for francophone women who have been through this kind of trauma. As the authors of a study on the situation of francophone refugees in Hamilton (Ontario) said: 'Survivors prefer to receive services in French but [French agencies] do not generally have resources in French or do not have access to French-speaking specialists in the specific field of trauma' (Diallo and Lafrenière 2007:57). In our study (Bassolé et al. 2004), the closest they came to obtaining help was from francophone services for victims of family violence whose staff on their own accord have developed an ability to respond to these situations through their knowledge of sexual assault and family violence issues. Major services, such as community health centres, which are generally attuned to these situations, provide French services in Ontario (Toronto, Ottawa, Sudbury, Hamilton, and Cornwall). Many professionals in these services, however, feel ill-equipped because of the newness of these issues. Moreover, they are so busy filling in the material and physical health needs of their clients, or so overwhelmed by the nature of the suffering, that they cannot, in their opinion, adequately serve the particular mental health needs of the most desperate women that come to seek help.

Many other women, however, were not so deeply affected by their experiences as to be unable to speak about their past, present, or future. Many were willing to tell their stories, although some of them did so for the first time with the research interviewers. In these cases, the issue of 'having somebody to talk to' was especially salient. A participant in the research, very aware that her past history of horrific rape and massacres had affected her mental well-being, sought help from an agency specializing in providing support to victims of torture. Not only was she not offered direct help in her mother tongue but not in French either. She had to go through a French-speaking interpreter, who translated her French into English. This experience was very discouraging for her, as she thought she could have expected some recognition of her second language by the agency. She also broke off the 'treatment,' as she thought this was not an effective way for her to heal. In fact, most women expressed surprise at the lack and invisibility of French services in a country that had been described to them as 'bilingual': 'For there are people, we do not know how to find them. That is the problem. Given the fact that here people speak English, you think that if I ask for something here, it will be in English. So [French services] should try ... I don't know ... they should try to become visible. That we can go to them without the path being so difficult.'

Many other women asked for the opportunity to express their distress among women who had undergone the same experience. To our knowledge, only a handful of agencies offer these services, most of them in large cities in Ontario. Most of the other services that could accommodate such interventions are located in settlement agencies that provide counselling or group work to the most recent newcomers and are precariously funded. Awareness of the effects of trauma on one's well-being is often overshadowed by the focus on clients' basic needs during the first years of settlement.

More important, however, was the fact that these newcomer women often do not know where to turn, even for the most basic needs of food, work, and housing. One of our participants discovered a community resource centre providing services in French by walking into a commercial mall and reading the agency's sign on the wall. Many others had to rely on the serendipity of meeting strangers able to tell them where they could get help. Some others used their established national network to become knowledgeable about potential help. As many said, however, this was not always the best source of information, especially when their 'modesty' was involved, meaning that issues of sexual assault, violence, and family difficulties could not be broached within their community without fear of ostracism.

Some women met knowledgeable professionals in their search for help, in particular health practitioners who are able to communicate in French. However, because these practitioners are not numerous and have to respond to an overwhelming demand, they are often not available. These encounters were seen as 'lucky' events, not to be relied on.

Generally, the help the most vulnerable women received was character-ized by these chance encounters.

Looking for a Place as a Francophone

One of the most salient points in our studies, however, was the idea that life in Canada did not correspond to what the women had expected, whether because they imagined Canada as a 'land of milk and honey' and were disappointed, or because they had hoped that in a bilingual country they would be able to work and communicate in French in their everyday lives. In essence, they found themselves in the same po-sition as other newcomers who could not communicate in either official language. They also thought that the 'selling of Canada' as a bilingual country was misleading. As usual, the intersection between different levels of discrimination left women puzzled regarding the reason why they could not access employment. One respondent wondered why she was not called for a job: 'Was it because I am Black? Was it because I am an immigrant? Was it because I don't speak English?'

Furthermore, most women encountered the everyday difficulties of speaking French in a predominantly English-speaking milieu that does not respond well to the plight of francophones. As another participant said: 'There are words you have to say [in English] and they don't un-derstand if you don't say the right word ... You are lost.'

The history of the relationship between francophones and anglo-phones plays a large part in this difficulty. Many women reported that as French-speaking persons, they could feel the brunt of the dislike some English-speaking Canadians express towards French-speaking people. One woman, for instance, analyses the many layers of discrim-ination that exist in her situation as a French-speaking immigrant in Toronto:

There is a hatred for francophones, and I felt it and I still feel it because my husband, in the end, he is one of them [who hates francophones]. He doesn't really like francophones. Well okay, maybe he says that because he doesn't want me to get too attached to the idea of going back to France. He tells me, well, anyway you know, [they're] 'frogs' you know ... Also, there is my mother-in-law who tells me that France is a worthless country ... that Canada is so much better ... and I know very well that it isn't true, but ... Well, it is true that I haven't lived here all of my life, but even I see the differences, and ... Ah yes, no, nobody likes French people. It is something

... In any case it is funny because it's what I used to say in France. I was subjected to racism because I was [nationality of origin]. And now, I'm subjected to racism because I'm French! Ah yes, it's clear and simple. I feel it. In any case, I feel it when I speak English. I have a big accent compared to everyone else. It isn't one [person], it's everybody.

The historical interplay between the French- and English-speaking people, specific to Canada, becomes blurred by the geopolitical colonialist history of France. In this case, the result is that this respondent was made to feel that she does not belong to any particular community, as she is marginalized as both a francophone and a French woman of foreign origin.

Some also felt that their French accents were not necessarily welcomed by native French Canadians, who sometimes did not display complete understanding of their language when spoken with a different accent. Moreover, the inability of many English-speaking Canadians to communicate in French was a subject of wonder, as the women we met were more than prepared to learn English as a third language. They concluded that French should be the second language of English-speaking Canadians, given the bilingual nature of Canada, as they were told it was.

On the whole, many women thought that the bilingual representation that has been created through the construction of the Canadian state was not properly reflected in their everyday lives, as they had expected. Most were engaged in language training in English and recognized the necessity to do so for the sake of their survival and the advancement of their children's education and future.

Belonging to a francophone minority outside Québec, however, allowed some women to forge a new identity, as they identified with the struggle of the native-born French-speaking minority. First, there was a clear consensus among some women that their situation as francophones was something that clearly impacted their lives and the reactions they encountered in their everyday interactions: 'I have the feeling that being immigrant and francophone means that it is too much (*que c'est quelque chose de trop*), that I ask for too much,' said one woman. But she continued: 'I do not know how to explain it, but it makes me rebel.' Clearly, the consciousness of being an 'outsider' to the dominant construction of what 'an immigrant woman' is in Canada contributed to the feelings of being displaced and inadequate. It also created feelings of anger towards these norms that ultimately could lead to women making an active claim of their position in the Canadian mosaic.

This rebellion has indeed translated into action for some: 'Since I have understood that the 'francophonie' is something important in Canada, I do not make any effort and I stand for that right,' says one woman. Women who expressed these feelings were the most 'integrated' women we have interviewed, as their identity formation was partly aligned with a socio-political process that was and might still be at the heart of a Canadian identity.

Knowing French was therefore not necessarily a 'bonus' for immigrant and refugee women living outside Québec who contend with the paucity of French services. Additionally, they experience the effects of the racialization of their group, whether in the French-speaking community or the English-speaking community. As a result, their social ties are often restricted to their own national community, with all the difficulties that it implies for women who face violence and upheavals in their family life or who are often solely responsible for maintaining familial harmony even under precarious circumstances.

On the other hand, some women are able to find a new place in the Canadian 'collective' by affirming their belongingness within francophone minority groups. Their minoritization is therefore a social location from where they (and their children) can find a new sense of purpose and meaning. This, we think, can be a shared space from which to grow and heal, as Spitzer (2008:11) also noted among francophone African women living in Alberta. However, as I have highlighted in the second section of this chapter, this place will always be a precarious place under present conditions. This is true for women, and women of colour in particular. The experience of belonging will depend on the capacity of the French-speaking community to accommodate the needs of strangers at a time when it is fighting for its own survival, on having Canadians recognize the linguistic duality of their country, and on the willingness of the state to extend the efforts of many generations of francophone women in the domain of health and well-being.

NOTE

1 Seventeen networks of professionals working in the broad field of health care have been created recently throughout Canada.

4 Enhancing Social Inclusion: Settlement Services in Relation to Lesbian, Gay, and Bisexual Newcomers

BRIAN O'NEILL AND KAMALA SPROULE

Introduction

Does Canada truly welcome lesbian, gay, and bisexual immigrants? This chapter focuses on the provision of immigrant settlement services and the social well-being of lesbian, gay, and bisexual (LGB) newcomers. Building on the holistic definition of health set forth by the World Health Organization (2006), the Public Health Agency of Canada (PHAC 2007a) identifies 12 factors that shape health, including education, employment, income level, and housing (see chapter 2, this volume, for further discussion). Particularly relevant to the well-being of LGB people are supportive social networks, inclusive social environments, and issues related to gender and culture, all of which are addressed by settlement services. Omidvar and Richmond (2005) have pointed out the value of comprehensive settlement services in promoting the inclusion of immigrants and refugees in Canadian society. They have argued specifically for services that address the needs of newcomers who are poor, non-white, female, and young. However, the settlement service needs of LGB newcomers have often been overlooked in the literature.

While LGB[1] individuals have the same range of health and social service concerns as do those who are heterosexual, they may also have needs related to isolation, lack of understanding, and discrimination associated with their sexual orientation. Recognizing the intersection of various markers of diversity and marginalization in reviewing literature on health and diversity, Weerasinghe and Williams (2002) highlight that non-English speaking, visible-minority, and LGB newcomers, among others, may share similar challenges in achieving and maintaining their well-being. Cultural and language differences in combination with discrimination based on racialized category, ethnicity, gender, disability, and sexual orientation can hinder newcomers' access to services. When they approach settlement services, LGB newcomers may encounter barriers associated not only with cultural differences but also with the heterosexism (Herek 2004; Walls 2008) that pervades society in general.

In this chapter we discuss same-sex sexual orientation and provide an overview of laws and attitudes regarding same-sex sexuality in Canada and in major source countries of immigration. Drawing on our exploratory study of settlement services in relation to LGB newcomers, we identify issues relevant to service delivery and present suggestions for enhancing the accessibility and responsiveness of services, and thus their potential for contributing to the well-being of immigrants and refugees.

Sex, Gender, and Sexual Orientation

In this chapter we make distinctions among concepts related to sexuality and gender. Following Health Canada's (2003) definitions, sex denotes the categorization of people as male or female based on biological differences, while gender refers to the socially constructed roles, qualities, and values attributed to males and females in a particular culture. As Spitzer discusses in chapter 1 of this volume, understandings of both sex and gender are influenced by ideologies related to various aspects of social organization – ethnicity and sexuality being particularly relevant to the focus of this chapter.

Sexual orientation is a socially constructed concept that emerged in discourses about sexuality in the 1970s referring to the focus of individuals' erotic interests (Weeks 2004). In Canada, and generally in the Western world, heterosexual sexual orientation is understood to be attraction between males and females; homosexual sexual orientation, attraction to members of the same sex; and bisexual sexual orientation, attraction to members of both sexes (Lee 2008). This one-dimensional conception rests on assumptions that there are only two distinct sexes and that erotic attraction is based solely on the sex of individuals involved. Clearly other dynamics are involved. For instance, in some cultures, attribution of sexual orientation is based on roles played in erotic interactions rather than the sex of participants (Huang and Akhtar 2005). In everyday life, sexual attraction and behaviour are influenced by many factors, including the age, appearance, and behaviour of participants, as well as the social context (Murphy 1997; Archer 1999). Our work is based on the assumption that sex, gender, and sexual orientation are independent, and that sexual orientation is not an indicator of sex or gender identity. For example, a person could identify as male, perform the masculine gender role as conventionally defined in his culture, and have same-sex sexual orientation.

There is evidence of same-sex eroticism in numerous cultures historically and currently (Churchill 1967; Diamond 1993; Scasta 1998; Crompton 2003); however, until Kinsey's pioneering studies of sexuality in the United States (Kinsey, Pomeroy, and Martin 1948; Kinsey et al. 1955), it was thought that same-sex sexual behaviour was an aberration. These studies suggested that 5 to 10 per cent of men and 3 to 5 per cent of women were exclusively involved sexually with members of their own sex for at least three years of their adult lives. In addition, findings indicated that an equal proportion of respondents were sexually attracted to members of their own sex, but did not act on these attractions consistently. More recent American studies continue to support these conclusions (Gates 2006; Hawkins and Stackhouse 2004). Surveys by Statistics Canada in 2003 and 2005 found that 1.9 per cent of respondents identified as gay, lesbian, or bisexual (Statistics Canada 2008). However, data regarding erotic attraction and behaviour were not gathered, and it can be assumed that the number of people who have some degree of same-sex sexual orientation is larger. There is less information regarding the incidence of same-sex sexuality in non-Western countries, but clearly it occurs widely (see Francour and Noonan 2004). For example, the International Gay and Lesbian Association is composed of LGB organizations in over 90 countries.

Identities Based on Sexual Orientation

Until relatively recently in Western societies, individuals' erotic inclinations were not a basis for ascribing identity. Rather, same-sex sexual activity was disapproved of in much the same way as was heterosexual 'immorality,' but not seen as a marker of identity. In northern European and American medical discourses of the late nineteenth century, individuals were labelled homosexual on the basis of their same-sex erotic attraction or behaviour, and were considered mentally ill (Weeks 2004). In resisting this stigmatization, during the twentieth century people who were sexually attracted to members of their own sex began defining themselves as gay or lesbian, embracing these designations as positive identities rather than psychiatric diagnoses (Altman 2004). In addition, some First Nations peoples adopted the term *Two Spirit*, based on complex conceptualizations of gender and sexuality, to refer to Aboriginal peoples who do not fit within rigid binaries of gender and sexuality (Cameron 2005). While Two Spirit people face many of the issues that LGB newcomers may encounter, we do not address their needs in this chapter as they are not migrants.

Coming Out

'Coming out,' integrating same-sex sexual orientation into one's identity and openly identifying as gay, lesbian, or bisexual, is seen as pivotal in the lives of LGB people (Todd 2006). This view is supported by evidence that successfully coming out contributes to psychosocial well-being (Halpin and Allen 2004). Horowitz and Newcomb (2001) have argued that rather than being an individual, intra-psychic process, same-sex sexual identity formation is to a large extent shaped by the broader social context within which it occurs. Given the relationship between individual identity and the social environment, coming out has also been used as a fundamental strategy for advancing recognition and acceptance of LGB people at the societal level (Warner 2002).

One thrust of lesbian and gay rights movements has been to pressure mainstream health and social services to become more responsive to LGB people in much the same way that they accommodate diversity in relation to ethnicity, gender, and ability. This approach, however, rests on assumptions that all people who experience same-sex attraction and participate in sexual behaviour with members of their own sex identify as gay, lesbian, or bisexual, and that they should reveal this information about themselves. In reality, many people do not come out, some due to fear of discrimination, while others do not identify as gay, lesbian, or bisexual despite feeling same-sex attraction or participating in sex with members of their own sex.

Cultural and social constructions of self and sexuality inform decisions regarding how much, what form, and where information about same-sex attraction should be revealed. Triandis (2001) distinguishes between people who live in collectivist and individualist cultures. He argues that members of collectivist cultures identify strongly with the group that they are part of, such as family or community, and conform closely to the dominant values and customs of the group. In contrast, members of individualist cultures are more independent of the groups they are part of and pursue their own personal goals and values. Of particular relevance to this chapter, many newcomers to Canada are from countries that have predominantly collectivist cultures, such as China and India, and may not come out because asserting an individual identity may contradict family and community expectations. Coming out both influences and is influenced by attitudes and laws in Canada and the countries from which newcomers have emigrated.

Canadian Attitudes and Legislation Relevant to LGB People

Herek (2004) defines heterosexism as '... the cultural ideology that perpetuates sexual stigma by denying and denigrating any non-heterosexual form of behavior, identity, relationship, or community' (16). In addition to overt assertion of negative views regarding same-sex sexual orientation, marginalization can be reinforced in more subtle ways, such as expression of positive stereotypes and paternalistic concern about anti-gay discrimination (Walls 2008). Heterosexism, similar to sexism and racism, influences and is reproduced by social institutions such as health and social services. Stereotypes that LGB people are mentally ill, potentially dangerous sexual predators, and unable to form stable relationships are especially relevant to service delivery.

Although historically, heterosexist prejudice has been widespread in Canada, over the past 30 years Canadians have become more tolerant of same-sex sexuality, with the majority now accepting LGB people (O'Neill 2006). Canadian legislation at the federal and provincial levels reflects these changes, recognizing rights to protection from anti-gay discrimination and receipt of equal treatment in services. Relevant to migrants, the provision of the Immigration Act that blocked the admission of LGB people to Canada was removed in 1977 (Willms 2005). Subsequently, in 2002, the Immigration and Refugee Protection Act (Bill C-11) was passed, allowing Canadians to sponsor the landing of same-sex partners and permitting persons persecuted on the basis of sexual orientation to claim refugee status. Clearly there have been significant improvements in attitudes towards LGB people; hopefully Canadians can move from the limited form of acceptance implied by tolerance to a more positive valuing of sexual diversity. While legislation mandates access to effective services irrespective of sexual orientation, as yet this goal has not been fully achieved in health and social services. Attitudes and legislation in some other areas of the world are less positive.

Overseas Attitudes and Legislation Relevant to LGB People

In 2006, China, India, the Philippines, and Pakistan were top sources of immigration to Canada (Citizenship and Immigration Canada 2007), and this pattern is expected to continue. Attitudes and laws relevant to same-sex sexual orientation in these countries are more mixed than those in Canada. Unfortunately, there is widespread denial and disapproval of same-sex sexuality in China (Ruan and Lau 2004), India (Nath and Nayar 2004), Pakistan (Kahn 1997), and the Philippines (Leyson 2004), although this is beginning to change.

With respect to overseas legislation, the 1948 Universal Declaration of Human Rights omits mention of sexual orientation, and some countries have opposed the inclusion of a prohibition against discrimination on this basis. Legislation relevant to same-sex sexual orientation varies widely around the world. Sex between people of the same sex is illegal in 86 United Nations member countries, with penalties ranging from imprisonment to death (Ottosson 2008). With respect to major sources of Canadian immigration, same-sex sex is legal in the Philippines and China, although in China laws are applied selectively to suppress such behaviour. Sex between men is illegal in India and Pakistan, while sex between women is permitted (Amnesty International 2006). In common with other countries that use sharia law, Pakistan retains the death penalty for sex between men. It is important to be aware of newcomers' possible pre-migration experiences in relation to attitudes and laws regarding same-sex sexuality, as they may shape the use and delivery of settlement services in Canada. Given negative attitudes and legislation in their home countries, it is understandable that some newcomers are fearful of disclosing their same-sex sexual orientation to service providers and may hold negative views regarding LGB people.

Service Needs of LGB Newcomers

Given the complexity of attitudes about same-sex sexual orientation and the fact that data regarding sexual orientation are not systematically gathered at the time of migration, it is not surprising that there is a lack of information regarding the settlement needs of LGB newcomers to Canada. There also is an absence of research regarding settlement needs specific to these populations, a gap this study aims to begin to address. We assumed in this inquiry that the demographic profile of LGB newcomers is similar to that of heterosexual immigrants in terms of age, gender, ethnicity, social class, disability, and other markers of social location.

We also assumed that LGB newcomers experience many of the issues that impact the well-being of native-born LGB Canadians. For example, internalized heterosexism can hinder development of self-esteem and establishment of supportive relationships (Pachankis and Goldfried 2004); and the stress of anti-gay violence and discrimination may contribute to mental health and addiction problems (Harper and Schneider 2003). Given that men who have sex with men account for the majority of people diagnosed with HIV/AIDS in Canada (PHAC 2007b), it is reasonable to assume that some gay and bisexual newcomers have complex service needs related to health. In this study we focused specifically on newcomers' needs relevant to settlement services, particularly those related to social support, one of the key determinants of health as noted earlier.

Settlement Services for Newcomers

Settlement services focus specifically on the social inclusion of newcomers. Funded by Citizenship and Immigration Canada (CIC), settlement services aim to '... facilitate the full and equal participation of all newcomers in Canadian society' (Canadian Council for Refugees 1998). Services are delivered by means of various arrangements across the provinces and territories, often through local ethno-specific agencies. Among other services, settlement programs provide referral and counselling, language skills training, orientation to life in Canada, and connections with mentors for support in adjusting to life in Canada. Values seen to inform best practices particularly relevant to LGB immigrants and refugees are promotion of access to institutions, inclusion, respect for individuals, and cultural sensitivity.

While there is a lack of information regarding the responsiveness of settlement services to LGB newcomers, a number of issues in the provision of health and social services to these populations have been identified that are relevant to the provision of settlement services. Out of fear of discrimination, some gay men and lesbians do not seek help, or, when they do, conceal their sexual orientation (Neville and Henrickson 2006; Ontario Public Health Association 2000). In withholding information related to their sexuality, clients may receive less than optimal service and professionals may remain unaware that they are serving LGB people (Brotman et al. 2002). Similarly, some service providers conceal their sexual orientation for fear of discrimination by colleagues and clients (Hughes 2004). The result is that their knowledge relevant to LGB issues is unavailable to colleagues and service users. Finally, there is evidence that some service providers lack knowledge and supportive attitudes regarding same-sex sexual orientation (Harris, Nightengale, and Owen 1995; Schwanberg 1996). This study of experiences and perceptions of LGB newcomers and settlement service providers aimed to shed some light on issues to consider specifically in relation to settlement services.

Description of the Study

We took a qualitative descriptive approach (Sandelowski 2000) to uncovering issues for consideration in the provision of settlement services to queer newcomers. The study was conducted in a large urban region in Canada that is a major reception centre for immigrants and refugees. We recruited newcomers for interviews by means of advertisements distributed to LGB community organizations as well as to personal acquaintances. We also sent letters to executive directors of agencies inviting the participation of administrative and front-line staff. Data were gathered using semi-structured interviews that explored perceptions of LGB newcomers' needs, experiences with services, and recommendations for change. We also asked service providers about agency policies and programs, including professional education relevant to serving LGB newcomers. Using qualitative content analysis (Hsieh and Shannon 2005), we examined interview transcripts for common themes.

The sample of newcomers included three lesbian immigrants, two gay male refugees, and one gay male immigrant. Two of these participants had emigrated from Malaysia, while the others came from China, Japan, Indonesia, and Chile. They were between 25 and 50 years old and all but one had post-secondary education. Three of these participants had arrived less than five years prior to the interviews, while the others had been settled in Canada for more than 10 years.

The sample of service providers included 11 women and seven men from seven settlement agencies. Within this sample, there was one gay man who had been a refugee from Mexico and another who had emigrated from China. Two of the service providers had been born in Canada while the rest came from China, Japan, India, Latin America, Africa, and Eastern Europe. All of the service providers except the refugee had been in Canada at least 10 years. These participants were between 30 and 50 years old, the exception being one who was 21 years old. All had post-secondary education primarily in the social sciences. Eight of the participants were in senior management positions while the remainder were direct service providers, including one volunteer. Given the small sample size, we recognize that other issues may have emerged had we spoken with more people. The points we discuss below are, however, worthy of consideration.

Identity and Coming Out in Various Cultural Contexts

To understand LGB newcomers' needs and agencies' responses to them, it is important to keep in mind the possible diversity of values and behaviours in relation to identity, sexuality, and coming out. As noted above, one issue is that newcomers may not identify as gay or lesbian despite their same-sex sexual attraction and behaviour. One queer newcomer noted that in some cultures '... sexuality is ... not a separate part of your identity ...' Even when people do identify as gay or lesbian, they may be reluctant to come out, in part because to do so may be seen as a reflection on their family and community. As a gay service provider commented:

> ... if you're from an individualistic community, it doesn't matter for you to stand up and be different from the community ... that drives the coming out perspective of the West. You have to come out, be honest ... be proud, and fight for acceptance. But if it's a more collectivist community, where the value is to be [harmonious] within the community, it is a risk to stand out, people do not want to stand out, they want to be part of the group ... in families, agencies and in community ... it's all right as long as you don't publicly acknowledge it.

Furthermore, coming out may contradict values in some cultural contexts. For instance, revealing that one is gay can be seen as conflicting with expectations to fulfill family duties such as having children. A sharp distinction may be made between what is kept private and what is shared with the community because of fear of creating scandal in the community. This need to preserve their image may inhibit discussion of gay-related issues when newcomers seek help from settlement services – venues that are seen as 'public' despite their promises of confidentiality. Furthermore, as a service provider noted, speaking openly about sexuality may also breach cultural mores, particularly because LGB issues may be understood as referring narrowly to specific sexual acts such as anal intercourse. A lesbian newcomer observed that in some ethnic communities there is a perception that there are no LGB people within their group. She commented, '... the minute you say "gay" it creates a particular image, usually very Western ...' She perceived that some newcomers believe that those who reveal their same-sex sexual orientation have given up their ethnic identity and taken on that of the dominant culture.

On the other hand, some newcomers resist pressure to be silent regarding their same-sex sexual orientation. Francisco Ibanez-Carrasco, a participant in this study, asked to be identified in reports by name as a gay, HIV positive, Latino man. He argued that it is important that heterosexist ideas be challenged. Therefore, rather than accepting being made invisible, he is proud of having gradually and successfully 'gone public' about who he is, and feels this is important for himself and others like him. Not all newcomers, however, come out in the Western sense when involved with settlement services, which impedes recognizing and responding to their needs.

LGB Newcomers' Settlement Needs

Participants believed that in addition to requiring services in the same areas as heterosexuals, LGB newcomers may have needs particularly related to their sexual orientation. Specifically, gay and lesbian immigrants and refugees may need help in overcoming isolation and in using mainstream services.

Overcoming Isolation

A key need identified by LGB participants was for acceptance and support within their cultural communities without having to conceal their sexual orientation. A gay newcomer described the isolation a newcomer may experience: '... because of ... language and the cultural perspective, it [is] difficult for [a newcomer] to meet people ... he's lonely, cannot find a boyfriend ... when immigrant services [are relevant to] sexual orientation is when he wants a relationship, but doesn't feel that he has a community.'

LGB newcomers may feel excluded from their communities in part due to their perception that oppressive laws and negative attitudes in relation to same-sex sexuality in the countries from which they emigrated may hinder their acceptance in Canada. A lesbian participant commented that there is considerable need for support around '... the emotional stuff ... self-hate, internalized and general homophobia.' Thus newcomers may be wary about being open about their sexuality, presenting a barrier in connecting with other queer people within their communities.

LGB newcomers expressed the desire to be connected with peers for social support as well as practical information. In major Canadian cities with large populations of recent newcomers, there are ethnic minority LGB groups that provide opportunities for socializing, as well as volunteer organizations that assist refugees and immigrants seeking admission to Canada on the basis of their sexual orientation. For example, Sher Vancouver and VariAsian are support groups for LGB Sikhs and people of Asian descent; ihola! is a Toronto group for gay Latinos; Helem is a Montreal group for LGBs of Lebanese backgrounds; LEGIT and Rainbow Refugees respond to refugees' needs. While such groups can provide peer support, LGB newcomers may still feel marginalized within their broader ethnic community.

Often newcomers look to 'mainstream' LGB communities in order to make social connections. Gay and lesbian participants articulated the wish that settlement services help them connect to both dominant-culture LGB communities for social support and practical information, as well as ethno-specific groups. In addition, newcomers may encounter racism within mainstream communities and feel excluded because of cultural differences. A gay settlement worker noted that it can be stressful for newcomers to participate simultaneously in ethnic minority and dominant culture LGB communities. Having to seek gay friends outside their ethnic communities can exacerbate the sense of isolation, interfering with the integration of newcomers' cultural and sexual identities.

Using Mainstream Services

It is always easier to access information in your native language, particularly when the topic is a sensitive and personal one. For instance, a settlement worker noted that newcomers who experience abuse from same-sex partners may need to be made aware of mainstream services for victims of violence. LGB newcomers may have particular needs related to health and immigration. For instance, Francisco Ibanez-Carrasco noted newcomers' need for information and support in relation to HIV / AIDS: '... sexual health issues don't come up properly in immigrant service organizations ... if you come from a region of the world where there is a lot of silence ... in terms of HIV, you can still get infected very quickly here ... people don't have the necessary networks, are forced to figure out all the many layers about sexual health and their sexuality here.'

Newcomers from societies in which same-sex sexuality is proscribed and hidden may be particularly vulnerable to HIV infection if they lack information and education on prevention methods. In addition, new-comers may need the support of a person from their own culture in accessing HIV services.

While the Immigration and Refugee Protection Act (Bill C-11) allows sponsorship of same-sex partners, a settlement worker noted that LGB newcomers may need to be made aware of this, and be informed about how it can be accomplished. The Act also allows individuals to seek refugee status on the basis of persecution in their home country related to their sexual orientation. Importantly, as one lesbian immigrant com-mented, seeking status on this basis can be anxiety-provoking because of fears about the impact of revealing same-sex sexual orientation.

Service Issues

Participants indicated that issues related to same-sex sexuality are sel-dom raised at settlement agencies. On the one hand, it appears that few newcomers present needs related to their sexual orientation when us-ing services, and on the other hand, most service providers do not ask about them. This pattern seems related to several aspects of the service delivery context.

Trust

One of the reasons newcomers may not approach settlement agencies for help relevant to their sexual orientation is that they do not feel safe in doing so. A gay settlement worker suggested that some newcom-ers would be reluctant to reveal sensitive personal information to what they perceive as 'official' organizations because of previous experiences in their homelands: '... where I came from, [in] government agencies ... confidentiality and respect are not guaranteed. I don't trust them ...' Service providers speculated that LGB newcomers may be particularly wary of coming out in an agency that focuses on serving their ethnic group out of fears that information about their sexuality would leak out to members of the community. Adding to such anxiety is the perception by a lesbian newcomer that heterosexism within her community might be reflected in the ethno-specific agency: 'I would not feel comfortable going to [a settlement agency]... because I don't feel [my] community is very open, especially since I attended that [anti-same-sex marriage] rally ... those people ... look like me. It was quite painful to see.'

Consistent with that observation is the deduction by a gay newcomer that 'colour-blind' agency approaches that claim to 'treat everyone equally' result in ignoring the presence of LGB people and a lack of sensitivity to their needs. The confluence of these influences makes it difficult for newcomers to trust settlement services enough to be open about who they are, and subsequently for agencies to become aware of the needs of this population.

Recognizing Needs

Individuals' attitudes as well as agencies' interpretation of their mission may influence recognition of newcomers' needs. For example, a gay newcomer described how an interpreter distorted his description of the sex-related issues for which he was seeking help: '... I realize[d], "No, that's not what I wanted to say" ... you have to help the interpreter if you know that she or he is not saying the truth, because sometimes they feel uncomfortable.'

He perceived that the interpreter's need to avoid explicit talk about sexuality caused her to translate his comments inaccurately. This man sensed a lack of understanding and acceptance when interacting with workers. It follows that if clients detect such reactions, they will be unlikely to be forthcoming about their needs.

Although service providers could see how information about clients' gender was relevant to the provision of settlement services, they questioned the significance of data regarding sexual orientation. Specifically, while recognizing that knowledge regarding the client's gender could be useful given that men and women might have different needs, providers could not fathom how information about a newcomer's sexual identity could be similarly helpful. If agencies assume that knowing clients' sexual orientation is immaterial to service delivery, they do not gather such information and thus conclude that such needs do not exist among the populations they serve. Further contributing to reluctance about addressing sexual orientation is service providers' worry about individual clients' reactions if such issues were to be raised, as well as trepidation about community reactions, particularly in terms of their effect on fundraising. They also wondered what implications for services would follow from an explicit commitment to address needs related to sexual orientation.

Enhancing Accessibility and Responsiveness

Participants' comments as well as the literature point to initiatives that services could undertake to support the settlement and integration of queer newcomers. These include shaping organizational cultures to be more inclusive of LGB people, and strengthening links among communities and services.

Shaping Organizational Cultures

A gay immigrant who worked in a settlement agency pointed out that values that newcomers bring from their homelands can influence organizational cultures to ignore the presence of people with same-sex sexual orientation. He commented: '... the [ethnic minority] community might criticize the [agency], so they'd rather ... be non-gay, non-controversial ... not have any programs or acknowledgement of gay people ... [the agency] can be quite progressive and caring about individual gay clients, but as an agency they don't say anything about that.'

To become more inclusive, settlement services could officially recognize the presence of queer people within their organizations and among populations they serve.

A lesbian newcomer suggested that formal acknowledgement of the participation of LGB people in agency programs would contribute to the creation of a safer environment in which service providers and clients could be open about their sexuality. She pointed out that this could be achieved by inclusion of references to sexual diversity in agency policies, program descriptions, publicity, and service delivery procedures. In addition, a service provider observed that '... a significant difference was having senior management who [were] openly gay ... other people see that.' Agency leadership can clearly contribute to making services more comfortable for LGB workers and clients.

Given the needs identified earlier with respect to using mainstream services, participants recommended that settlement agencies make information about discrimination, sexual health, and abuse in same-sex relationships available in various languages. They also advocated use of gender-neutral language and provision of opportunities for clients to self-identify their sexual orientation during intake practices if they choose to.

Staff Development

Bringing about change in organizations in relation to any issue can be challenging, and this is particularly true when addressing LGB issues given the pervasiveness of heterosexism. Both service providers as well as newcomers emphasized the importance of education for agency staff regarding LGB issues in general, and also more specifically in relation to settlement and integration. A lesbian newcomer pointed out the value of training that is culturally appropriate: '... the fact that different communities express their queerness in different ways ... when you just learn about gay and lesbian [issues] in a North American context, you think that all people are gay in this way, when folks from your own community might not relate to gayness in that way.'

Furthermore, she felt that it was key that LGB issues be integrated into all aspects of staff training rather than isolated in a separate workshop.

Strengthening Links among Communities and Services

Service providers argued that support from newcomers' communities is necessary for settlement services to become more inclusive of LGB people. They advocated fostering dialogue within newcomer communities regarding sexuality, heterosexism, and homophobia. They also saw the building of bridges between settlement services and queer organizations as an effective approach to increasing inclusion. A service provider described the positive impact of LGB people volunteering in settlement agencies: '... it's good to have gay ambassadors ... I know an Asian guy who volunteers for [a settlement agency] ... he's out, and they love him ... it's an educational process, they ask him questions, they're comfortable ... he is a part of the community.'

A gay service provider's experience was that collaborating in service delivery builds capacity in both settlement agencies and LGB community services. On the other hand, a lesbian newcomer pointed out that LGB community organizations are not always that welcoming of immigrants and refugees in part because of racism.

As another lesbian newcomer stated, enhancing the inclusion of LGB people in settlement services is fundamentally motivated by a commitment to social justice. The goals of helping to integrate newcomers in Canadian society and of respecting individual differences with cultural sensitivity need to be embraced by settlement services in relation to the unique needs of LGB newcomers.

NOTE

1 Although transgender people face marginalization similar in some aspects to that encountered by LGB people, their needs are distinct from those of LGB people and are not addressed in this chapter.

5 The Fatherhood Experiences of Sudanese[1] and Russian Newcomer Men: Challenges to Their Health and Well-being

DAVID C. ESTE AND ADMASU TACHBLE

Introduction

The *2010 Annual Report to Parliament on Immigration* highlighted the key immigration activities that took place in 2009. The number of permanent residents admitted into Canada in 2009 was 252,179. These figures are consistent with the government's intention to have a balanced immigration plan to ensure that the labour needs of the country will be met. Meanwhile, family reunification will continue to be fostered, and the humanitarian principles of refugee protection will be honoured (Citizenship and Immigration Canada 2010).

There were 247,243 newcomers admitted into Canada as permanent residents in 2008. Of these, 63.9 per cent (149,072) were Economic Immigrants and Their Dependents, 22.5 per cent (65,567) were designated Family Class, 9.3 per cent (21,860) were Protected Persons Class (Citizen and Immigration 2010). The foreign-born population increased by 13.6 per cent between 2001 and 2006. According to the 2006 Census data, 19.5 per cent of Canada's total population was born outside of the country. Statistics Canada (2007) reported the top three countries of origin as China (155,051, or 14 per cent), India (129,140, or 11.6 per cent), and the Philippines (77,888, or 7 per cent).

Calgary, the site of this study, also experienced considerable growth in its foreign-born population during the period 2001 to 2006. There were an estimated 252,800 foreign-born residents in the city in 2006, a 28 per cent increase from the 197,400 reported in 2001. These figures represent 23.6 per cent of the Calgary population in 2006 and 20.9 per cent in 2001. According to the 2006 census data, Calgary as a metropolitan area was the fourth largest in attracting newcomers (5.2 per cent of the estimated 1.1 million newcomers who ventured to Canada between 2001 and 2006), and with its strong economy, it is highly likely this trend will continue (Statistics Canada 2007).

Gender and Immigration

From a gender perspective, the terms *gender* and *immigration* tend to be associated with women's experiences. This has been an important movement in recognizing that health, social, and other forms of integration may be differentially experienced by women due to issues of power, cultural norms for gender roles, and reproductive health, and their positions within families. As a number of chapters in this volume illustrate, there is the need for continued emphasis on research into women's experiences of immigration; however, this chapter draws attention to the corresponding need to understand the experiences of men. It is no longer acceptable to assume that all men equally share positions of power. As will be evident from the voices of the Sudanese and Russian fathers presented in the following pages, these men face significant challenges in Canadian society, not only as fathers but also as immigrants or refugees in a new context. Hence, it is paramount that we examine our constructions of gender and the importance of better understanding the intersection and influences of gender on the immigration experience for both men and women. By paying attention to this issue, we will have a heightened understanding of the complexities associated with the adaptation experiences of newcomers (Rose, Preston, and Dyck 2002).

Immigrant and refugee male adults come to Canada with multiple identities, experiences, and roles, one of which may be paternal. Using the experiences of newcomer Sudanese and Russian fathers in a major Canadian urban centre, this chapter examines the challenges they encounter and how they may impact not only their own health and well-being, but also that of their families. The next section provides a brief review of Sudanese and Russian immigration to Canada, followed by a review of existing literature on the experiences of immigrant and refugee men as fathers. A description of how the study was conducted is then presented, followed by a summary of the major findings. This section is followed by a discussion of our final conclusions.

Sudanese and Russian Immigration to Canada

Years of internal conflict served as the primary reason for the migration of the Sudanese to Canada over the past 15 years, the majority of whom came from Southern Sudan. Subjected to harsh challenges such as severe drought, oppressive behaviour including mass killings, and environmental destruction perpetuated and sanctioned by the national government, it is estimated that over half a million Sudanese have fled to other African countries (Ethiopia, Uganda, Chad, Kenya) (Both 2003). Thousands of children and youth were left orphaned. Describing the civil war, Both states that '... the country (Sudan) has continued to be economically backward with peripheral areas in deterioration and millions of people dying of starvation in a very rich country in terms of agricultural potential and mineral resources. The natural revenue has always been allocated for military build-up to quell the Southern rebellion by force' (3).

It is estimated that 15,000 to 20,000 Sudanese reside in the Greater Toronto Area. Simich et al. (2005) comment on the community in that city: 'The population is internally very diverse in ethnic, religious, and social terms, including urban professionals, international students, and rural peoples from all regions of Sudan who have been arriving in Canada in steadily growing numbers since the early 1990s' (11). They also discuss the Sudanese community in Ontario: 'Overall, the Sudanese population in Ontario is relatively young, moderately educated, and largely underemployed. The majority of Sudanese in Ontario are government-assisted refugees (GARs). The majority have come directly from refugee camps' (11).

The majority of the approximately 7,500 Sudanese who reside in Calgary are government-sponsored refugees who fled civil strife in Sudan (personal communication, Wek Kuol 2005). A major integration challenge for this population is employment. Individuals with a university education or trained in the trades are usually working in low-skilled, low-paying jobs. Although language is a major barrier to employment, discrimination appears to be a key contributor to the issue of underemployment. The majority of Sudanese who have settled in Canada are from the Southern Sudan where the majority of the population is Christian. This is reflected in the study's sample as all of the participants are of this religious faith.

The Russian Jewish community has resided in Canada since the end of the nineteenth century. According to Cohen (2001), there have been several strong waves of Russian immigration to Canada during the past 100 years. At the turn of the twentieth Century, economic crises precipitated a mass migration of individuals from Ukraine to western Canada. From 1918 to 1930, Russians attempting to escape persecution during the post-revolution era migrated to this country. A smaller wave settled shortly after the end of the Second World War.

From the late 1960s to the end of the 1980s, members of the Soviet Jewish community migrated to Israel, some of whom later relocated to Canada. Since the early 1990s a group of successful and highly qualified specialists from Russia described as the 'professional wave' came to Canada in search of employment that matched their skills and knowledge (Cohen 2001). According to Statistics Canada, in 2001 approximately 50,000 Russian Jews resided in Canada with the largest concentrations in Toronto and Montreal. Smaller communities exist in Vancouver, Calgary, Edmonton, Halifax, and Ottawa. It is estimated that between 70 and 75 per cent migrated to Canada after an initial settlement in Israel. In Calgary specifically, immigrants from Russia constituted one of the high-growth newcomer communities from 1992 to 2002. In fact, this group ranked ninth in terms of countries of birth for newcomers in 2005 (City of Calgary 2007). Despite the relatively small sample size of the Russian community in Calgary, estimated to be approximately 5,000 individuals (personal communication, Gayla Rogers 2008), six of the 14 Russian fathers who participated in this study were Jewish.

Fathering Roles

In North America the role of the father has continuously fluctuated over time. He has offered moral guidance; served as the breadwinner; been a sex role model, nurturer, and co-parent; and provided marital support (Stearns 1991; LaRossa 1997; Cabrera et al. 2000; Lamb 2000). The shifting conceptualization of the father could be attributed partially to the number of women in the workforce, rising rate of unemployment among men, growth in the feminist movement, and the desire by men to be more involved with their children (Stearns 1991; Bouchard 2003). The shift in the construct of the place of the father in the family, however, did not mean a total shift as we moved from one period to the other. In multicultural societies such as Canadian and Russian, there may be cultural and sub-cultural variations by which parents perceive their family roles and responsibilities, and these factors undoubtedly shape expectations as to what it means to be a father (Marsiglio et al. 2000; Lewis and Lamb 2003). A cross-cultural understanding of fathers, therefore, requires sensitivity to the function of men within the family. Despite the key role fathers play in the family setting, research on fathers appears to be marginalized and the service needs of male parents are 'generally an afterthought' by researchers (O'Donnell et al. 2005:395). The following section provides a brief overview of the migration process with focus on the primary reasons why people migrate and a review of pertinent studies that examined the experiences of immigrants and refugees as fathers.

Literature Review

The contemporary era is characterized by the unprecedented movement of people from one corner of the globe to the other. Such movement of people could take place on an involuntary or voluntary basis, although, as argued in the introduction of this volume, the boundaries between voluntary and involuntary migration can be somewhat indistinct. The United Nations High Commission for Refugees (2003) estimates there were 20 million displaced people who were forced to live in neighbouring countries as refugees. Furthermore, Rowe and colleagues (2000) state the number of voluntary migrants who leave their homelands in search of better life and working conditions (mostly to North America and Western Europe) in a given year far exceeds the number of refugees.

People generally relocate for two reasons: to look for greater economic opportunities to improve one's standard of living; and to experience social, religious, and political freedom and stability that might be denied in their home country (Christensen 2001). Those looking for better opportunities initiate the movement of their own free will, and their actions involve a certain level of planning, while those in search of an accepting political climate to protect their beliefs, values, and lives are forced to make a sudden departure. Whatever the case, moving means leaving that which is familiar for some place that is different in many ways (Hulewat 1996). Immigrant fathers who have left familial and cultural settings must adapt to a new context and reorganize their lives, often requiring them to change values, expectations, norms, and behaviours, including the perceived role of the father. Individually and collectively, these challenges may impact their health and well-being.

Economic provisioning is considered to be a central feature of a father's role in most segments of society (Featherstone 2003), the one 'fathers perceive as their fundamental role' (Bouchard 2003:8) as evidenced by their 'vulnerability and distress when they fail to fulfill' (7) this duty under different circumstances. To fathers, the ability to provide their children with 'food on the table, a warm place to live, stability, a solid place in the community, and good prospects for the future' (7) is considered vital. It is the role that immigrant and refugee men, however, find difficult to discharge when underemployed or unemployed (Cabrera et al. 2000; Clark, Shimoni, and Este 2000; Shimoni, Este, and Clark 2003).

One of the few studies that examined paternal engagement in immigrant and refugee families in Canada was conducted by Shimoni, Este, and Clark (2003). Twenty-four immigrant and refugee fathers of preschool children from the former.Yugoslavia, South America, South Asia, and China (Hong Kong and the Mainland) were interviewed. Their average length of stay in Canada was 2.75 years. Questions focused on their understanding of the meaning of being a father, the values and principles that guided their practice, and their perceptions and experiences on being a father in Canada. More specifically, the challenges encountered in the new environment, and understanding how Canadian society facilitated their practice of fatherhood were addressed. Commentary was offered on how struggles with unemployment and underemployment impacted them emotionally. It was apparent to the authors that despite this barrier, the fathers were not at risk for disengaging from their children: '...we saw a group of fathers from four different cultures who are positively engaged with their children as they face the struggles of acculturation, language acquisition, and employment ... we repeatedly saw stress related to unemployment and underemployment' (565).

Appreciation for parent education opportunities in which they had participated or a desire and need to learn more was evident (Shimoni, Este, and Clark 2003:566), a direct result of the increased child-rearing responsibilities fathers experience in Canada.

Bhandari, Horvath, and To (2006) conducted a participatory action research project involving eight Canadian men from six different countries. The participants shared their experiences and knowledge on integration issues impacting men in Canadian society from which the authors created a questionnaire that was administered to 30 men from 12 different countries. These respondents identified settlement and adaptation to life in Canada and barriers to employment as their two major challenges.

Grant and Nadin (2007) in their study focused on the experiences of 180 skilled immigrants from Asia and Africa who experienced difficulty having their foreign credentials recognized. Although most had completed advanced post-secondary training and held positions requiring a high level of skill prior to relocating to Canada, many were unable to obtain equivalent work and were employed in jobs for which they were overqualified. Grant and Nadin (2007) comment on the impact of the employment challenges experienced by skilled immigrants: 'Of course, living with un/underemployment is stressful for most individuals but it is particularly so for skilled immigrants because it exacerbates acculturative stress and prevents immigrants from achieving full economic adaptation defined as "full economic participation" in the economic life of Canada' (144).

A study by Strier and Roer-Strier (2005) on the perceptions and experiences of 15 Jewish immigrants from Ethiopia and 15 from the former Soviet Union, now in Israel, exhibited both change and continuity. Fathers in both groups maintained core cultural values and simultaneously adopted new ones to facilitate integration into their new environment. Both acknowledged increased participation in raising their children and in supporting their spouse. The authors acknowledged the variation in conceptualizing the impact of immigration on the fathering experiences of these two groups. Fathers from the former Soviet Union contended that immigration to Israel enriched their family role. Conversely, Ethiopian fathers maintained the settlement process jeopardized their place in the family. Strier and Roer-Strier suggest that such differences may be attributed to the ecological differences of the countries of origin and to the higher levels of systemic racism experienced by the Ethiopian fathers.

Methodology

This study utilized what Patton (2002) describes as the pragmatic approach to qualitative research. Despite the fact that there are several 'paradigms' in qualitative research, it is acceptable for researchers not to use a specific qualitative approach such as grounded theory or phenomenology. Patton describes what he means by pragmatism: 'My pragmatic stance aims to supersede one-sided paradigm allegiance by increasing the concrete and practical methodological options available to researchers and evaluators. Such pragmatism means judging the quality of the study by its intended purposes, available resources, procedures followed, and results obtained, all within a particular context and for a specific audience' (72).

Schatzman and Strauss (1973) echo Patton's position, as they are primarily concerned with strategies to collect and analyse data collected in the field. They state: '... field research is a methodological pragmatist. He sees any method of inquiry as a system of strategies and operations designed – at any time – for getting answers to certain questions about events which interest him' (7).

Sample

Given the focus of the study, it was determined that a criterion sampling strategy would be most appropriate to identify and select fathers to participate. This type of purposeful sampling involves the selection of participants on the basis of preconceived criteria. Hence, based on the lead author's previous study exploring the experiences of immigrant and refugee fathers, recruitment was guided by two criteria: (1) a minimum of up to six months and a maximum of 10 years residence; and (2) fathers with children up to 12 years of age.

Selection of Newcomer Communities

A number of factors contributed to the decision to focus the study on Sudanese refugee and Russian immigrant men. The Sudanese community has emerged as the largest African newcomer community in Calgary over the last decade, yet very little research exists on this population in the city. One of the authors (Este) is well connected with the Sudanese community in Calgary through his participation in other studies; this was perceived to be his advantage with respect to the merits of the study and the recruitment of participants. The influx of Russian newcomers from Russia and Israel resulted in a sizeable increase of this community in the 1990s. Like the Sudanese, there is virtually no research on this group, and this was, therefore, the major reason for selecting this community. The lead author is also well known to the agencies that assisted in the recruitment of Russian fathers.

Recruitment

Three non-profit organizations in the city of Calgary were approached to assist with the recruitment of participants. The Calgary Immigrant Aid Society (CIAS) and Jewish Family Services play an important role in assisting in the settlement and adaptation. The third agency, the New Sudan Society of Alberta, works directly with members of the Calgary Sudanese community.

Information pertinent to the study, purpose, and rationale for the study, the selection criteria for recruiting participants, and the expectations of participants in the research process were presented to key agency personnel by the research team.

Demographic Profile

At the time of the interview, the 20 Sudanese refugee men who participated in the study had resided in Canada for no longer than 10 years. Nine had arrived since 2000, eight were Canadian citizens, 11 were landed immigrants, and one did not share his status. Fourteen of the Sudanese fathers possessed some post-secondary education, nine of whom were university graduates; one did not have secondary school education. Fourteen were employed, two were seeking employment, and four were students. They ranged in age from 25 to 57. All of the men were of the Christian faith from Southern Sudan where the Christian population experienced persecution and oppression by the Islamic Sudanese who primarily resided in the northern part of Sudan.

The sample from the Russian community consisted of 14 men from the former Soviet Union who immigrated to Canada between 2000 and 2005. Their ages ranged from 27 to 50, the majority of whom were under 40. The Russian fathers held at least a diploma or a certificate from a college. Five graduated with a bachelor's degree, five held a master's degree, three had a diploma or certificate, and one possessed a doctoral degree. Twelve respondents worked full time; the remaining individuals were employed part-time and attending university. Seven participants were employed in either the construction or health fields; the balance worked in the services sector.

Data Collection

The 2003 Shimoni, Este, and Clark study on the experiences of immigrant fathers, as well as commentary provided by other sources, assisted in the creation of the interview guide. During the interviews, which ranged from 40 to 90 minutes, participants were asked to respond to questions on the meaning of fatherhood, the values that guide their behaviour as fathers, how they learned to be a father, the nature of their interactions with their children, aspirations for their children, decision-making in the family, benefits gained from their move to Canada, and the challenges they encounter as fathers in a new society.

To ensure consistency on how the interviews were conducted, the Sudanese men were interviewed by a male member of the community with a graduate degree in social work and considerable experience as a research interviewer. The Sudanese interviews were conducted in English; however, the interviewer spoke the same languages as the respondents (Dinka or Arabic) and could therefore interpret questions or concepts into their first language. The Russian interviews also were conducted by a graduate student in social work who was familiar with the agency from where the men were recruited.

Data Analysis

Given the nature of the research design, an inductive data analysis method was used. Patton (2002) states '... inductive analysis involves discoveries, patterns, themes, and categories in one's data. Findings emerge from the data' (453). Lincoln and Guba (1985) define data inductive analysis as 'a process for making sense of field data' (202).

After the interviews were transcribed, research team members read the transcripts several times. The lead author identified categories and themes, which resulted in the creation of an initial coding framework that served as the foundation for the subsequent in-depth analysis and a more robust coding system. The data analysis was facilitated by the use of Atlas.*ti*, a software program for the management and analysis of textual data through coding and recoding, organization of families of codes, and retrieval of information. To strengthen inter-coder reliability, random interviews were coded manually by the lead author and then compared to the analyses of the co-author. The next section of the chapter presents some of the major results of the study. Particular attention is placed on the challenges faced by the participants in carrying out their role as a father and how these barriers may be impacting their health and well-being.

Experiences of Fatherhood in the Canadian Context

Meaning of Fatherhood

When questioned about the meaning of fatherhood, respondents from both groups expressed notions of responsibility, commitment, and care. The majority contended providing for their family was their major priority. One Russian participant stated, '... to take care of my children ...

my family.' The following words from a Sudanese father also capture the essence of this sentiment: 'As a father, you have to take full charge, full responsibility of your kids in terms of providing the services that are essential for them.' However, some participants encountered difficulties fulfilling this priority.

Assuming the role of the teacher educating their children on how to be 'good' citizens with a strong sense of right and wrong also emerged as an important paternal duty, '... teaching them my mother tongue and respect to other people and teach them how to interact with other people' (Sudanese father). This was reinforced by one of the Russian participants as he maintained, 'It is more important to be a good person in this world.'

Being a protector for their children was also identified as a primary responsibility. One Russian father commented: '... to provide safety for my daughter.' For a Sudanese father, fleeing his conflict-ridden country and coming to Canada was perceived as a major benefit: '... at least I am safe and I do not feel anything life threatened.'

Guiding Values

Discussing the values that guide their behaviour as fathers, Sudanese respondents consistently stressed the value of ensuring that their children are respectful: 'You have to show your children how to get along with people, how to give them [the children] respect, and show them how to respect other people.' For the Sudanese participants, the importance of their culture and traditions emerged as a major value that guided their behaviour as fathers: 'The behaviour of the father is guided by old African traditions as well as the community tradition. One has to follow all the traditions.' Another strong value for the Sudanese was the overwhelming importance placed on ensuring their children were respectful and well mannered: 'From the place I came from and the way I was brought up, I have to teach my children how to respect other people.'

Values such as the importance of education and one's family were also identified by the Russian fathers. For the Russian fathers, the importance of the family unit emerged as a primary value. As two fathers, respectively, remarked: 'First of all, the family unit is not only very important but the most important thing ... probably everything is less important than relationships in the family,' and 'It is the relationships [within the family] ... good relationships and understanding each other.'

Consistently, both groups of fathers stressed the importance of their children getting a good education: 'The most important thing is that they have to go to school to study ... I will try my best to support them so that they can get a better education and get a good job when they finish their studies.' One Russian father remarked, 'I am ready to give my child a good education.'

Aspirations for Their Children

As noted, one of the primary reasons individuals migrate to Canada is to ensure their children will have better educational opportunities that will in turn lead to employment to provide economic security. Fathers from both groups strongly reinforced this sentiment. One Russian father remarked, 'I want her to go to university after high school. It is very important for her to become a professional.' Another participant from the same community stated, '... if you want your kids to get a college or university degree, you have to send them outside of Russia where they would be able to complete high school and then go to university.'

The following words from two Sudanese fathers mirror the hopes expressed by their Russian counterparts: 'I always tell them they should pursue their education, they have to finish their education. Secondly, I always tell them that they should have ambitions in life ... having a career,' and 'I am really hopeful that when they become adults they will begin to provide for themselves and will be responsible citizens.'

The latter father also expressed the hope his children 'will get better work than the work' he and his wife currently hold. The future well-being of their children definitely appeared to be a major preoccupation for both groups of fathers.

Interaction with Their Children

Fathers from the Sudanese and Russian communities interact with their children in a number of ways, since spending time with them was deemed important: 'If we go outside together, camping or barbecue, we do it together and she likes to go fishing' (Russian father); 'I sit with my daughter to do housework or we share the television' (Sudanese father).

Other activities included visiting friends, going to parks, reading to their children, and going for walks. The amount of time spent with their children, however, was contingent upon the type of job held and hours of work. One Sudanese father stated: 'In Canada as an immigrant, I do not have time for the family because all the time I just work, work, sleep, and there is no time you can enjoy, even with your family.' Some of the Russian fathers also felt they did not have enough time to interact with their children.

Challenges Impacting Fathering Role

The major challenge facing immigrants and refugees in their efforts to integrate into Canadian society is the lack of recognition of their foreign credentials. This issue is well documented in several studies and reports (Ngo and Este 2006; Wayland 2006; Longitudinal Survey of Immigrants 2003; Austin and Este 2001; Basran and Zong 1998). The Longitudinal Survey of Immigrants (2003) noted the following in its discussion of the major obstacles newcomers confront when entering the labour force: '[For new arrivals with foreign credentials] the most critical hurdles faced when trying to find employment were lack of experience in the Canadian workforce and difficulty in transferring their qualifications. Each of these obstacles was cited by 26 per cent of newcomers who had foreign credentials and reported at least one problem when trying to enter the labour market' (33).

In their project that involved immigrant men, Bhandari, Horvath, and To (2006) reported the following: 'A participant discussion concluded that foreign university degrees and work experience are regarded as worthless by agencies and Canadian employers. Additionally, barriers such as inadequate language proficiency and/or discriminatory hiring practices often hamper the economic performance of immigrants' (143).

The issue of being underemployed impacted both the Sudanese and Russian fathers. However, comparatively speaking, it emerged as being extremely problematic for the men from the Sudan: 'My work does not match the experience and education I got before I came to Canada. I was expecting a better position than the one I am now doing. I am just working as a labourer, a physical job, a meat cutter, and I have wasted more than 20 years of studying' (Sudanese father).

Another Sudanese male who held a degree in mechanical engineering completed in the Sudan commented, 'I am doing just a surviving job, that upsets me a lot.' Some of the Sudanese fathers commented on the treatment they received in their work environment and the impact of such behaviour: 'Some may just insult you for no reason as it is very normal at my place of work ... someone may annoy you and then you come home not happy'; 'Many of us are working in meat plants that are oppressive and take advantage of us. At these workplaces, we are subject to name calling by white workers.'

Some of the Russian fathers also experienced underemployment: 'I am an electrical engineer but in Canada I work only using my hands, nothing using my head and I cannot work with my head ... My education is a university degree, a bachelor's degree, and I want to work in my profession.' Not surprisingly, fathers from both communities expressed frustration with their underemployment status. In the words of a Sudanese father: 'We do not have opportunities to gain good jobs despite our educational credentials. It seems we are relegated to secondary status because of the colour of our skin. This causes considerable stress on us as individuals and our families.'

A Russian father expressed his unhappiness: 'I want to spend time with my family, my wife and my daughter; however, I have to work many hours because I need the money.' As a consequence of their employment situation, some of the men expressed frustration with their inability to provide all of the things needed by their families, particularly their children: 'As long as you are underpaid you do not feel good, and all the things that you need for your children you do not get so you are really under pressure and one can get distressed' (Sudanese father); '[In Canada] it is not easy to make money. Making money is not easy' (Russian father).

It was apparent that providing for their families was extremely important; however, due to limited opportunities, they were forced to take jobs where their knowledge and skills are underutilized. Hence, the message of working hard and obtaining a good education did not translate into well-paid, meaningful employment for these men. Being underemployed with low-paying jobs appeared to impact their self-esteem and self-worth.

Lack of Social Support

Both groups of respondents commented on the lack of social support as fathers in Canada. Some expressed difficulty adjusting to their new environment without this support: '... the tough part is that it is only me who takes care of my family ... But if it is back home, I do not see anything that is tough in taking care of the family because the responsibility of the family is not only you alone. All relatives are part of this responsibility.'

In comparing his situation in Canada, one Russian father comment-ed, '... there is nobody here [family] to help us ... I do not have my parents ... We take care of everything ourselves.' Another stated, 'We do not have any relatives here; we do not have any friends.' A Suda-nese father responded: '... back home there is all the people to visit and we go to parties together, and we find lots of people, friends, other relatives, and others. But here we are few people so this makes things sometime difficult for me and my wife.' However, fathers from both groups identified where they and their families received social sup-port. The primary sources included fellow community members and community-based organizations such as those serving immigrants and families. One Russian father remarked: 'I say community support is very good. For example, since we came to Canada, Jewish Family Ser-vices in Calgary helped us a lot and take care of us.' In discussing the support he receives from the Sudanese community in Calgary, a father stated the following: 'Sometimes when there are difficulties we go to the Sudanese community and then they provide us with anything we need.'

Role Change

A change reported by 12 of the Sudanese participants was the sharing of household tasks. As one respondent said, 'We share the kitchen. I do not wait for her to prepare food for me. I can do it, prepare it for myself, but in the Sudan that does not happen. A man does not go into the kitchen.' Role change of this nature was not noted by the Russian fathers.

Discussion

Beginning in the early 1990s and continuing throughout the decade, Russian and Sudanese immigrants and refugees represented new groups settling in the city of Calgary; however, research on their settle-ment and adaptation is virtually nonexistent. This chapter is focused on the experiences of Russian and Sudanese newcomer men as fathers in Canadian society. In particular, the challenges these fathers encounter and how they impact their health and well-being represent the salient contribution to this volume.

The experiences of immigration may be compounded by gender expectations, including men's traditional roles as breadwinners and heads of families. Concerns associated with underemployment and unemployment unsurprisingly emerged as the dominant issue. The underemployment status of a majority of the study's participants is clearly related to the lack of recognition of their foreign credentials. This issue is documented in several studies and reports (Ngo and Este 2006; Wayland 2006; Austin and Este 2001; Basran and Zong 1988), and is an ongoing problem that deeply impacts the ability of newcomers to integrate into Canadian society.

Bhandari, Horvath, and To (2006), in their project involving immigrant men, reported that one of the major obstacles identified were the barriers in finding professional employment: 'A participant discussion concluded that foreign university degrees and work experience are regarded as worthless by agencies and Canadian employers. Additionally, barriers such as inadequate language proficiency and/or discriminatory hiring practices often hamper the economic performance of immigrants (143). The following comment clearly captures the emotional impact of underemployment: 'Sometimes emotionally, it affects me. I feel I do not do well because I do not feed my family as head of the family. This sometimes affects me emotionally and makes me feel bad' (Sudanese male).

The self-worth and self-esteem of Sudanese men appears to be negatively impacted by underemployment. The Sudanese come from a culture that some writers (Hynie 2008; Triandis et al. 1988) describe as collectivist in nature. Hynie (2008) comments on the salient characteristics of this type of culture: 'Collectivist cultures tend to stress group harmony, obedience, and strictly hierarchical relationships. Individual desires are subordinated to the well-being of the collective and individual differences from the ingroup are repressed' (3).

In cultures with strong collectivist values, Hynie (2008) asserts that men in the family are responsible for their family's economic upkeep. She also maintains that men typically engage in marketing and labour outside the home and handle the families' finances. Coming from a society where men are expected to be the primary provider, some fathers claimed it is difficult to fulfill this role because of their inability to gain meaningful and well-paid employment. As a result, they may view themselves as unsuccessful fathers and husbands. Two Sudanese respondents voiced the following: '... back home where I was raised and where I came as an adult, there is too much pressure to work. If you do not work, you are not a valuable social member because without work, even what you say could be invalid' (Sudanese male); ... basically work is what counts. Your name and your person ... is worthy of nothing if I do not work' (Sudanese male).

With limited employment opportunities, Sudanese fathers must endure such behaviour that, combined with their underemployed status, may result in considerable stress and feelings of alienation or marginalization in a country that proudly declares itself 'multicultural.'

For the Russian men, lack of meaningful employment to provide some financial stability appears to result in frustration and worry: 'In Canada, it is not that easy to make money; making money is not that easy' (Russian father); 'I hope that I can find a job and eventually get myself everything that I need and provide my family with all that they need without any problem' (Russian father).

For some of the Sudanese fathers, racism and discrimination emerged as an issue. The question of how racism impacts the health and well-being of its victims has been garnering increased attention in the scholarly literature (Harrell 2000; Rollock and Gordon 2000). Writers such as Dobbins and Skillings (2000) and Harrell (2000) claim the impact of racism may be viewed as a clinical syndrome. Describing how racism afflicts its targets, Harrell (2000) states: 'Racism can traumatize, hurt, humiliate, enrage, confuse, and ultimately prevent optimal growth and functioning of individuals and communities' (42). One Sudanese father described the persecution he endures at work and the impact of such behaviour: 'Some [whites] just insult you for no reason as if it is very normal at my place of work ... someone may annoy you with their comments, then you come home not happy.'

The absence of social support provided by family members and friends prior to migrating to Canada was identified as a challenge for the participants. In some instances, this necessitated greater involvement with their children. The absence triggered feelings of social isolation and the lack of a sense of belonging. One Russian father stated, '... there is nobody here [family] to help us ... I do not have my parents ... We take care of everything ourselves.' (For further discussions of social support and health, see Hyman et al., Simich, and Spitzer, this volume.)

The Sudanese men in particular described the gender role changes they experienced as fathers in the Canadian context. These changes included becoming more actively involved in the raising of their children and taking on more household activities. Such changes represent movement from the specific gender roles in their home country.

The issues identified by the fathers in this study impact their health and well-being. Collectively, the effects of underemployment, lack of social support, and feelings of isolation may contribute to depression and feelings of alienation and marginalization. If Canadian society does not seriously intervene to address these problems, particularly in the area of labour market integration, the talents of these men will be wasted. Hence, a major objective of the nation's immigration policy – the need to attract newcomers to ensure the Canadian economy will continue to prosper – will be negated.

NOTE

1 Data collection took place prior to the establishment of the Republic of South Sudan on 9 July 2011.

PART 2

The Sequelae of Suffering

6 The Mental Health and Well-being of Immigrant and Refugee Women in Canada[1]

ILENE HYMAN

Introduction

Immigration is an increasingly important component of population growth in Canada, and ensuring the mental health and well-being of immigrants represents an important national priority.

The first part of this chapter presents an overview of existing literature on the health of immigrants in Canada, raising important questions about determinants of mental health among immigrant women and what contributes to an increased vulnerability over time in a new country. The second part adopts a comprehensive framework to identify and examine the determinants of immigrant women's mental health. The chapter concludes with a summary of the main determinants of mental health, highlighting the importance of examining intersections between gender, ethnicity, and migration.

The Health of Canadian Immigrants

In 2006, 251,649 immigrants made Canada their home (Statistics Canada 2006). According to the 2001 census, first-generation immigrants represented 18.4 per cent of the total population, and 39 per cent of the population were first or second generation. Recent immigrants – those arriving in Canada between 1991 and 2001 – represented 6.2 per cent of the total population (Statistics Canada 2003a). Canadian immigrants are extremely heterogeneous with respect to source country, length of stay, immigration class, ethnicity, racialized status, and socioeconomic status, factors that affect health (Statistics Canada 2003b).

Many reports and articles have shown that upon arrival Canadian immigrants experience a health advantage compared to the Canadian-born population (Hyman 2007a; Hyman 2004; Ali, McDermott, and Gravel 2004; DesMeules et al. 2004; Newbold and Danforth 2003; Perez 2002; Chen, Ng, and Wilkins 1996a,b; see also chapters 1 and 2, this volume). The healthy immigrant effect refers to the observation that immigrants (both male and female) are often in superior health to the Canadian-born population when they first arrive in Canada, but lose this health advantage over time. The healthy immigrant effect is believed to result in part from a self-selection process in which people who are able and motivated to move do so, and those who are sick, disabled, and in institutions do not. It is also the result of immigration procedures that select the 'best' immigrants on the basis of education, language ability, and job skills – characteristics that facilitate social and economic integration, go hand in hand with healthy lifestyles, and exclude immigrants with serious medical conditions.

Compared to the Canadian-born population, Canadian immigrants have a lower prevalence of chronic diseases, and lower rates of mortality and morbidity from all causes (see Hyman and Jackson 2010, and Hyman 2007a for a review). However, many of the studies reviewed showed these rates converged over time with those of the Canadian-born population, indicating that initial good health is no guarantee of good health in the long term. Mental health has been defined as 'the capacity of each and all of us to feel, think, and act in ways that enhance our ability to enjoy life and deal with the challenges we face' (Health Canada 2006:2). This definition conveys mental health as a positive sense of emotional and spiritual well-being that respects the importance of culture, equity, social justice, interconnections, and personal dignity.

The Mental Health of Canadian Immigrants

Arrival and resettlement in a new country often involves a period of significant readjustment and stress (Canadian Task Force on Mental Health Issues Affecting Immigrants and Refugees 1988; Canadian Council on Multicultural Health 1989). Some theories emphasize the negative and stressful effects of this process on immigrants' health, while others propose that immigrants are a self-selected and resilient group who are less likely to experience psychological problems (Beiser 1990).

Overall, the literature suggests that Canadian immigrants initially experience fewer mental health problems than their Canadian-born counterparts. For example, Ali (2002) used data from the Canadian Community Health Survey to examine the healthy immigrant effect among Canadian immigrants in terms of their mental health. After adjustment for age, length of stay, and other demographic characteristics, the risk of experiencing depression was lower for recent immigrants (0-9 years) compared to non-recent immigrants (10+ years) and the Canadian-born population. Beiser (2005) critiqued the cross-sectional nature of this dataset, but still found the findings plausible due to the rigorous selection processes and to the observation that aging may be a more potent risk factor for mental health among immigrants as compared to non-immigrants.

Suicide rates have also been used as an indicator of migrant mental health. Kliewer and Ward (1988) investigated factors influencing suicide rates among 25 immigrant groups in Canada and found that the suicide rates of immigrants converged with those of the Canadian-born population. Among immigrants from low-risk countries (countries with lower suicide rates than Canada), suicide rates increased compared to those of Canada, and among immigrants from high-risk countries, suicide rates decreased. Malenfant (2004) used Canadian Vital Statistics and the World Health Organization data to compare age-standardized suicide rates among immigrants overall, and by country of birth with those of the Canadian-born population. He found that suicide rates for immigrants were approximately half those of the Canadian-born population, and gender differences were less pronounced than among the Canadian-born.

Other Canadian studies examined the mental health of specific immigrant communities, highlighting the possible need to consider ethnicity and racialization as well as migration and refugee status. For example, the prevalence of depressive symptoms was found to be higher among elderly Chinese and Taiwanese immigrants than among the general elderly population in Canada (Lai 2005, 2004). Refugees have been shown to experience higher rates of certain chronic diseases than either other immigrants or the Canadian-born (Redwood-Campbell et al. 2003), especially post-traumatic stress disorder (Li and Browne 2000; Fowler 1998; Weir 2002; Beiser and Wickrama 2004; Fenta, Hyman, and Noh 2004).

There have been, however, relatively few longitudinal studies examining changes in immigrant mental health over time. Although Ali

(2002) suggested that the healthy immigrant effect may apply to mental health, a 10-year longitudinal study of mental health among Southeast Asian refugees found that the risk of depression decreased over length of time in Canada (Beiser 1999). On the other hand, findings from the Pathways and Barriers to Health Care for Ethiopians in Toronto project suggested that the risk of developing depression increased after a few years and reached its maximum at approximately 15 years post-migration (Fenta, Hyman, and Noh 2004).

Compared to Canada, there was more evidence from the U.S. literature that immigrants experienced fewer mental health problems compared to their U.S.-born counterparts but increasing time in the United States was associated with increasing rates of mental health problems (see Gee et al. 2006).

Mental Health and Gender

According to the Canadian Task Force on Mental Health Issues Affecting Immigrants and Refugees (1988), immigrant and refugee women have greater mental health needs than their male counterparts; however, few Canadian studies have specifically examined the mental health of immigrant women and/or made comparisons with Canadian-born women or immigrant men.

Franks and Faux (1990) found higher rates of depression among women of four ethnic immigrant groups (Chinese, Vietnamese, Portuguese, and Latin American) than among women in the general population. More recent arrivals had the lowest depression scores, suggesting that a group's past hardships make their present conditions seem more tolerable in the short run. Literature reviews on childbearing and mental health cited high rates of post-partum depression and depressive symptoms among immigrant women relative to their native-born counterparts (Stewart et al. 2008; Zelkowitz et al. 2004; Vissandjée et al. 2001). A review of Canadian research on immigrant and refugee women's health identified psychiatric symptoms attributable to trauma and multiple trauma such as rape as important mental health issues for many refugee women (Mulvihill and Mailloux 2000). Preliminary findings from a Tamil mental health study indicated that one-third of respondents had experienced traumatic events, and rates were higher for immigrant women than for immigrant men (Beiser, Simich, and Pandalangat 2003).

Among the community-specific studies comparing the mental health of immigrant men and women were studies of elderly Taiwanese and Chinese immigrants to Canada (Lai 2004, 2005) and a study of Korean immigrants to Toronto (Noh et al. 1992). These studies found higher prevalence rates of depression among immigrant women than men. However, a survey of Iranian immigrants to Canada found no difference in depression rates by gender (Safdar and Lay 2003). Beiser (1999) found that Southeast Asian refugee women were more likely than their male counterparts to experience depression in the later follow-up period, while men exhibited symptoms earlier in the follow-up.

It seems clear that gender differences in mental health vary by culture, country of origin, ethnicity, and other factors. It has also been suggested that gender differences in mental health are more prominent in high-income, industrialized countries, where the rate and ratio of depression among women compared to men is generally about 2:1. On the other hand, in low-income countries, gender differences vary and many report no differences in rates (Culbertson 1997). The mixed evidence of gender differences between immigrant men and women may be a reflection of this heterogeneity in trends around the world. In the studies reviewed above, gender differences in mental illness are either comparable to that of the Canadian-born population or else smaller. Rates of mental illness among immigrants, however, are sometimes higher than those of the Canadian-born, especially among elderly Asian migrants, refugees, and non-recent migrants.

Fewer Canadian studies have examined the intersections of health, migration, gender, and poverty. This represents an important omission considering rates of depression are higher among women relative to men and among those with lower income relative to those with higher income. Newbold (2005a,b) used longitudinal data from the National Population Health Survey to assess changes in self-assessed health in four Canadian immigrant arrival cohorts over time. Findings showed that all immigrant cohorts rated their health as worse than the Canadian-born population, and there was evidence of declines in self-assessed health in every cohort and at each follow-up point. Although nativity was not a significant predictor of self-assessed health, with the inclusion of interaction terms for gender, nativity, and income, findings suggested that female immigrants and low-income immigrants were at greatest risk of transitioning to poor health status.

Similarly, Smith, Matheson, and colleagues (2007) used Canadian Community Health Survey data to examine interactions between gender, length of stay, and income and mental health. Their findings supported previous findings that depression is more prevalent among women, non-recent immigrants, and individuals with low-income. Findings also highlighted critical intersections between gender, poverty, and length of stay, such that female low-income, non-recent immigrants were four times as likely to have depression compared with their male counterparts.

Moreover, there is a growing literature on the effects of precarious immigration status on health. In their review of the literature on this topic, Magalhaes and colleagues (2010) found that non-status migrants may be at particularly high risk for negative health and mental health consequences, and that the precarious nature of migrants' lives may exacerbate existing health issues. Caulford and Vali (2006) described the effect of not having health insurance on immigrants and refugees (including claimants) using Scarborough Hospital Clinic data: the majority of attendees were female and had experienced deficiencies in prenatal care. Oxman-Martinez and colleagues (2005) examined health indicators and access to health care for women with precarious status (including sponsored, temporary residents, caregivers, and women with irregular status, i.e., no legal papers, but not refugee claimants). Financial barriers to health services (e.g., lacked health insurance, receipt of welfare, and poor housing) intersected with socio-cultural variables to increase women's vulnerability. Bannerman and colleagues (2003) noted the 'runaround' that uninsured people typically experience when trying to access services. In some cases, individuals experienced long waiting lists, racism or offensive treatment, rude remarks by staff members, or they were denied services altogether. Frustration over these factors combined with a lack of information in general about services led to eventually giving up and not receiving the much-needed care.

Summary

The literature reviewed suggested that immigrant and refugee women in Canada generally experience a higher risk of mental health problems relative to immigrant men, and that their risk of experiencing these problems increases with age and length of stay. Although literature is limited, important intersections were observed between gender, ethnicity, racialized status, poverty, and length of stay that raise questions about the determinants of mental health in this group. For example, are gender differences in mental health among immigrants determined by the same factors as among the Canadian-born population? Do changes over time in the determinants of immigrant women's mental health contribute to their increased vulnerability? The remainder of this chapter explores whether these findings can be explained by examining gender-based contextual variables such as social support, discrimination, and lack of access to economic resources.

Determinants of Immigrant Mental Health

According to the Canada's Population Health model, many broad determinants, including gender, income, and social status, employment and working conditions, health practices, social and physical environments, and culture, influence the health of all Canadians (Health Canada 1994). Many of the determinants of mental health lie outside the health care system and are influenced by other sectors such as the economy, education, and housing (Government of Canada 2006). The literature on the determinants of mental health amply demonstrates that mental health is the result of complex interactions between genetic, biological, personality, and environmental factors. For example, 'long-term changes in brain function can occur in response to factors in the environment such as stimulation, experiences of traumatic or chronic stress, or various kinds of deprivation' (Health Canada 2002:22). Poverty may increase the risk of exposure to chronic or traumatic stress, one of the strongest correlates of mental health status (Stephens and Joubert 2000). When combined with genetic predisposition, these factors greatly increase the likelihood of developing a mental illness (Health Canada 2002).

It has been suggested that the process of immigration and resettlement may influence immigrant health and mental health indirectly via determinants of health and mental health. More recently, however, our literature review of the determinants of immigrant health provided strong evidence for considering determinants of immigrant health outside the Population Health framework (Hyman 2007b). The review provided ample evidence that determinants such as resettlement stress, racism, and existing government immigration policies also affected the health of Canadian immigrants.

Other Canadian research highlights the importance of examining intersections between gender, ethnicity, length of stay, and health (Vissandjée et al. 2007; Boyd and Grieco 2003; Meadows, Thurston, and Melton 2001; Weber and Parra-Medina 2003). For example, immigrant and refugee women may be at risk for mental health problems due to their disadvantaged and marginal status in society compounded by social isolation, lack of socio-economic integration, and differences in access and power (Weber and Parra-Medina 2003).

There is clearly a need for a comprehensive framework to examine immigrant women's mental health in Canada that considers both traditional determinants of health as well as determinants of health related to the *migration context* (e.g., racism, migration policy, and resettlement stress) and intersections between gender, poverty, and length of stay. One such framework, adopted by the Victorian Health Promotion Foundation in Australia (Vic Health), focuses on three determinants of mental health: social inclusion, discrimination and violence, and access to economic resources (Rychetnik and Todd 2004). To this end, the Vic Health framework seems a promising way to examine the determinants of immigrant women's mental health in Canada. For the purposes of our review, the social inclusion determinant was broadened to include social support and social capital, and henceforth will be named 'social environment.'

Findings

Social Environment

This determinant encompasses the constructs of social support, social capital (and social networks), and social inclusion. Although there is some overlap between these constructs, each is described here in terms of its impact on immigrant women's mental health.

SOCIAL SUPPORT
Health Canada (1994) describes social support in terms of social networks that include families, friends, and communities that help people solve problems and deal with adversity, as well as in terms of a sense of mastery and control over life circumstances. Research has consistently demonstrated that social networks and social ties have a beneficial effect on mental health outcomes, including stress reactions, psychological well-being, and symptoms of psychological distress including depression and anxiety (Kawachi and Berkman 2001).

Less research has examined the effect of social support on the mental health of Canadian immigrant women. This is partly because only limited information on social support has been available from national and provincial health surveys. For example, studies using these population health databases often used marital status as a proxy for social support (McDonald and Kennedy 2004; Newbold 2005a,b; Vissandjée et al. 2004). However, for immigrants, sources of social support often extend beyond the marital relationship or even the nuclear family. (Further discussion can be found in the final section of this text on Communities, Social Capital, Resilience, and Empowerment).

Data from immigrant-specific surveys conducted in Canada suggest that social support is an important determinant of immigrant health. For example, in his study of Southeast Asian refugees, Beiser (1999) demonstrated that an early period of elevated mental health and illness risk was not universal but appeared only among immigrants lacking personal and social resources (e.g., a significant personal relationship and the presence of a similar ethnic community). This led the author to conclude that social support needs to be incorporated into models explaining mental health during resettlement. Lack of social support and unsatisfactory marital relations were two of the three factors found to be significantly and independently associated with depression among pregnant immigrant women (Zelkowitz et al. 2004).

Much of what we know about the relationship between social support and immigrant health has been obtained from qualitative research studies, notably the Multicultural Meanings of Social Support Project (Stewart et al. 2004). Examining the meaning of social support from different perspectives, social support was found to play a major role during the transition period by enhancing coping, moderating the effect of stressors, facilitating access to needed employment and services, and promoting health and well-being (Simich, Beiser et al. 2005; Simich, Mawani et al. 2004). Simich, Beiser, and Mawani (2003) also examined the role of social support as a determinant of immigrant and refugee well-being. Among the types of support needed that were identified were: accurate information about the cities in which they were destined to live, informal sources of social support to meet the social support needs that formal government programs could not, and affirmational support from immigrants who have successfully adapted, as well as familiar others and family/friends. Of particular concern was the finding that an immigrant's need for social support often contributed to a secondary migration, away from areas of economic opportunity.

It is also clear that some government policies have contributed to delays in family reunification, reducing access to important sources of social support. In a review of the literature on policies affecting immigrants, newcomers who experienced extended family separation often found family reunification to be an unexpected and extremely difficult barrier to their settlement (Wayland 2006). The negative health outcomes of prolonged separation include emotional distress and post-reunification stress on the family (Canadian Council for Refugees 2004).

Still, it is important to recognize that despite research documenting the negative impacts of reduced social support and social isolation on the mental health of immigrant women (e.g., Ahmad et al. 2004), several studies challenged the tendency for researchers to portray immigrant women as passive victims of social processes. According to Guruge and Collins (2008), 'the fact that most immigrant women eventually lead successful lives is a testament to their strengths and resilience' (13).

The results of a qualitative study of South Asian women's management of health and illness suggested a framework that acknowledged immigrant women as skilled and knowledgeable agents who make use of both traditional and Western biomedicine in their management of family health problems (Dyck 2004). Similarly, findings from another qualitative study of immigrant women from five ethno-cultural communities challenged existing stereotypes of Asian women and suggested that women adopted diverse and independent strategies to maintain well-being (Wong and Tsang 2004).

SOCIAL CAPITAL

Social capital is emerging as a key social determinant of health and aspects of mental health such as common mental illnesses, happiness and well-being, and self-assessed mental health status (Pevalin 2002; Pevalin and Rose 2002; Rychetnik and Todd 2004; Putnam 2001; see also Vissandjée et al., this volume). Social capital has been defined in various ways, including the features of social networks such as social engagement, norms of reciprocity, and interpersonal trust that facilitate community and social participation to achieve mutual benefits including health (Putnam 1993), and the resources available to individuals and communities through their social relationships (Kawachi et al. 2004). A number of scholars argue that there are two main types of social capital: 'bonding' (or the horizontal tight-knit ties between individuals and groups sharing demographic characteristics); and 'bridging' (or the ties that cut across communities/individuals). Among immigrants, it is the dynamic interplay between the two and the sharing of resources within the networks that is believed to contribute to social capital (Kunz 2003).

Little research has been conducted on social capital and immigrant health in Canada. One study, using data from the 2003 General Social Survey (GSS), examined which aspects of social capital were considered to be important to the perceived health of immigrants (Van Kemenade, Roy, and Bouchard 2006). They found that the size of a network with strong ties was positively associated with health for women in the general population, immigrants, and low-income men; however, this association was stronger for immigrants as compared with other groups. Reciprocity in social relationships was associated with good health among both immigrant and non-immigrant women, but the relationship was stronger among immigrant women. Kazemipur and Halli (2000) suggested that living in a poor neighbourhood with people of similar ethnic origins may be beneficial to immigrants in terms of facilitating integration and reducing stress, because less racism and cultural incongruity is experienced.

SOCIAL INCLUSION

A socially inclusive society is defined as one in which people feel valued, their differences respected, and their basic needs met so they can live in dignity (Rychetnik and Todd 2004). According to the Government of Canada's (2006) report on mental illness, 'belonging to a supportive community contributes to good mental health by providing support in times of crisis, grounding in one's cultural roots and opportunities for creativity' (12). As with social support, studies consistently demonstrate that people who are socially isolated experience greater mental health risks.

Many immigrant women in Canada experience reduced social networks, difficulty securing employment, and linguistic, geographic, and economic barriers to necessary resources. Marginalization, a sense of being overlooked, categorized, or misrepresented, has been found to be a central feature of Canadian and British immigrant women's relationships with others, affecting their ability to access and mobilize resources for health (Lynam and Cowley 2007).

Settlement policy consists of a variety of programs and services designed to help newcomers become participating members of Canadian society. However, most of these services focus on the early stages of settlement and fail to recognize the intermediate and long-term settlement needs of immigrants, particularly immigrant women. A literature review identified several needs or concerns emerging later in the resettlement process, such as language and skills training for women, discrimination and social exclusion, the adoption of health risk behaviours, lack of access to appropriate and affordable housing, culture shock, and intergenerational issues (Hyman 2007b).

Freedom from Discrimination and Violence

As implied by its heading, this determinant encompasses the constructs of discrimination and violence, both collective trauma and intimate partner violence.

DISCRIMINATION

Racism is defined in terms of the practices or attitudes that have the effect, whether by design or impact, of limiting an individual's or group's right to the opportunities generally available to the public because of attributed rather than actual characteristics (Abella 1984). This implies that racism is not only an attitude but also the specific actions that result from this attitude which impact upon, marginalize, and oppress some people. 'Racial discrimination' refers to differential or unequal treatment on the basis of racial characteristics that may occur as a result of stereotyping, prejudice, and bias. Subtle and subversive forms of racial discrimination have been identified as the most common ways in which racialized people experience unequal treatment (Ontario Human Rights Commission 2008).

Although there are many forms of discrimination (e.g., due to racialization, ethnicity, gender, or sexual orientation), by far the largest body of evidence addresses the effects of racial discrimination on health. Several studies (mostly non-Canadian) demonstrated negative associations between racial discrimination, health, and mental health (Paradies 2006; Gee 2002; Harris et al. 2006; Williams et al. 2003). There was also ample evidence from the U.S. literature that racialized groups, particularly Blacks and Hispanics, did not have equal access to health care, had more unmet health needs, and experienced worse health status (American College of Physicians 2004; Bhugra, Harding, and Lippett 2004).

It has been hypothesized that racism indirectly influences health through differential exposure to determinants of health – for example, restricting socio-economic mobility, contributing to differential access to resources – while effects such as trauma, stress reactions, and lowered self-esteem may directly impact on health (Harris et al. 2006; Brondolo et al. 2003). The relationship between racism and socio-economic status is complex in that racism restricts its attainment for members of racialized and ethnic minority groups; meanwhile 'race' itself is an antecedent and determinant of socio-economic status (Williams 1999; see also chapter 1, this volume, for a discussion of race as a social construct).

Racism is often compounded by sexism and xenophobia, and related sources of social exclusion; for example, unemployment, poor housing, and residence in a low-income neighbourhood. Although many of the 138 empirical studies on racism reviewed by Paradies (2006) found that the prevalence of self-reported racism was higher among males, this was not always the case and variations by setting were observed; for example, service provision and employment. Gender-based discrimination and sexual harassment in the workplace also impact on the mental health of immigrant women in Canada (Ahmad et al. 2004; Farmanova-Hayes, Rose, and Vissandjée 2006; Meadows, Thurston, and Melton 2001; Zelkowitz et al. 2004).

Although a recent mental health report recognized that mental health is associated with social issues such as racism and discrimination (Government of Canada 2006), few empirical studies have examined the impact of racism on the health of Canadian immigrants. Data from the Korean Health Study demonstrated that 85 per cent of respondents had experienced racial discrimination and that, after controlling for other variables, perceived discrimination was associated with depressive symptoms (Noh and Kaspar 2007). Using data from the Southeast Asian refugee study, Beiser (2006) identified racial discrimination as a predictor of depression among Southeast Asian refugees; however, early integration militated against discrimination and also against depression. A study conducted by Women's Health in Woman's Hands Community Health Centre found racism to be a risk factor for physical health and stress among female youth of colour (Ali, Massaquoi, and Brown 2003). De Maio and Kemp (2010) used data from the Longitudinal Survey of Immigrants to Canada (LSIC) to explain the decline in physical and mental health status over four years. As previously reported, physical health status declined from 43 to 23 per cent reporting excellent health, and the proportion of new immigrants reporting depression or sadness increased (5% to 30%). Of note, participants who reported experiencing discrimination or unfair treatment were significantly more likely to experience deterioration in physical and mental health status.

There was some evidence from the United States that perceptions and experiences of discrimination among immigrants from Africa, the

Caribbean, Mexico, and other Hispanic countries (e.g., Puerto Rico, the Dominican Republic, and South American countries) increased with length of stay (see Gee et al. 2006). This has been attributed to a greater recognition of discriminatory behaviour, as well as increased exposure to discrimination over time. It has also been proposed that discrimination and 'Othering,' a process of marginalization, disempowerment, and social exclusion (Grove and Zwi 2006), better explain why immigrant health deteriorates over time than socio-cultural factors such as changes in health behaviours and social support. Viruell-Fuentes (2007) found that second-generation Mexican immigrant women in the United States experienced more pervasive and cumulative exposure to 'Othering' than the first generation. Gee et al (2006) also found that length of residency in the U.S. moderated the relationship between discrimination and health, such that the association between discrimination and mental health problems was stronger for non-recent as compared to recent immigrants.

VIOLENCE

Violence includes collective trauma – the instrumental use of violence by people who identify themselves as members of a group against another group or set of individuals in order to achieve political, economic, or social objectives (e.g., refugees) – and interpersonal victimization, violence largely between family members and intimate partners (Rychetnik and Todd 2004). Each is discussed here.

COLLECTIVE TRAUMA

Refugees represent a unique subgroup of immigrants with specific health needs. Unlike immigrants, refugees may have experienced long-standing problems prior to migration, including lack of access to curative and preventive health care, the direct and indirect effects of war, and the psychosocial effects of war trauma and refugee camp internment (Canadian Task Force 1988). Survivors of trauma are at a higher risk of developing emotional disorders. Documented health problems include an increased risk of mortality, infectious diseases, and mental health problems such as post-traumatic stress disorder and depression (Beiser 2006; Canadian Task Force 1988). Refugee survivors of torture are often ill-prepared and vulnerable to life stresses during post-migration. Qualitative evidence suggests that excessively long waits in the refugee-family reunification process contribute to health risks for family members, emotional distress, and stress of the family post-reunification (Canadian Council for Refugees 2004). There is also research that suggests that a high proportion of independent immigrants to Canada have also been exposed to political violence (Rousseau and Drapeau 2004).

Most of the studies reviewed suggested that pre-migration stresses exerted a negative effect on refugee health; however, the duration of this effect was not clear. For example, Southeast Asian refugee data demonstrated that the effect of pre-migration stress on mental health, such as the severity of conditions in a refugee camp, was salient only in the short term (six-month post-migration); post-migration stresses and the availability of personal and social supports were stronger predictors of mental health in the long term (10 years post-migration) (Beiser, Cargo, and Woodbury 1994; Beiser and Hyman 1997; Beiser 1999). As previously mentioned, the risk of developing depression among Ethiopian refugees was low during the first few years of resettlement, but increased after a few years and reached its maximum at approximately 15 years post-migration (Fenta, Hyman, and Noh 2004).

INTIMATE PARTNER VIOLENCE (IPV)

The WHO defines violence as the intentional use of physical force or power, threatened or actual, against oneself, another person, or against a group or community, that either results in or has a high likelihood of resulting in injury, death, psychological harm, mal-development, or deprivation. Studies have consistently shown that women, compared to men, experience higher rates of disability and illness, battery and sexual assault, depression, post-traumatic stress disorder (PTSD), and suicide attempts (see WHO 2002). Men, on the other hand, have higher rates of alcohol abuse and completed suicides (Astbury 2001). These gender differences reflect, in part, differences between women and men in predisposition to some mental illnesses, and differences in social conditioning. However, women's increased risks of adverse mental health outcomes are also attributed to a wide range of adverse consequences disproportionately experienced by women: poverty, discrimination, violence, low social status, and traditional female gender roles (Astbury 2001; Patel et al. 1999).

Data from the 1996 General Social Survey were used to examine the prevalence of and help-seeking behaviour for IPV among Canadian immigrant women. Findings suggested that the risk of IPV among immigrant women in Canada increased with length of stay (Hyman et al. 2006). This may be because risk behaviours associated with IPV, such as alcohol and drug use, increase with length of stay (Chen, Ng, and Wilkins 1996a; Hyman 2002; Perez 2002) as a result of alienation from traditional support systems, perceived discrimination, and acculturative stress. A study of Ethiopian immigrants in Toronto identified post-migration changes including loss of social support, income and status, and changes in gender roles as impacting on marital relationships both positively and negatively (Hyman, et al. 2008). Prevailing community norms that perpetuate gender inequality and male domination and post-migration stresses were identified as key determinants of IPV in the Tamil community (Hyman and Mason 2011).

Access to Economic Factors

There is an established literature demonstrating strong correlations between poverty and mental health – particularly psychiatric disorders such as schizophrenia and personality disorders, but also anxiety, depression, and substance abuse (Health Canada 2002). Although many studies have found that socio-economic status is inversely related to the development of mental health problems, the relationship between poverty and mental health is complex. Two theories have been proposed to explain this relationship. According to the indirect association theory, individuals with mental health problems may 'drift' into poverty. Direct association between poverty and mental illness implies that the social experience of low-income individuals increases the likelihood that they may develop a mental illness. For example, living in poverty may lead to a lack of opportunity and consequently to hopelessness, anger, and despair (Health Canada 2002). Features of poor neighbourhoods such as physical deterioration and crime may inhibit the development of social cohesion (Government of Canada 2006).

There is ample documentation that immigrants and racialized groups in Canada are disproportionately poorer than the population as a whole. Of particular concern, however, is the fact that recent immigrants are not catching up economically, as did their predecessors. Poverty rates for recent immigrants have increased substantially since 1980 (Picot and Hou 2003; Statistics Canada 2003c). Despite the fact that immigrants arriving in the 1990s were the most highly educated cohort of immigrants to date, the wage gap relative to their Canadian-born counterparts has increased (McIsaac 2003).

Employment is seen as crucial because it provides essential income as well as psychological benefits in terms of a recognized role in society and a sense of personal and social identity. Research shows that unemployment is a significant risk factor for not only the physical and psychological health of immigrants but also for a host of related and unrelated negative life events as well (Aycan and Berry 1996; Reitz 2005; Tang, Oatley, and Toner 2007; see also Spitzer, this volume).

Much of the literature on patterns of immigrant employment in Canada highlighted the negative impact of racialization. Recent immigrants to Canada, many of whom are racialized, are less likely to have full-time employment, are over-represented in lower-paying and lower-status jobs, and receive lower salaries than other Canadians (Galabuzi 2005; Ornstein 2001, 2006; Raphael 2007). Using census data (1996-2001), Teelucksingh and Galabuzi (2005b) found substantial income and labour market participation gaps between racialized and non-racialized earners, even when educational attainment was taken into account, as well as gaps between racialized men and women.

There is evidence that integration processes are different for women than for men (Basran and Zong 1998; Das Gupta 1996; Espiritu 1999), yet integration theories do not always consider gender (Tastsoglou and Preston 2005). Findings from the Longitudinal Survey of Immigrants to Canada (LSIC) suggested divergent patterns of labour force integration for male and female migrants, such that six months post-arrival a lower proportion of women than men were in the labour force (Statistics Canada 2005). In other words, women may not follow a linear trajectory of socio-economic integration. Traditional gender ideologies and gender-based divisions of labour emphasizing the role of women as homemakers, providing at best a supplementary income, result in immigrant women being unable to take advantage of official language training programs available only to recent immigrants, diminishing their prospects for meaningful employment and confining them to poorly paid jobs. At other times a reversal of traditional gender roles occurs, wherein women settle earlier than men and take up the first job available.

While socio-economic integration is largely influenced by individual skills and experiences and couples' weighing of the advantages and disadvantages of employment versus costs of childcare, neighbourhood factors such as the availability of childcare and/or access to language training programs may also be important facilitators or barriers to socio-economic integration of immigrants, particularly for women. Problems with the lack of coordination of English as a Second-Language (ESL) or French as a Second Language (FSL) policies, the need to fund programs longer and disparities in adult ESL/FSL programs remain.

This may help to explain why English fluency was a significant determinant of both depression and employment among Southeast Asian refugee women in British Columbia (Beiser and Hou 2001). Using the same dataset, these authors also learned that when women were able to participate in formal language training, they benefited even more than their male counterparts.

Summary/Discussion

The literature reviewed suggested that determinants related to the social environment, discrimination, violence, and access to economic resources all contributed to the mental health and well-being of immigrant and refugee women in Canada.

Literature on determinants related to the social environment confirmed that immigrant women require high levels of social support and strong social networks to maintain themselves and their families in good health. Existing government policies, however, often fail to address social support issues emerging later in the resettlement process. More research is necessary to identify what aspects of social support and social capital are important to immigrant health and well-being, and how these vary by gender and length of stay.

It seems clear that determinants related to discrimination and violence pose significant risks for the mental health of Canadian immigrant women. Although there was a dearth of Canadian research on discrimination and mental health and gender differences were not always examined, the studies reviewed implied that the effects of discrimination on mental health are substantial and may increase over length of stay. Although pre-migration trauma continues to exert an effect on the mental health of some refugees, most of the studies reviewed suggested that post-migration stresses exerted a greater effect on mental health. In fact, resettlement stress (defined as a range of post-migration resettlement stresses including poverty, unemployment, perceived discrimination, and family problems, etc.) has consistently been shown to be a major predictor of immigrant mental health (Beiser 1999; Fenta, Hyman, and Noh 2004; Tang, Oatley, and Toner 2007). Contrary to popular belief, it was shown that many of the determinants of mental health such as financial stress and social isolation did not decrease, but increased, with length of stay (Hyman and Dussault 2000). Also, the experience of IPV poses a real and substantial threat to the mental health of Canadian immigrant women, and it was clear from recent research that the risk of experiencing IPV increased with length of stay.

Most of the studies reviewed under determinants related to economic access demonstrated that Canadian immigrant women were more likely than their male counterparts to experience barriers to socio-economic integration, and, as a result, were less likely to have access to economic resources. Recent immigrants to Canada were also more likely to experience disparities in income and employment compared to previous cohorts, which undoubtedly increased their likelihood of experiencing economic disparities over time. The fact that many Canadian immigrant women continue to be primarily responsible for the home and children means that they are unable in the short term to access ESL and other settlement services that would help them to achieve socio-economic integration in the long term.

The findings presented in this chapter help to shed some light on why recent literature shows female low-income, non-recent immigrants experienced the highest risk, relative to their male counterparts and to Canadian-born women, of developing mental health problems and of transitioning to poor health (Newbold 2005; Smith et al. 2007). These women are more vulnerable to determinants of mental health such as lack of social capital, marginalization, IPV, and lower socio-economic status than immigrant men and Canadian-born women. Additionally, they are more susceptible to heightened discrimination than Canadian-born women. Many of these determinants increase with increasing length of time in Canada, and may only worsen if the slower economic catch-up of recent immigrants persists.

These results also present a challenge to Canadian settlement agencies, health and social service providers, and policy makers. For example, they support the development of policies and programs that impact on settlement beyond the first few months after arrival in Canada, and to specifically address issues of social support, discrimination, violence, and access to economic opportunities. Developing programs and policies that focus on the determinants of immigrants' mental health as outlined in this chapter will help to ensure the continued good physical and mental health of newcomer immigrant and refugee women and men in Canada over the long term.

NOTE

1 The author gratefully acknowledges the contribution of Sarah McDermott and Marie DesMeules to the first part of this chapter on mental health.

7 Gender-Based Interpersonal Violence and the Challenges of Integrating in Canadian Communities

W.E. THURSTON

Many women who immigrate to Canada have faced or will face gender-based violence. In this chapter, the experience of interpersonal violence (IPV) is foregrounded and placed in the context of institutionalized abuse and systemic racism. The policy community in Canada that advocated for and operated services for women who experienced IPV originated from the women's movement. One of the challenges faced by immigrant women has been finding culturally competent services, but another challenge is the lack of gender analysis within the larger organizations that provide settlement and integration services. Women repeatedly demonstrate, however, that given the basic necessities of life such as housing, food, and personal security, they will access services and strive to make a better life for themselves and their children. The voices of immigrant women bring important perspectives and are welcomed in a renewed debate on how to make gender-based IPV less common in Canadian society.

In this chapter I explore these issues, beginning with an overview of the theoretical approaches that inform my analysis. Next, I review the literature on IPV and describe the results of a multi-city study on immigrant women, homelessness, and IPV. I conclude with a discussion of the policy response and the possibilities that participatory policy making holds to help support the efforts of foreign-born women to create a rewarding and healthy life for themselves in Canada.

Introduction

This chapter is based on two conceptual frameworks. The first is an ecological model for understanding gender, migration, and health (Thurston and Vissandjée 2005). The second framework is for understanding the development of public policy, particularly health policy (Thurston et al. 2005; Thurston, Scott, and Vollman 2004). It is important to relate these two frameworks because the way social problems are understood and talked about affects how they are acted upon (Caragata 1999; Connell 1994; Deetz and Mumby 1990; Fairclough 1992).

The ecological model for understanding gender, migration, and health relates the determinants of population health commonly discussed in Canadian health policy (Public Health Agency of Canada (PHAC, 2007d), health research (Dunn and Dyck 2000), and health program development (Sent et al. 1998; Vissandjée et al. 2001) to women's experiences of migration over time. Thus, it is argued that migration should be added to PHAC's 12 accepted determinants of population health: social support networks, biology and genetic endowment, personal health practices and coping skills, healthy child development, education, income and social status, employment and working conditions, social environments, physical environments, health services, gender, and culture. Migration is conceptually distinguished from culture. Culture is understood to be a socially constructed set of beliefs, practices, and norms that may be relatively stable but are very fluid in application and everyday experience. The ecological framework incorporates the intersections of micro-, meso-, and macro-level factors, all of which act upon or are resisted or accommodated by the individual. The micro-level includes the cognitive and behavioural characteristics of individuals. The meso-level includes characteristics of groups and organizations, and the macro-level includes the state as well as social institutions such as gender, religion, and culture that shape our everyday lives. Migration, like culture, is an experience of individuals that is shaped by meso- and macro-level policies. Who is accepted as a migrant and what shapes the migration experience differs, like culture, by place, class, gender, and other social and material characteristics. The migration experience requires a variety of transitions that may, or may not, stress the cultural practices of a group, but which will most certainly require psychological and social adaptation, and in many cases physical adaptation to different climates and food supplies, and therefore will affect health.

Migration experiences take place over time and include experiences pre-migration, during settlement in a new country, and post-migration (Thurston and Vissandjée 2005). One of the experiences of migration is self- and institutional identification as an immigrant. Some people refer to themselves as a second-generation immigrant, meaning they were born of parents who immigrated to the country, while others may reject such a classification. In terms of settlement or integration, there is no clear demarcation of how long this will take individuals or groups (see chapter 1, this volume, for further discussion).

The framework for development of public health policy (Thurston 2007; Thurston et al. 2005) draws our attention to the idea of policy communities where social problems are discussed and analysed and potential solutions are identified. Policy communities are composed of people who share a common interest. Membership can vary, as can the degree of consensus, connections among players, and resources to facilitate work. Policy communities that are composed of loosely affiliated organizations and individuals with few formal coalitions or networks will likely be less able to respond with a strong unilateral voice when opportunities arise for policy or program development; for instance, when a government department decides it is 'time to do something' or a funding body creates a grants program for immigrant services. The policy development literature, however, stresses that policy development is not a linear process and the work of a policy community is only one factor that impacts outcomes. Another important consideration is that policy changes, reflected in program changes, can happen at the operational level of an organization, such as a health authority, and policy communities may have success there when higher-level formal policy change is harder to achieve (Thurston et al. 2005).

Migration and Gender-Based Interpersonal Violence

Gender-based interpersonal violence (IPV) is defined by the United Nations Declaration on the Elimination of Violence Against Women as: 'any act of gender-based violence that results in, or is likely to result in, physical, sexual or psychological harm or suffering to women, including threats of such acts, coercion or arbitrary deprivation of liberty, whether occurring in public or private life' (United Nations 1994: Article 1). Three decades ago, the terms *wife abuse* or *wife battering* were common (Thurston 1998). It is important not to assume that everyone is talking about the same thing when discussing IPV, and to spend some time clarifying the concept (Ashcraft 2000; Eliasson and Lundy 1999). There are legal definitions and these vary among countries, but there are also different social norms, and countries vary on whether IPV has become a recognized social problem as opposed to a personal, family, or individual, private problem. It has only been since the 1960s that the Canadian women's movement succeeded in bringing IPV into public policy discussion (Eliasson and Lundy 1999).

Alarmingly high numbers of women around the globe experience abuse and violence at the hands of loved ones, particularly boyfriends and husbands (Garcia-Moreno et al. 2006; World Health Organization 2002). In 1999, approximately 8 per cent of all women in Canada reported experiencing at least one incident of spousal violence within the previous five years (Canadian Centre for Justice Statistics 2003) and this dropped to 7 per cent in 2004 (Canadian Centre for Justice Statistics 2005). Slightly more than half of Canadian women (51 per cent) have been victims of at least one act of physical or sexual violence since the age of 16 (Statistics Canada 1993). Rates of physical abuse of women from other countries using a variety of methods and definitions vary – Barbados (30–50 per cent); Zambia (40 per cent); India (22 per cent); and Mexico (57 per cent urban, 44 per cent rural) (Heise 1993; Heise et al. 1994) – but suggest the widespread and serious nature of IPV (Garcia-Moreno et al. 2006). In some countries there are forms of IPV that are socially sanctioned (e.g., honour killing, genital mutilation) (Javed and Gerrard 2006), and women do not always escape these practices upon migrating to Canada.

Given these statistics, it is no surprise that women migrate to Canada with partners who have already been abusive and that some IPV starts in Canada after migration. Statistics from 10 years of operation of the Brenda Strafford Centre, a second-stage shelter[1] for women and their children fleeing IPV in Calgary, Alberta, showed that among the women for whom citizenship was known, on average 34 per cent had immigrated to Canada from another country. This was a percentage disproportionate to their representation in the population of the City of Calgary, as statistics showed that the proportion of the general population of Calgary who had emigrated from another country in 2001 was 21 per cent (City of Calgary 2003). Over-representation of immigrant women in the second-stage shelter should not be interpreted as excess IPV within immigrant populations. First, the sample is biased and not representative of either immigrant or non-immigrant women who experience IPV. In addition, there are other explanations that will be discussed in this chapter.

A study of immigrant women's experiences of IPV and homelessness was done in Calgary, Winnipeg, and Halifax (Thurston et al. 2006). Twenty-four immigrant women were recruited in Calgary (64.9

per cent), 10 in Winnipeg (27.0 per cent), and three in Halifax (8.1 per cent), and were interviewed three times over six months. The majority of women interviewed were between the ages of 30 and 39 years (52.9 per cent), were separated or divorced (88.8 per cent), and had children living with them (80.6 per cent). The women came from 26 countries of origin, and the most commonly reported length of time in Canada was five to less than 10 years (27.0 per cent), with the next being three to less than five years (21.6 per cent). Most of the women immigrated with their spouses but some came to Canada on their own or with their family of origin. Some of the latter group married or had relationships with Canadian citizens. The majority of participants (48.6 per cent) were Canadian citizens, while 43.2 per cent were landed immigrants, and the remaining participants had other sorts of status (e.g., refugee, student). This trend was seen in Calgary, but in Winnipeg the majority of women were landed immigrants. Calgary had women who were refugees, while Winnipeg did not. Due to the small number of participants, the immigration status of Halifax women will not be disclosed.

From this and other studies, we learned that all women who experience IPV, including women who have migrated, have much in common. Women talk about a continuum of IPV, as described in the United Nations definition (United Nations 1994).

Levels of reported family violence varied greatly, from those who had experienced relatively low levels of verbal abuse to reports of years of severe physical and psychological violence that led to hospitalization. Most women reported levels of abuse and violence between these extremes. Most women in our study were abused by an intimate partner, usually a spouse. Several women were abused by other members of their family or their partner's family. Women reported physical abuse (slapping, kicking, punching, choking, physical abuse while pregnant, use of weapons), sexual abuse (sexual control, sexual assault), verbal abuse (insults, name-calling, swearing), emotional or psychological abuse (harassment, manipulation, stalking, threats of violence or death threats towards the woman and/or the children), social abuse (social isolation, control of social contact), spiritual abuse (restricting access to religious services), and financial abuse (abuser controlling all finances) (Thurston et al. 2006:19–20).

Women often did not label their experience as IPV, or know that Canadian society had labelled it as such and that there were services to specifically address IPV. While it may be assumed that this is more likely to happen among immigrant women, the evidence suggests otherwise. Many Canadian women express the same challenge after first speaking to a counsellor about their experiences. Landenburger (2007) discusses the denial of abuse among both women and their friends and family. In addition, it should be remembered that nearly half of the women in this study had been in Canada between three and 10 years. They expressed many of the same fears that women who experience IPV generally express.

Other reasons women stayed in abusive relationships were language barriers, lack of independent income, fear of being separated from children or children being taken by child welfare authorities, concerns about living independently, or shame about disclosing the family violence. Shame about leaving the family unit was a particularly compelling factor, keeping them from seeking emergency services for their injuries or prompting them to attempt suicide: 'One night I was really, really depressed and I was up at three o'clock in the morning. There is no other way to survive. If I did live separate or I'll leave my kids. It's a big shame because of our culture, because of our own community and all these things. It's better to commit suicide and I took all the medication' (Thurston et al. 2006:21).

The women described efforts to isolate them socially and emotionally. The reasons for fleeing and seeking help were also the same as expressed in many other reports from women fleeing IPV – an escalation of the violence and fear for their lives, and/or a perception that the children were at risk of violence or suffering from the violence. The women expressed similar experiences as those of all women fleeing IPV in trying to get services and instrumental assistance such as income and housing.

Institutionalized Abuse and Systemic Racism

As in the ecological model described above, Lorber (2005) describes gender as a social institution: 'Gender's thrust is structural in that it orders the processes and practices of a society's major sectors – work, family, politics, law, education, medicine, the military, religion, and culture' (15). Thus our state institutions and practices continue at best to covertly reflect a history of misogyny and discrimination against women, and, at worst, to continue in either overt or covert discrimination against women. Women fleeing IPV in Canada have repeatedly identified treatment they received in the justice, health care, and social service systems as further victimization (Audy 1994; Rigakos 1995; Varcoe

2001). While the violence prevention policy community has achieved remarkable reforms in the justice sector, with special courts and trained sympathetic staff, much remains to be done in that sector (Rigakos 1995). Even more change remains to be accomplished in other sectors. The health sector, for instance, has been one of the last to recognize that health professionals have a role to play in prevention of IPV (Thurston and Eisener 2006).

Women who have migrated to Canada experience inequity compared to men in the negative impacts of migration policy, in the gendered nature of work in Canada, and in access to settlement assistance such as language training (Boyd and Pikkov 2005). Faced with lack of recognition of their professional qualifications or having no special training, and raising young children, women migrating to Canada enter a gendered work environment that also judges their accents and behaviours through a racialized lens (Graham and Thurston 2005; Helly 2004).

Immigrant women fleeing IPV confront all the challenges of institutionalized abuse and systemic racism. In the context of feeling like 'the Others' (Javed and Gerrard 2006:37), as compared to 'real citizens' (38), immigrant women struggle with the decision to confront the abuse and the potential this has for social exclusion from their ethnic community, discrimination against their husband in the legal system, and dealing with poverty: '[Members of my community] are not good support, as they are blaming me. They are not saying that the man was wrong, they are putting everything on the woman and it's your fault ... I'm supposed to go back to my husband's place for the sake of myself and my children' (Thurston et al. 2006:22).

In the study *Immigrant Women, Family Violence, and Pathways Out of Homelessness*, Thurston and colleagues (2006) found that the key causes of persistent and repetitive housing insecurity among immigrant women who had experienced IPV were systemic in nature: the availability of safe and affordable housing, transportation, neighbourhood safety, low wages, social assistance rates, barriers to language acquisition, availability of culturally safe services, and the immigration process. The woman's health status was the key individual-level factor linked to her housing situation by limiting her ability to work or make other decisions. A woman's health status, of course, is affected by the experiences of abuse and of discrimination (Campbell et al. 2002).

Removing the barriers to safety and security for immigrant women who have experienced IPV will require the collaboration of several sectors. In particular, the immigrant service agency sector has a service role to play in education, identification, referral, and support. The IPV service sector (shelters, educational and special programs) is required to develop cultural competence and to provide equitable services to immigrants. Other sectors, such as justice and health, equally need to understand IPV (Thurston, Cory, and Scott 1998) and cultural competence and safety (Anderson et al. 2003). Much work has been done on cultural sensitivity, that is, on understanding that groups of people have deeply valued norms and traditions that affect their behaviours. Cultural competence builds upon cultural sensitivity and involves understanding that differences in norms and traditions are common and not dependent on racialized status, country of origin, or individual characteristics of others; therefore, each of us brings culture to the table and we need to communicate to avoid cultural misunderstanding, especially when providing services. Cultural safety requires attention to cultural competence – beginning with critical self-reflection, imbalances in power relations, disparate socio-economic realities, and the outcomes of historical relations – the culturalist underpinnings of policies and procedures, and the composition of staff (Brown et al. 2009; Wilson and Neville 2009). Unfortunately, analysis of gender and culture are not mainstreamed at the operational level of the health system, although at the governance level some health ministries and authority boards state that the health of women, or sub-populations of women, is a priority (Horne, Donner, and Thurston 1999; Donner et al. 2001; Thurston and Eisener 2002).

Participation of Immigrants in Policy Development

The role of ethnic minority and immigrant-serving organizations is particularly discussed in the literature concerning participation of immigrants in health policy development. They are considered essential to the processes of community development (Rice and Prince 2000) and health care (Thomson 1993; Fisher et al. 1991) for ethno-cultural minorities. These organizations play an important role in offering their members a sense of belonging to a particular ethno-cultural or social group (Kirrane 1995). Recognized as a relevant form of public participation (Heiley 2001), they represent structures within the community systems (Thomson and Kinne 1998) where people come together and establish organizations that perform different tasks and provide all kinds of services (Cooper 2000; Rice and Prince 2000). Through services they provide, they meet their members' special needs, and in addition help to avoid fragmentation and reduce inequalities that exist between the majority and the minorities in a diverse society (Kirrane 1995; Rice and Prince 2000). Aside from providing direct services, these organizations serve to monitor and critique the government with the goal of improving programs and policies (Alcock and Christensen 1995). Public policy making represents a process that involves policy makers operating within the governmental arena, as well as a diverse set of people or constituency groups with special interests that function outside the government, pressing government for their demands and influencing the public policy making process (Nakamura and Smallwood 1980, cited in Rist 1994). Ethnic minority and immigrant organizations represent forces operating outside government that influence the process of policy making (Kirrane 1995; Cooper 2000).

Organizations are essential to the development of collective power and shared values and ties, and provide members with experiences of power (Speer and Hughey 1995). The relative proportion of organizational assets among settlement and immigrant-serving agencies dedicated to women's needs may speak to the capacity or willingness of the larger community to attend to these needs. In Canada the availability of settlement services specifically designed for immigrant women has much to do with the uneven distribution of migrants across the land; smaller towns have fewer resources for developing specialized programs. Baukje and Wachholtz (1999) explored some of the barriers faced by abused immigrant women in accessing justice services in New Brunswick and concluded that the main barrier was the lack of services specifically for abused immigrant women, particularly in small rural communities.

In a study of participation of immigrant women in IPV health policy development in Calgary, Thurston and colleagues (2004a,b) learned that there were few connections among the key sectors: the immigrant-serving sector, health sector, and IPV-serving sector. There was doubt expressed that immigrant-serving agencies were asking women broadly about IPV. As a former staff member of an immigrant-serving agency stated, '[There is] a sense that there are other issues much more pressing for the immigrants than family violence; therefore, why would we need to spend time on those issues given that people come to us for different reasons, and much different than those (chuckle) to do with family violence.'

And there was acknowledgement that cultural integration has not necessarily moved from the front lines of the IPV service sector to management. As one shelter manager commented: 'I think as in most, as in many organizations, once you move up into administration and management it's still by and large dominated by white middle-class women, and, you know, I'm not sure that that's always the most valuable place to get some of the information [about immigrant women's needs] that you're asking for.'

The study could not assess whether the lack of connections was preceded by or resulted in a lack of consensus on what the policy agenda might look like, but there was little consensus across the sectors. Respondents from immigrant-serving agencies described 'the problem' primarily in terms of access to health care – ineffective health care sector responses to immigrant health must be addressed before IPV and health policy can be broached. An IPV service manager did not even see the health sector as having a role in addressing IPV beyond provision of mental health services. The respondents in this study discussed a number of barriers to building relationships so that a policy community could develop. These barriers included: working in single issue 'silos,' the need to build trusting relationships, and perceptions that immigrants only needed to be at the table if there was a 'cultural' issue.

Conclusion

Immigrant women who experience IPV face many challenges and losses on top of having left their country of origin and often their support networks. However, not all losses are viewed negatively and many women find opportunities in Canada they would not have otherwise had: 'I feel secure here. I made this decision [to leave my husband]. I can't make in my country so I was in my country, I never ever can make this decision and this is a big advantage for me to came here (laughter) ... I say to myself yeah, I was lucky because I feel I can leave this man' (Thurston and Eisener 2006:30).

Importantly, women display reserves of resiliency and coping strategies that enable them to protect themselves and their children (McLaren and Dyck 2004; Graham and Thurston 2005; Javed and Gerrard 2006). With assistance from advocates for secure housing, income, and services they can lead healthy and fulfilled lives. The challenge is for all sectors to work to incorporate cultural safety and a deep understanding of gender-based IPV into the daily practices of their staff so that they can provide immigrant women with the advocacy that is needed.

NOTE

1 Primary-stage shelters take women and their children in crisis and have relatively short length-of-stay requirements. Second-stage shelters take women from the primary stage and permit longer occupancy. The length of stay at the Brenda Strafford Centre was six months.

8 Liminality and Mental Well-being among Non-Status Immigrant Women

LAURA SIMICH

Introduction

Many personal and social determinants of health contribute to experiences of stress among immigrants (Beiser 2005), but one factor that has been understudied is immigration status as a legal and social marker. Status designations such as 'immigrant' and 'refugee' that once clearly implied voluntary and forced migration, respectively, have become less distinct as patterns of migration become harder to define and control. Psychosocial implications of immigration status for health are even less clear, but some research suggests that immigration status is associated with health disparities in immigrant-receiving countries (Gagnon 2002; Gagnon et al. 2007; Sundquist 1995; Silove et al. 1998). Increasingly restrictive public policies that limit access to citizenship, health insurance, and health care for immigrants tend to legitimize such inequities, but neglect health and human rights (Fassin 2005; Ku and Matani 2001).

Among those most negatively affected in Canada are non-status immigrants. Called 'undocumented' or 'irregular' immigrants elsewhere in the world, they may include asylum seekers awaiting immigration decisions and visitors with expired visas, who, for a variety of complex reasons, must circumvent regular immigration procedures in the countries in which they reside (Jordan and Düvell 2002). Although non-status men and women both may face uncertainty and hardships, non-status women may be especially disadvantaged by lack of access to health care, social services, and legal channels, since they tend to have greater or even sole responsibility for childcare and family well-being and fewer options when struggling against violence and abuse. They are not, however, lacking certain strengths.

Although more notorious in the United States and Europe, the non-status immigrant population has grown in Canada, but empirical studies have been slow to emerge. Discussions of the needs of non-status migrants and fundamental health and human rights tend to occur in 'politically charged environments' (Watters and Ingleby 2004:550). Prejudices against non-status immigrants are reinforced by popular discourse that endorses 'good' versus 'bad' images of immigrants, and positions non-status immigrants as threatening to society. This 'Othering' process creates an 'us versus them' way of thinking that is inimical to public health promotion (Grove and Zwi 2006). Research and well-informed discussion is needed in Canada, because there is currently little information regarding the profile of non-status migrants.

In the United States, undocumented immigrants accounted for one-third of the total increase in the number of adults without health insurance between 1980 and 2000 (Goldman, Smith, and Sood 2005). North of the border, accurate population figures are impossible to obtain. Unofficial statistics collected by labour unions estimate that at least 200,000 non-status workers are employed in the underground economy, but the figure may be much higher. Officially, Canada uses a working estimate of about half a million unauthorized immigrants, still a relatively small but growing proportion of the 30 to 40 million non-status immigrants worldwide (Papademetriou 2005). Of the nearly 250,000 refugee claims adjudicated in Canada since 1997, 60 per cent have been rejected, and many claimants remain in the country without health insurance, adding to the numbers of immigrants in Canada with inadequate access to health care (Caulford and Vali 2006).

What are the realities of living without status? Using the analogy of migration-as-rite-of-passage, one American anthropologist has described living without legal immigration status as a liminal existence (Chavez 1992). In a prolonged condition of liminality that often lasts for years, non-status immigrants remain on the threshold of an incomplete social transition, stuck in arrested anticipation of legal incorporation into a new society. Everyday life is marked by ambiguity regarding social entitlements and personal security. Moreover, being in transition suggests inherent uncertainty about the future, potential for psychological distress, and heightened self-awareness (Turner 1967). Recent studies have suggested that women in such precarious situations may be particularly vulnerable (Anderson 2004; Oxman-Martinez et al. 2005), but little mental health-related research has been conducted directly with non-status immigrants (for a survey of research on the mental health status of immigrants with legal status in Canada see Hyman, McDermott, and DesMeules, this volume). This chapter therefore contributes to our current knowledge of this understudied population by providing a glimpse of hidden mental health concerns and personal responses to liminality among Latin American women living without legal immigration status in Toronto.

I begin with an overview of the health challenges faced by non-status immigrants and of the notion of health security. Following, I describe the study we conducted with non-status immigrants in the Toronto area that brought into focus the consequences of liminal, precarious immigration status on health and well-being.

Health Security and Non-Status Immigrants

Health issues are unexplored in the non-status immigrant population, but due to its size, the issues are likely significant for host countries and for underserved non-status immigrants themselves. Non-status immigrants are generally working members of society, but they do not share fully in society's health and social benefits. They typically have significant health needs that are not being met (Gushulak and MacPherson 2000), such as perinatal care and treatment for workplace injuries (Anderson 2004; Caulford and Vali 2006). Non-status immigrants tend to surface in deprived urban areas where other immigrants concentrate, and to be more ill when they do seek services (Reijneveld et al. 2001). When they seek health care in emergencies, they not only face linguistic and cultural barriers like other immigrants, they must also shoulder the high costs of paying for treatment and hospitalization on their own. Service providers in the United States, Europe, and Canada testify that non-status immigrants have unmet needs for health care due to lack of knowledge of their basic rights and fear of being turned away and deported (Berk and Schur 2001; Chauvin and Parizot 2006; Nyers 2006; Torres and Sanz 2000). They are often excluded from comprehensive primary health care by eligibility rules as well as the limited capacity of community clinics that may accept them as clients.

Working typically as cleaners and caregivers, non-status women hold stressful, unsteady jobs for lower pay than legal workers and are afraid to report exploitation (Mehta et al. 2002). Immigrant women, who tend to have lower levels of language proficiency than men, may also be more disadvantaged in navigating the health care system. Given their special needs for gynaecological services, contraceptives, and pregnancy care, along with childcare responsibilities and the potential need for services to cope with abuse and violence, it is reasonable to assume that non-status women have high unmet health care needs, including mental health.

The few studies that exist of emotional distress among non-status migrants demonstrate reasons for concern, although they have not specifically highlighted women's issues. One study of 'illegal' Irish immigrants working in the United States found that they had both positive and negative feelings about their lives, but they felt particular stress related to being illegal (Aroian 1993). In Australia, policies of deterrence and detention have been reported to add significantly to the mental distress that unauthorized asylum seekers experience (Silove, Steel, and Watters 2000). Another study of asylum seekers in Europe found that they experienced three overwhelming negative feelings: lack of control, a crisis of identity brought on by criminalization, and a sense of isolation from supportive social networks (Koser 2000).

The concept of health and well-being used here is broad, as in the World Health Organization (WHO) definition of health as 'a complete state of physical, mental and social well-being, not merely the absence of disease,'[1] but it goes somewhat further. The emphasis here is on health security, which refers to personal safety, protection from health risks, and access to health care. First used in the United Nations Development Program Human Development Report of 1994, the idea is that security is not exclusively tied to nation states, but is interpreted subjectively as a quality that people experience in their everyday lives (Lammers 1999). Health security for individual immigrants or societies cannot be achieved through obsolete containment and control approaches common in public health (MacPherson and Gushulak 2001), particularly with respect to mental health. In the case of non-status migrants, the concept draws attention to the interaction of pre-migration circumstances in the country of origin and post-migration social and environmental contingencies that underlie health disparities and affect mental health. This approach is relevant to non-status women immigrants for whom personal safety and protection from health risks is embedded in intersecting oppressions associated with gender, in addition to classed, racialized, ethnic, and legal identities extending from the country of origin to Canada. As we see in this chapter, health security for non-status women is often defined by the intersection of personal, social, and legal concerns. Exploring perceived health security from their perspective also privileges the subjective experiences of women's well-being and may uncover previously unrecognized realities.

Study Methods

For this study of experiences and health care needs, a research team led by Dr Simich interviewed clients who defined themselves as 'non-status' at a downtown Toronto community health centre.[2] The main research objectives were to understand what it means to be 'non-status' and how living without status affects mental well-being and social integration. No previous research had been conducted with this immigrant group in Toronto when the study began, although community advocacy activities had begun when interviews were conducted in 2004 and 2005, perhaps helping some non-status immigrants feel safe enough to come out of the shadows.

Qualitative descriptive methods were used to explore and to understand personal experiences of study participants (Denzin and Lincoln 2000; Sandelowski 2000). The Research Ethics boards of the University of Toronto and the Access Alliance Multicultural Community Health Centre, which serves immigrants and provided a supportive interviewing environment, both granted the study prior ethics approval. Researchers discussed the study population and relevant issues in Toronto with an advisory group assembled by the community health centre. Preliminary key informant interviews with members of immigrant service, labour, legal, and faith-based organizations helped to gather background information and to develop a purposive sampling frame for subsequent interviews. We decided to concentrate on recruiting Spanish-speaking participants to form a more homogeneous sample for analysis and because they were the predominant linguistic subgroup of non-status clients at the clinic. However, non-status immigrants are found in many ethno-cultural populations in Canada. The study sample was mostly female, composed of eight women and three men (see Table 1). Gender imbalance in the sample is not surprising; women in general seek health care in higher proportions than men, and 66 per cent of clients attending another Toronto health clinic for uninsured migrants were also female (Caulford and Vali 2006).

Two Spanish-speaking former staff members of the community health centre recruited participants through clinic and community networks by distributing information letters in Spanish that described the purpose of the project and emphasized confidentiality. As expected,

Table 1
Description of Study Sample (Women Only)

Demographic variables		Number of participants
Country of origin	Argentina	1
	Costa Rica	2
	Ecuador	2
	Mexico	2
	Peru	1
Age range	20–30	2
	30–40	3
	50–60	2
	Over 60	1
Legal status upon arrival (before loss of status)	Refugee Claimant	4
	Visitor's Visa	4
Marital status	Married	4
	Single	2
	Separated	2
Number of children under 18 in household	0	1
	1	1
	2	4
	3	1
	4	1
Educational level	Professional / University	
	All or part of Secondary	4
Occupation in Home country	Professional	4
	Management/Clerical	2
	Self-employed	1
	Labour	1
Occupation in Canada	Labour	6
	Unemployed/unpaid	2
English proficiency (self-reported)	Good	1
	Fair	4
	Poor	3

recruitment was initially difficult due to the inherent reticence of non-status migrants, but eased as trust was established. Recruiting was intentionally abbreviated in 2005 to avoid unwelcome exposure of those who feared the stepped-up deportations occurring at the time. The final sample size was adequate for study purposes and qualitative analysis, although a larger sample including more men and other ethno-linguistic groups would be desirable to ensure data saturation in future studies.

The women were eager to share their personal experiences, although they showed more emotional distress than the men who were interviewed, sometimes weeping and revealing traumatic experiences that they had no previous opportunity to discuss. Interviewers did not press for details for ethical reasons, but offered support and referrals for counselling if desired. The assurance of confidentially was especially important to engage participants, but the opportunity to give personal testimony about the experience of living without status during an interview was also compelling.

Open-ended, semi-structured interview questions were asked to help uncover unanticipated issues, but the following topics were included in all interviews: pre-migration experiences, arrival and settlement in Canada; the immigration process, the impact of being non-status on work and family; social support; and health status and health care experiences. The interviews, conducted with the help of trained cultural interpreters provided by Access Alliance, averaged 1.5 hours, and were audiotaped with participants' permission. Participants received honoraria of $25 and public transportation expenses.

Spanish-speaking research assistants transcribed the taped interviews and verified the accuracy of translations. Using NVivo analytic software, the research team coded and discussed the transcripts. In the first analysis, the coding framework followed the interview topics for comparability across cases. In the second phase of analysis, researchers regrouped categories into theoretically defined stages of the migration process (i.e., pre-migration, transition, and post-migration), noting situations and emerging themes related to psychosocial stress and liminality.

We analysed the interviews using the anthropological paradigm of liminality as discussed by Chavez (1992) in his studies of the lives of illegal Mexican immigrants in the United States. Applied to migration, this paradigm comprises three phases: first, separation (pre-migration and leaving home); followed by a transitional or liminal phase (migration and initial settlement in the new society); and, finally, social incorporation (full settlement and social integration). In reality, this is a complex, non-linear process, but it suggests a way of understanding the stress and ambiguity experienced by non-status migrants, who are by definition caught at the cusp of a social status transition that may never be completed.

The central phase of liminality is characterized psychologically by disorientation, indeterminacy, suspense, and heightened self-awareness. For non-status immigrants, liminality is a more ambivalent and culturally complex process than 'acculturation' because de facto and de jure experiences of adaptation and social integration are contradictory. Some challenges, such as having to learn the language of the receiving society, sustaining social ties, and finding employment, occur commonly among immigrants. For these women however, there was also the overriding fact of being non-status. Paradoxically, for the non-status women in this study, present insecurity and future potential both affected their sense of psychological well-being.

Study Findings

An overview of findings is presented here before specifically highlighting some psychosocial issues associated with liminality. Discussions of study participants' reasons for migration, selected health issues, examples of stigmatizing encounters with the immigration system, and perceptions of health care have been discussed elsewhere (Simich 2006; Simich, Wu, and Nerad 2007). Reasons for migration among non-status immigrants are worth noting here, however, because non-status immigrants tend to be conflated with 'queue-jumping' economic migrants, 'bogus' asylum seekers, 'undeserving' refugees, or even terrorists, by media and political interests in Europe, Britain, and elsewhere (Jordan and Duvell 2002; Sales 2002; Watters and Ingleby 2004; Fassin 2005). As Sales (2002) points out, mistrustful attitudes legitimize a punitive system of social support and promote intense social exclusion. The question is, how do non-status immigrants cope psychologically with the discrepancy between the public view and their self-image?

In this study, reasons for migration, whether forced or voluntary, were generally expressed as hopes for a better life, and these women were not exceptional in this regard. Although economic instability was sometimes an additional 'push' factor in their decisions, the primary aim of emigration was not to obtain material benefits. Rather, participants, both male and female, sought increased personal security; they sought to escape threats or acts of violence such as rape, sexual violence, police harassment, and political threats against self or family members. Two women came in hopes of obtaining better medical care for their small children, but they and their family members were also seeking refuge from what they described as violent, life-threatening situations.

One woman came to join a long separated husband, but encountered unexpected personal and legal barriers upon arrival.

All study participants had entered Canada legally and had attempted to follow correct immigration procedures. At the time of the interviews, the women were legitimately waiting for immigration decisions, yet they were fearful of being deported. Of the four women who entered legally on visitor's visas that had since expired, one was still waiting for family sponsorship to be approved, one was awaiting a visa renewal for lack of other options, and one had legally sound reasons to apply to stay in Canada on 'humanitarian and compassionate' grounds. The last woman had taken refuge in Canada on a visitor's visa due to lack of knowledge of the correct refugee application procedures. After more than two years – just before our interview – she had finally received legal status as a woman in need of protection from sexual harassment by police in Mexico. Those remaining women who had entered Canada as asylum seekers were technically 'in the system' waiting for their refugee claims to be heard or for previously unsuccessful appeals to be adjudicated and finalized. Despite ongoing involvement in the legal and immigration systems, all study participants labelled themselves 'non-status.' All women were employed on the margins of the economy, working in one or more low-paying manual jobs in janitorial services, factory work, or informal caregiving without job protection, employment benefits, or health benefits, despite most having obtained university or professional education and having held managerial or 'white collar' jobs in their home countries.

All participants reported emotional suffering from chronic stress, depression, and family separation. Two women revealed traumatic experiences of sexual abuse in the home country for which they had not received any treatment or counselling; other women only hinted at such experiences. Several reported developing stress-related physical conditions such as persistent headaches, sleep problems, and increasing symptoms of diabetes. (See also chapter 2, this volume.) Although some expressed the desire for professional psychological help, most participants actively used personal coping skills to overcome mental distress. Notably, they universally rejected the stigma of criminalization, asserting their own sense of morally upright behaviour in having migrated to Canada. They made concerted efforts to lead productive and socially meaningful lives.

Beyond the individual emotional health effects of being non-status, the greatest impact was on their families, particularly the increased

Figure 1. Liminality and mental well-being among non-status immigrants: Qualitative elements of stress, stigma, and social control

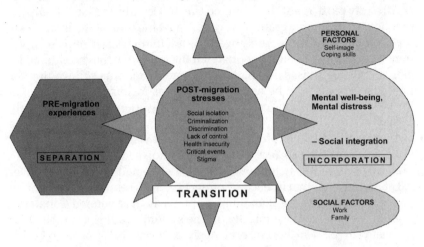

stress for their children. All but one of the women interviewed (a 62-year-old) had at least one child under the age of 18 in the household. Typically, some members of the family had legal status, but not all, creating differential access to health services and contributing to worries about family separation if those without status were not permitted to stay in Canada. Most participants reported having good social support within their immediate families, but limited support from extended and non-family acquaintances. Some women cultivated strong, discrete social ties with neighbours and other acquaintances.

The women's comments presented below illustrate many of the psychological challenges of liminality, but they also express potential for gaining new perspectives and hope. Specifically, they describe three paradoxical themes or contradictory feelings. First, women articulate a sense of insecurity that deeply affects mental health, coupled with a sense of potential self-realization; second, they recount experiences of economic exploitation, yet partial social incorporation through social ties and their own contributions; and third, they reveal that caring for family can be simultaneously a source of stress and a means of coping.

Many of the women spoke with a mixture of fear and self-defining defiance about how they were affected by being non-status. One middle-aged woman from Ecuador said of her situation, 'You don't have that security. You're always afraid, because for someone who doesn't have status and who gets caught, it's like they caught a thief, a criminal. It's terrible. I've lived it. I've felt it. It's a crime to work to want to help your family!'

A woman from Argentina described an encounter with condescending border authorities who mocked her ability to speak English, which initially saddened her but eventually fuelled her self-esteem and perseverance. She explained:

> When I got out of Immigration two officers were watching me. Today I realize that they were saying, 'She doesn't speak English,' and they laughed in my face! I decided if I spoke more slowly they would understand me, so I said, 'My husband is coming for me,' and they laughed, and told me that I would have to leave. This is what helps me to continue fighting, because I realized that the fact that I don't speak English doesn't make me unable to do things. Listen, I've done things that I feel personally proud of. Every time that I do something, I always remember those people who laughed at me right in front of my face.

Most of the women had worked in middle-class occupations in their countries of origin and described their working lives in Canada with a sense of loss and injustice. For example, one described how she worked 'cleaning offices, and I have work cleaning in a school, cleaning the classrooms. It's very hard. It's very hard for me to talk about this, because we all [voice becomes emotional], we are professionals from our countries.' When asked about relations with co-workers, she replied, 'I have met different classes of people. Some of them are very racist. Just because we are from Latin America they think that we will go along with everything that they say, everything that they tell us to do.' She continued with a mixture of hope and resignation, 'You know, the kind of work that I do is not a problem any more, because I have accepted it as a step that I have to go through. I know I have time, for me, to become a professional as I was.' But, as she declared that this step was 'for her kids,' her voice wavered and she began to cry.

When describing the contradictions of having to work without benefits or recognition, most women felt a sense of indignation because of their work ethic and perceived contributions to society. When threatened with deportation, a woman described how 'They took away my social insurance card, they took away my work permit, they took everything!' Despite her deportation being stopped on legal grounds, she explained that it was difficult to 'go forward.' As she explained, 'If I don't have a social insurance number, I can't work. Many people don't want to give work without a social insurance number and those who do hire without it exploit people.' Nevertheless, she had not quit her job cleaning buildings as she was told to do, and, using a false social insurance number, she filed her tax return within the week.

The majority of women described exploitation on the job. One woman from Costa Rica reported 'a very ugly experience.' She had worked a night shift for nearly two weeks, and then found a second, daytime job that was better for her children. The first employer demanded 15 days notice and refused to pay her for the time worked. 'Obviously they knew I don't have papers,' she said, 'so they took advantage of me. They knew that I couldn't complain. They said no, because I didn't follow the laws here.' When she pointed out that they were not doing things legally by giving jobs to people without papers, they responded angrily, saying that 'people without papers should appreciate what we're doing because we give them jobs.'

The women also noted unethical practices by employment agencies. One observed, 'People here illegally who get work through agencies don't make the same as everybody else, because those agencies keep a certain amount of money. They take advantage of people. I know people who have worked like that for a month. They don't pay them and they say, "Where are you going to go and complain?" I don't think that's right. It's not human.'

Despite feeling exploited in Canada, the women demonstrated concern for the welfare of others. Some worked as caregivers and hoped to have futures in social service. One woman from Mexico held multiple jobs, working in janitorial services, cleaning houses, and picking up children from childcare centres. She also worried about her elderly neighbours. 'I am needed by the seniors,' she explained, 'because the lady is suffering from Alzheimer's and her husband has Parkinson's disease.' Her own personal strengths and cultural norms compelled her to lend a hand in spite of her own insecurity.

As for social support for themselves, many of the women had someone in whom they could confide, their immediate families or small circles of friends, but maintaining support networks was sometimes challenging. Liminality intensified their moral sensibilities although it undermined individual control, and it awakened a sense of communitas, or feelings of equality and common humanity. One woman from Peru described not having many friends and keeping a low profile. Yet, when she reflected on the impact of living without status, she identified strongly with others and attempted to protect women and children in the same situation. She said:

> I think that they are scared. Sometimes I see this as my own future. Like, there is this family living in the basement of the house where I live. When they talk about their situation, I place myself in something that will come if I get a 'no' answer [from immigration authorities]. In their case, their child can't attend school because they are afraid. The husband works in construction. She stays at home. I try to find out about places where they don't ask about immigration papers or anything, so she can go out and have something to do. I have always tried to bring her here [to the community clinic]. I think because of her husband now she is trying not to talk to me too much. I always have told her, listen if you have an emergency you have a place to go.

Some women actively pursued new social relationships and recreated social networks to normalize their lives. One woman from Argentina recalled, 'The first friend that I made, apart from a Colombian friend that we had, was Iraqi. I'm not sure how we do it, but still we communicate by telephone. We participate in everything, everything that we're invited to. Friends, we have a ton, my husband through soccer, my daughter through dance. Entire families. We do not have family here. We are just my husband, my two children, myself, and one cousin, but we see [this community clinic] as another family. I cook for them when they have parties. And for people who get deported or for newcomers, I have been to the airport to see what I can do for these folks. There's always someone to help.'

A woman from Costa Rica described her new friendships with housemates as important in helping her to carry on: 'Women newcomers from other countries, we help each other a lot. For instance, they help me a lot with my children. I helped them when they just arrived and they had to go places. I help as much as I can and they help me as much as they can. We are like five sisters. People get closer to you even though they don't belong to your bloodline. Many situations in life make you feel that those people are your family.'

As we can see, most of the women are socially integrated in Canada through limited, but helpful social networks. Their uncertain immigration status does not allow them to become officially or economically integrated; they obtain only marginal employment and are often exploited, but they try to normalize social life as much as possible.

The balances among stress, coping, and mutual support are less publicly, but more poignantly expressed through effects on the family. One woman from Ecuador who had anticipated being sponsored as an immigrant by her sister was disappointed to learn upon arrival in Toronto that immigration laws had changed and sponsorship by siblings was no longer possible. More than laws had changed; from her perspective, her family's loyalties were altered by Canadian society. She went to work temporarily in the United States, leaving her son in Canada and sending her earnings to support him, but her sister felt little obligation to help. 'The mentality here is different,' she learned. 'In the first few days everything's okay, but then you have to fend for yourself. Here in Canada there's a lot of independence. It's a matter of self-interest.'

Attaining different immigration statuses also divided family members and created bureaucratic nightmares for parents. For example, the brother of one woman who sought refuge in Canada had come 14 years ago after trouble with police in Peru, and, after seven years in Canada, was finally accepted as a refugee. The woman, conversely, was working and living a comfortable life in Peru and not planning to emigrate at all, until she had a confrontation with terrorists and was forced to flee. She was pregnant at the time of the interview, but was too distressed to talk about her husband. On arrival in Canada, she said, 'I didn't know what to do. I carried my 15-day-old baby and I needed to take him to doctor and I didn't know where to go. Thank God the nurse from the hospital gave me a hand.' Unlike her brother's successful refugee claim, her own claim was denied, leaving her status and her child's future in limbo. She maintained that, 'Sometimes I feel like I don't have the right to feel sick. My parents on are my side, but it seems like I have to be the strong one.' Worries about her children were paramount. 'Even though the children are Canadian, to receive medical attention they are always asking about my status, my papers. If I decided to stay illegally here, everything is going to be cut off for me and my children, because there is an expiration date on the health card. I won't have a chance to renew it. To renew theirs I have to show them mine. It worries me that they might get sick in the middle of the night, because I won't be able to take them to the hospital. What am I going to do?'

Worries about how to protect her children if she were deported also weighed on the mother from Argentina who had come to Canada to seek refuge and to obtain medical care for a small son with a serious kidney illness. Her story illustrates some of the effects of liminality and its precipitous, disorienting impacts on children and adults. One underlying problem she identified is the immigration agreement between Canada and the United States, which detains and deports refugee claimants en route to Canada. What happens to the children when adults are deported? 'That's just it,' she answered, horrified. 'I know what has happened to many people from my country. I know the children are put in jails with offenders, just like anybody else, because they think this is an offence.'

Like parents everywhere, her greatest interest was the health of her two children, and she was grateful for the clinic and the temporary health insurance she had as a refugee claimant. But even so, she witnessed her children's health beginning to suffer: 'I was working from morning to night,' she explained. 'My son started showing signs of stress, because the situation in which we were living was very uncertain. We could not make plans for the future, because we didn't know what the future was. Between this insecure situation and my husband without work, the situation in my house was one of nervousness. My husband doesn't like to be without work. He was desperate. We realized that these things were affecting our son, who started to show signs of depression and bedwetting. Thank God, my son plays football. My husband volunteers as a coach, and this helped to support him. It was a distraction from all the problems in my house.'

Coping with the family's insecurity also affected the older daughter, who 'had to become the one who cared for her brother. We didn't have any other options.' Reflecting on how her daughter reacted to life events, the mother said, 'In the beginning, I think she was like all children; she didn't want to accept being here. But after three months she started to speak English, and she did a ton of things that I think back there she couldn't have, and wouldn't have thought to do. She dances in a group, she takes painting classes after school, she participates in everything that she can at school. She brings home excellent report cards. But when she found out about the negative decision from Immigration, she cried and cried. Her best friend told her she could hide in her basement. She was crying and asking me, "Why can't the people from Immigration ask me? Why do they have to make decisions for me? I don't want to leave." Poor thing, the truth is she's the one who has had to grow up the most.'

When asked what she herself does to cope, the mother said she worked to avoid having too much time to think. She liked to imagine a future in Canada, which felt to her 'like two arms that support my son's health. I dream of my children fulfilling their dreams, and myself as an elderly woman, happy and tranquil.' Her brief reverie ended with a recollection of her family's past and current circumstances: 'My son lost a kidney in my country because they didn't want to operate on him, so this is my fear about leaving. What if there is a problem and he loses his other kidney, what will we do?' This thought revived painful memories and more fears. She paused to take a deep breath and then said:

> Sometimes I feel that it's too much. Sometimes I think I just can't do any more. Many times, before I got married, I had depression. One year, I was hospitalized twice. Sometimes I fear that I will return to that same state. My whole childhood was very sad, my adolescence was terrible. The only thing that was important to me was my mother and I lost her. The only thing I have now is my husband and my children. So, I always think that if I have to go back there, I believe that would be the end of everything for me. I love my country, but I feel a lot of rage about everything that happened to me there.

But she shook herself and continued: 'They told us that Canada doesn't want anyone who is sick, and we presented to them our son's problem. I don't believe that it would be good to have another sick person.'

Conclusion

To summarize, liminal experiences of non-status immigrants affect health security and contribute to mental distress, but complex personal and social coping strategies alleviate some of the suffering associated with the prolonged, uncertain transition. While 'being non-status' is stressful, the liminal state also confers self-awareness, new perspectives, and a sense of solidarity or communitas. Study participants expressed a sense of feeling stigmatized as non-status persons, but they also protested criminalization. Moreover, the sense of being treated unfairly was counterbalanced by the sense of moral right. Non-status migrants also endure stress from social challenges common to other immigrants' experiences in Canada, including underemployment, discrimination, and family separation, but with additional barriers. They face greater uncertainty about the future and more restrictions on health care access than other immigrants do, which exacerbates and hinders helpful responses to mental anguish.

Despite added worries about their families' futures, non-status immigrant women carry on working and caring for others, doing what they can to increase their sense of security and well-being. Many of the women, in particular those who had suffered from sexual violence in their home countries, felt grateful for the safety and personal security accorded to them in Canada due to more prevalent respect for women's rights. Their gender roles as mothers, wives, and caretakers, however, created additional burdens and affected strategic decisions. The women lack control of the future, but everyday acts of protecting and providing for others confers a sense of self-esteem and personal agency. Like many immigrants, the women suffered from unaccustomed social isolation in their new environments, but many received and provided strong social supports within the family. Most women actively sought ways to recreate helpful social networks, and because they perceive themselves as contributing socially and economically, they can almost imagine having status and future well-being in Canada.

Perhaps it is appropriate to conclude this chapter about the experiences of non-status immigrant women with the plea for understanding, with which one woman ended her interview. She said:

> They [Canadians] don't know how we are treated. They don't really know who we are. What I would like is that they understand how we are treated, what we are doing, what we are paying. And I would like that they stop seeing us as intruders who are taking advantage. I would like you to show them, to show them everything, the way that Immigration treats us, the way that they take our money and the kind of opportunities that they give us. I would like them to know how we live. That we have to live with doubts. That we have to lie sometimes so that we are not found out. And that they understand, not only my children, but all the children, the Dreams and the ambitions they bring to this country.

NOTES

1 Preamble to the Constitution of the World Health Organization as adopted by the International Health Conference, New York, 19 June–22 July 1946; signed 22 July 1946 by the representatives of 61 states (Official Records of the World Health Organization, no. 2, p. 100) and entered into force 7 April 1948.

2 Dr Simich gratefully acknowledges the help of Access Alliance Multicultural Community Health Centre; the Dean's Fund, Faculty of Medicine, University of Toronto; and the non-status women and men who came forward to share their personal stories and experiences. Fei Wu, Mary Roufail, and Julie Mooney provided valuable research assistance.

9 Social Suffering and Witnessing: Exploring the Interface between Health Policy and Testimonial Narratives of Canadian Afghan Women

PARIN DOSSA

Introduction

It is well recognized that trauma and suffering have become a systemic part of our global reality that bears significant impact on the health and well-being of individuals, communities, and peoples. Yet scholarship has only begun to address the *interrelated* questions on the events surrounding trauma and how they are articulated from the bottom up, which includes body language,[1] for a layered approach to effect structural change (Douglass and Vogler 2003). Social scientists have identified different vantage points. Behar (1996) suggests that we adopt the position of a vulnerable observer so that we can feel the pain of the 'far-out lives' (7). Das and Kleinman (2001), on the other hand, argue that we cannot fully grasp other people's suffering. The least we can do is witness their stories. 'In the end we can say that while the ownership of one's pain rests only with oneself ... no one speaking on behalf of the person in pain has a right to appropriate it for some other use ...' (29). Farmer (2003) and Kleinman and Kleinman (1997), on the other hand, spell out the geopolitical script to establish the link between social and political factors and life stories. The authors draw our attention to institutional responses that accentuate rather than alleviate one's pain.[2] The scholarly literature on trauma remains polarized, as substantively we have not been able to resolve the gap between the geopolitics of trauma and human agency, with its focus on ownership and also recovery, to forestall victimization. Scheper-Hughes' (1992) point of intervention is to suggest a middle path, but this too is problematic as it leads to a division of labour where scholars generate theory and the research participants provide the data (Hill-Collins 2000; Dossa 2004).

I propose an approach where the latter are given central space on account of the fact that the sufferers' voices are often silenced in the dominant discourses, especially if they are women (Ross 2001; Todechini 2001). I argue that this is a crucial first step. A second step is to foster a dialogue between the women and the stakeholders, where women are recognized as producers of context-specific knowledge. I wish to show that it is through this dialogue that we can affect paradigm shifts in policy, from charity to entitlement. I propose a third step to heighten the need for the policy shifts. I argue that it is necessary to establish politicized and global connections between the lives of the women in their homeland and in the diaspora. This connection is muted to advance the political agendas of more powerful countries.

In this chapter I engage with the above issues through a reading of testimonial accounts of Afghan women from a low-income housing area in metropolitan Vancouver. The narratives form part of a larger study that examined the impact of displacement and migration on the health and well-being of Afghan women. Health status of younger and older women has been extensively researched on the grounds that these women are doubly disadvantaged. Being a woman and being old are considered a social burden (Lock 1993a). There is negligible research on racialized women who are subject to intersecting inequalities. Their lives may be read in the context of *social suffering*, a term that suggests three scenarios: existential suffering, institutional responses, and re-making of worlds by those who have been victims of social violence and war (Das and Kleinman 2001).

In the way of a modest beginning, I want to suggest a contextualized and layered reading of one woman's testimonial narrative. I use the term *testimonial* in an expanded sense. While I focus on the story of one woman that captures the experiences of her cohort – this is what makes it testimonial – the voices of the ones that follow are not necessarily excluded. As I show below, opening up the boundaries of a text constitutes one means through which we can witness stories of suffering.

I set the stage by introducing the study I conducted with Afghan women in the Vancouver area, and offer the testimony of 'Meena.' Contextualizing the pre- and post-migration experiences of Afghani Canadian women, I unpack the multiple and embodied meanings of Meena's narrative and conclude with a call for active witnessing of social suffering to move towards the healing of women's wounds.

The Study

The testimonial account presented here comes from in-depth narrative interviews with 15 Afghan women from a residential area in Burnaby that we refer to as Valley View for the purpose of confidentiality. In the same vein, names and identifiable markers of the women have been changed. Women participated in two to three interviews. Five more women participated in a focus group session. The women determined the interview schedule depending on their willingness to continue with their stories or whether they felt that other women would fill in for them. This mode of collective storytelling is common among oppressed groups (Dossa 2004). Originally we had planned to interview aging Afghan women, but younger women came forward and stated that they considered themselves to be old. War and displacement had deprived them of their adulthood. The women were Convention refugees as defined by the 1951 United Nations Convention Relating to the Status of Refugees. Some had completed elementary school while others had mid-range education (high school through to Grade 12). In addition, some women completed short courses sponsored by non-governmental organizations in social work, midwifery, and other health-related fields. Their length of time in Canada ranged from two to 12 years, giving insight into their settlement experiences from an early to a relatively later period in their lives. In the interview sessions, we invited women to tell the stories of their lives using an aide memoir that included topics such as being a newcomer in Canada, work and everyday life, encounters with social and health providers, and managing health and illness. Group interviews were designed to encourage dialogue and discussion among women themselves as well as between the women and other parties (an indigenous service provider, a researcher, and a research assistant).[3] All the interviews were conducted in the women's first language of Dari, and were subsequently translated and transcribed by two research assistants, one Afghan and one Iranian.[4]

Meena's Story: Laying Out the Context

Meena came to Canada in 1998 with her second eldest daughter. Like other women in our study, she came from another country (India) where she lived for seven years with her husband and five children (four daughters and a son). Meena had lived through war and civil strife since 1979, when the then-Soviet Union invaded Afghanistan. A decade of Soviet presence (1979–1989) meant that Afghanistan became the battleground for the Cold War. The United States provided arms and ammunition to several hundred anti-community jehadis (resistance fighters) to drive out the Russians, converting Afghanistan into a landmine (Cooley 1999). During the time of the Soviet Occupation, 1.5 million Afghans lost their lives, 2.5 million were injured, and 1.1 million were internally displaced. Out of the 5 million refugees, 2.6 million lived in camps in Pakistan and Iran where the living conditions were only marginally better than what was found in war-torn Afghanistan (Brodsky 2003).

This is what Meena has to say about her country: 'All our houses were bombed. Several bombs came to our neighbourhood. I am not saying that the situation was bad only for us. No, for everybody in that area. When they bombed a neighbourhood close to us, 18 families were killed.' She continued: 'Who cannot be happy in their own country? Who likes to be homeless and confused? Who? Don't you like your home country? Everybody likes to live in their home country so far as there is peace, food, and happiness' (interview data). Note how Meena engages the reader through the use of the words 'who,' 'you,' and 'everybody.' As I show below, it is in this broader social context that Meena acts as witness to her own story.

Meena related that her family had to flee Afghanistan to avoid the abduction of her daughter by a Mujahideen (a fundamentalist, anti-Soviet faction that ruled with an iron hand from 1992 to 1995). Following an incident when a bearded man came to the house at 2:00 a.m. asking for her daughter, Meena's husband sold their house at a low price and used the money to get fake passports for India. Their eldest daughter, who stayed in Afghanistan to continue her work as an airline hostess, supported the family for a year until the Taliban forbade women from working outside home even if they were supporting families. Meena's husband left the family in search of work and she lost regular contact with him. Meena and her second eldest daughter were accepted into Canada on the grounds that she was a 'single mother.' Her other daughters got married. When Meena came to Canada, she sponsored her husband; five years have gone by and the couple is still separated despite the fact that the judge has accepted his application. The separation has caused her a lot of agony. In response to our question on health, Meena observed: 'This [my health] depends on my need for my husband. He needs me and I need him. He is my husband. He is depressed. So all my depression is about this. My illness is about this. I have cried and cried, shouted and screamed, but no one has listened to me until now' [meaning the time of the research interview, November 2003]. Meena's everyday life is governed by her concern that her husband is not with her.

Speaking through the Language of Everyday Life

Feminists have endeavoured to document the everyday lives of women, highlighting two issues. First, women's everyday activities have been rendered invisible for the benefit of the capitalist system. Without women's unpaid work within the private sphere and low-paid/ghettoized work in the public sphere,[5] the male-oriented, market-based system would have suffered (Fraser 1989; Smith 1984, 1987). Gendering of everyday life is then of interest as it reveals the workings of the larger system within a localized space. Second, women's engagement with the materiality of everyday spaces has brought into relief numerous ways in which they subvert the system – an aspect that is critically important as it contains seeds of social change (Dossa 1988).

Everyday life then featured high in our interview schedule. What was foremost in our minds was the image of a busy woman carrying a double load. But this aspect was not of interest to Meena, although she looked after her two-year-old granddaughter and cooked for three people (her daughter, her son-in-law, and herself) and did all the cleaning. As we have seen, Meena's everyday life was filled with one worry: that of the separation from her husband. In her words: 'I have become ill. I have got blood sugar. I am sick because of my stress for my husband. He is my husband. We lived together. He is in India. He is sick as well. He is worried, lots of pressure. I went to my doctor. She wrote a letter that I am sick. I am worried. I long for my husband and I am sad. I gave them the letter. I have got depression. Doctor said so twice. We have sent them letters but I do not know why nothing happens.'

Meena stated that they have taken all the necessary steps that would facilitate her husband Mohammed's immigration to Canada. Meena has paid up the government loan she received for her air ticket to Canada, she has obtained a letter of employment for her husband from an Iranian shopkeeper, who is a friend, and she has submitted all the necessary documents. The latter includes a medical certificate attesting to the fact that spousal separation has made Meena sick. The only response she got from the immigration office over the past five years is: 'today, tomorrow, today, tomorrow, so we do not know when he will come.'

Attending to her wounds has become part of Meena's everyday routine. The term *wounds* is of value, as it blurs the boundary between her diagnosed illness (high blood pressure and diabetes) and her pain and suffering caused by over two decades of war and violence brought about by the rape of Afghanistan – this is how the women in our study viewed the situation. This violation has been expressed in the form of wounds on the bodies of women. Meena speaks from her wounds when she says she is sick because of her diabetes and the stress of missing her husband: 'I have become ill. I have got blood sugar. I am sick because of my stress for my husband.' Her illness then cannot be reduced to clinical diagnoses where the socio-political context is silenced. Meena is on medication, placing the onus on her to get well. Societal institutions are absolved from responsibility.

Meena is not the only one who tends to her wounds on a day-to-day basis. Consider the following two scenarios pertaining to their experiences in Afghanistan relayed by Leila and Salima, respectively.

> I was at home once. We had made some food. I told my son to go to the bazaar and buy something. He left and I went to wash my hair. I had washed all the clothes and cleaned the house. A boy from the neighbour came and said, 'Lady. Your son was taken from the road. They put him in a car and left.' I put on my burqa and ran to the streets. I did not know where to go. The car had stopped somewhere close to get other boys, 10 to 11 years old. So I found the car and told that man, 'Dear father, please. I will go on my knees but do not take my son.' He said: 'No. We have to.' And I have seen so many things. Our sons and children beaten and slashed on the streets. So much cruelty we have seen. No one can believe.

The poignancy of this event is highlighted by the disruption of what we regard as ordinary activities: cooking (Leila) and going to the bazaar for a missing ingredient (son). It shows how war and violence enter civil space, the end result of which is drastic displacement of people and loss of civilian lives. Although Leila's son returned, it did not lessen her trauma as she witnessed his friends being 'beaten and slashed on the streets.'

Salima stated: 'God knows that we have seen the killings of people, our neighbours, other people, relatives, see them dying in their situation. I have suffered so much. Still, when I see someone without a leg, I suffer for that person. But what should we do. Go where?'

With the onset of violence, there did not seem to be any safe space left for the women and their families to continue living everyday lives as they had known them. Every single woman in our study had multiple stories [of their homeland] that they remembered on a daily basis for the simple reason that their wounds have not healed even in their new country of settlement in Canada, which they consider a 'heaven.' Neglect and institutional insensitivity to their pain and suffering have given rise to more wounds that have become embedded in the bodies of the women. It is from these wounds that they tell their stories. Yet, the women worked hard not merely to survive but to live. Meena, for example, went for walks and to the library, as she loved reading. She also went to Surrey by bus. Being a kindergarten teacher in Afghanistan, she wanted to babysit other children for pay. The extra money would help her with household expenses, including her medicine. But she was afraid to do this job, as she was told that if she dropped the baby, owing to her dizzy spells, she would be sued.

Other activities that formed part of the women's routine included going to a makeshift mosque on Fridays, participating in the Afghan women's drop-in programs (organized by a resource-deprived community centre), and keeping in touch with relatives in other parts of the world. But all these activities may be considered 'peripheral,' as they did not address fundamental issues that the women were confronted with in their new homeland. As shown below, women's everyday lives were filled with emptiness that on the surface could be attributed to their experiences back at home. Here are two accounts, from Meena and Nargis, respectively.

> They took everything from us. Everything was destroyed, even our homes were bombed. Three or four times we had bombs in our house ... For a minute all our houses were shaking. Mirrors got broken and shattered glass came like rain on our head. Blood everywhere and people were dripped in blood because of all those ruins. So we had very bad situation in Afghanistan. Many people lost their legs, hands, and other body parts.

Nargis stated that they lived in misery:

> No electricity, no lamp, nothing. You cannot see. You are scared. All the noise, all the bombs over our head. So I had also illness at the time. My legs did hurt. So we had so much misery. We had no choice but to leave the country leaving everything behind: our house, furniture, rugs, china, our life there.

It is important to note that stories of suffering can be pathologized, given our institutional framework. Kleinman and Kleinman (1997) make two points. First, 'their [sufferers'] memories (their intimately interior images) of violation are made over into *trauma stories*' (10, original emphasis) by institutions that deal with asylum seekers. Second, in the hands of medical professionals, these stories/real life events are converted into images of victimization – a passive stance. Based on these observations the authors pose the question: 'We need to ask, however, what kind of cultural process underpins the transformation of a victim of violence to someone with a pathology?' (23). For Kleinman and Kleinman a step forward is to ensure that local participants are included in the process of policy making and the development of programs.

This laudable goal, I argue, cannot be fully accomplished without listening closely to what the participants have to say about their experiences of suffering and pain. This listening is not merely confined to words. This does not mean that we underestimate the power of words. The women in our study made good use of words to build vivid images: 'shattered glass,' 'dripping of blood,' 'missing legs and hands,' 'grief in my body,' and many others. But we must also acknowledge that words do not fully capture experiences of pain and suffering. Furthermore, words and stories of marginalized people are not valorized unless they resonate with the language of the dominant group. Hill-Collins (2000) puts it this way: 'Oppressed groups are frequently placed in the situation of being listened to only if we frame our ideas in the language that is familiar to and comfortable for a dominant group. This requirement often changes the meaning of our ideas and works to elevate the ideas of dominant groups' (vii).

To avoid the situation of diluting their experiences of suffering or risk the possibility of having them appropriated by institutions, the women in our study took on the stance of wounded storytellers – a position that allowed them to witness their own stories. It is at this level that the women sought to engage the reader/researcher so as to effect multilayered change ranging from small acts to large-scale solutions. The emphasis is not on the expert (anthropologist or health and service provider) assuming the position of a witness – a top-down approach – but on ethical listening with its bent towards *speaking with* our research participants and *not for them*. The issue is to let the participants represent their own worlds in as much as this is made possible in a research setting. It is in this vein that I looked at other modes of communication used by women in our study, primary among which was that of telling stories from the wounds.

The Wounded Storytellers: 'Afghanistan has been destroyed'[6]

People tell their stories from the wounds when words fail to capture their experiences of pain and suffering. Rather than being individual acts of narration, the stories, notes Frank (1995), contain narrative truths suppressed by the dominant language. Stories make it possible for sufferers to position themselves as witnesses to their suffering, inviting audiences to reciprocate by becoming witnesses in turn. This is what gives the story from the wounds its power.

As Frank (1995) expresses it, 'What makes an illness story good is the act of witnessing that says, implicitly or explicitly, 'I will tell you not what you want to hear but what I know to be true because I have lived it' (63). For Frank, the reclaiming of a voice begins with the body that in turn creates the self which connects with people who may be motivated to effect change within their spheres of influence. It is in this context that I will focus on an ethnographic moment[7] to show how stories from the wounds can be acts of self-witnessing with the intent of engaging others.

'I can talk, I am not afraid of anything.'

Meena's statement says more than what appears on the surface. To begin with, it is an act of breaking out of structural silence, as people do not ordinarily say 'I can talk' or 'I am not afraid of anything.' The women in our study have been silenced, not because they cannot speak, but owing to our failure to listen to the larger narrative that implicates us (the First World) in the destruction of Afghanistan – the painful face of the country. How does the First World represent Afghanistan?

Afghanistan made headline news on two occasions: the invasion of the country by the Soviet Union (1979), and a second invasion by the United States and its allies (post-9/11). Following the departure of the Soviets in 1989, and the overthrow of the Taliban in 2001, Afghanistan has receded into the background, a wounded country. As one woman expressed it, 'It is the fate of Afghanistan that it is forgotten so quickly. The country has been destroyed from the outside and no one cares. Is this fair?'

Not to see the painful face of Afghanistan is morally wrong, as it was the Cold War between the two superpowers, and of late the United States' war on terrorism, that have destroyed the country. During the time of the Soviet occupation, the United States armed and trained the jehadis (fundamentalist anti-Soviet resistant fighters). The fighters received no training in governance. And this is what our research participant had to say:

> Afghanistan has lived with killings, and war, and suffering. We, all of us, are homeless, and kids who should be educated are homeless and in mountains and deserts. All of them have been involved in criminal roles. Today Afghanistan has been involved in so many crimes and drugs. What is the reason? All these countries [foreign powers] made this happen. I mean we in Afghanistan, we did not make the weapons. Who would put the guns in their hands? Someone needs to do that in order for people to fight and kill each other.

The situation was compounded by United States foreign policy that aimed to create a military force within the country so that it could engage in low-intensity warfare that protected its own soldiers and kept the cost low. Low-intensity warfare claims the lives of civilians, but this has not concerned the foreign powers. The fact that over a million Afghans have died as a direct result of more than two decades of war is of no consequence. United States' soldiers (including allies) are given full honour in case of death (Cooley 1999).

The Mujahideen and the Taliban, the two regimes that brutalized the people of Afghanistan, emerged from the U.S.-trained military force of the jehadis. Although Taliban members were trained in Pakistan *madrassas* (religious schools), they were supported by the United States, which had taken Pakistan under its wing (Cooley 1999). These 'monsters' – the term used by the women – were created by foreign powers and were not integral to Afghanistan. It is interesting that the women referred to members of these regimes as 'people with no human eyes' and 'scary faces' – indicating that they were not Afghans in the cultural sense of the word. They were foreigners created by outsiders. The American war on terrorism now involves rooting out the jehadis it had helped to create. The arms and ammunition that it placed at their disposal makes this task difficult, coupled with the fact that the resistance fighters have their own agenda of establishing an Islamic fundamentalist government. As the United States and its allies have had difficulty identifying particular 'terrorists,' they continue to wage their war on

Afghanistan as if everyone is a terrorist. Several hundred civilians have lost their lives in the indiscriminate usage of arms, all of which come from outside the country (Cooley 1999; Goodson 2007).

The larger story that would implicate the world powers for reducing Afghanistan into an armed camp, void of even a basic infrastructure, remains untold. Instead the hegemonic narrative in circulation is that United States invaded Afghanistan to liberate its people, and especially women, from the cruelty of the Taliban. That this regime was brutal to women is without question. Women were not allowed to leave their homes without being accompanied by a close male relative. Furthermore, they were not permitted to attend school or work outside the home. Interactions with males, neighbours, shopkeepers, and doctors were forbidden. The sounds of women's shoes and their laughter were not to be heard in public spaces. These restrictions, 'along with the harsh and unpredictable physical punishment for breaking these rules, did the most physical and psychological damage' (Brodsky 2003:101). The Taliban regime, however, did not spring from the native soil although it wore the garb of Islamic fundamentalism. Misinterpretation of Islam, or for that matter any religion, occurs in times of crisis when men feel the need to wrestle for power. As Meintjes, Pillay, and Turshen (2001) have argued, the struggle for power is gendered and the first targets are invariably women. Women are subject to bodily and structural violence in times of war and civil strife, the aftermath of which is worse.

It is this untold story of the destruction of Afghanistan, its painful face, and its aftermath as it unfolded on Canadian soil, which the women endeavoured to narrate through their wounds. Like the Black South African women who told their stories using socially valorized metaphors of domesticity (Ross 2001), our research participants were aware of the need to use alternative modes of communication that would ensure that their stories are heard and not denigrated. Telling an untold story also means engaging in an act of self-witnessing. To leave this task to others would mean risking appropriation of their stories. Witnessing, as opposed to mere observation or participation, is an engaged activity. When one witnesses one's own story, an engaged and sensitive listener can be drawn into the story. This process can be achieved if we live in the story rather than just listen to it (Frank 1995). It is in this spirit that we can understand Meena's[8] words cited at the beginning of this section, and it is in this spirit that I continue with her story. It is important to note that though each woman focused on her own experiences, the collective story remained in the forefront. This was a natural outcome of the women's experiences of war and violence.

Referring to the death of her husband, Nargis stated, 'I was in pain, a lot of pain, but I was not alone. Everybody lost someone, brother, sister, mother, father, son, daughter. It was war. Everyone got killed there. People got killed in huge numbers.'

A common thread in all the stories was the destruction of Afghanistan. Meena bemoans the fact that it will not be in her lifetime or the lifetime of her children that Afghanistan will be the country as she had known it before it had to bear the wounds of war. She recalled the happy times when they lived in peace and had 200 guests at weddings – a mark of good times. 'Now they [the United States] say there is peace in Afghanistan [angry tone of voice]; even if there is peace in Central Afghanistan, there is war in the four corners of the country ... Who likes to be homeless and confused? Who? Don't you like your home country?' (She cries.)

Afghanistan carries multiple scars evident in the destruction of buildings, loss of lives, disabled bodies, and dislocation of people. The women in our study carry these scars on their bodies and it is from this space that they tell stories that are at once individual as well as collective. This impulse is also found in the work of the Revolutionary Association of the Women of Afghanistan (RAWA). Mariam, a RAWA supporter, has this to say: 'RAWA has felt the pain and the miseries of the people of Afghanistan, especially its women, and that is why they can be the real representative of the women of Afghanistan. I don't think that other women can be the true defenders of women in Afghanistan, like so many who have not spent their life among people, who have not experienced the bitterness of the society with their skin, bone, and flesh' (cf. Brodsky 2003:145).

It is from the skin, bone, and flesh (wounds) that the women in our study told their stories, and this is the reason why they must witness their own stories. On our part, we need to learn to listen (to unlearn the privileged status that we assume as experts) so that we do not dismiss the multiple ways in which women speak, and likewise we do not dismiss women's own initiatives to effect change, however small those changes may be. Here are three examples that Meena shared with us.

CITIZENSHIP TEST

I get dizziness. My eyes do not see well. I have done the citizenship test twice but I have failed. I have read, borrowed all the books for citizenship

test. I read them but I get dizzy . . . How can I do this test? I have gone to
the judge twice. They asked me questions and I answered but then they
told me to study more. I failed. So you know if one is sick, nervous, and
sad, how can one not fail?

Meena's illness cannot merely be explained by the medical diagnoses of high blood sugar. This is evident in the fact that she talks about
her illness, in this passage and throughout her narrative, in relation to
grief ('There is so much grief in my body') and sadness. Her husband's
absence is making her feel lonely and depressed, but this is not an indi-
vidualized issue. In the context of geographical breadth and historical
depth, Meena's spousal separation is caused by war and violence in
her country – war and violence brought about by foreign invasions.
Afghanistan's pain would be less if these invasions were short-lived,
but this is not the case.[9]

The women in our study talked about the destruction of their country from the time of the Soviet invasion (1979) to the present. They also
included Iraq to make their point. 'Now [2004] they want to liberate
Iraq. But look at the women and kids getting killed or disabled. This
is not liberation. Bush has destroyed the world' (Meena). Our research
participants were not content to talk only about Afghanistan. This is
because they had the experience of migrating in the aftermath of war
to the First World, which must be held accountable for its actions in
Afghanistan. As a settler society and as the long-time ally of the United
States, Canada is not an exception, although it presents itself as a kinder
and a gentler nation that could not possibly engage in any kind of violence (Razack 2000). The women were left with the task of establishing a connection between the violence they experienced in Afghanistan
and the misery and neglect that they are subject to in Canada. Meena's
'failure' at the citizenship test implicates the society that has failed to
heal her wounds.

In her account of the citizenship test, Meena provides one message:
she failed the test twice because she is sick. But her sickness/wounds
tell a larger story. She is unable to pass the citizenship test because society (the international community) has failed her on two fronts: in Afghanistan and in Canada. It is her wounds that establish the linkage
between the two. She bears the wounds of a war-torn country and she
bears the wounds of an indifferent host country.

Wounded storytellers initiate their own process of healing, not only
through the act of telling the stories of their lives, but also identifying
strategies that allow them to live as opposed to merely survive. Given

their vulnerable position in society – this is the reason why they are wounded – these strategies point to spaces and areas where change can be effected. They also bring into relief the fault lines of society. It is important to take note of both aspects if we are to work towards incremental change from the grass-roots level.[10] It is in this context that I present the second example.

SCATTERED SPACES: LIBRARY/CLINIC/BUS

When Meena discovered that there was a public library in her neighbourhood, she was overjoyed. On one occasion, when Meena was walking to the library, she met an Afghan woman who advised her not to go as she may contract SARS. The woman told her that the librarian had advised her to keep away from crowds because of her age (she was only 56 but looked older). In the eyes of the librarian this woman looked 70, as did 58-year-old Meena. 'So I came back. Now I will not go there this Monday, but next Monday I will go to the library for sure.'

Afghanistan is not any closer to achieving peace though the United States claims it has liberated Afghanistan. In a televised speech in 2004, then-President George W. Bush stated: 'That nation [Afghanistan] is a world away from the nightmare of the Taliban.' The fact that the librarian wanted to 'protect' these seemingly elderly women from biological disease, but had no insight and could do nothing to help these women alleviate their social suffering speaks volumes to the way in which exclusive focus on the diseased body masks and silences social pathologies.

The library incident brings home two points. First, Meena's neighbourhood contacts are limited to people from her own community. A superficial explanation would be that Meena does not speak English. Overlooked here is the structural factor that there are barely any ESL classes available for Afghan women in Valley View.[11] The premise at work is that these women are not breadwinners, and therefore any investment would be a waste. Such is the thinking prevalent in a market-oriented society. Second, despite Meena's 'illness' (the dis-eased social body), she has taken the initiative to find a public place and engage in an activity that she enjoys. Meena's initiative must be built upon, as it brings to light 'a lively engagement between people and place' (Dyck, personal communication; see also Dyck 1998, 1995) – a building block for positive change.

Social marginalization does not translate into passivity. Adopting a pragmatic stance, marginalized people remake their worlds even if this means taking small steps one at a time, as Meena's narrative has revealed. These strategies are of value, as they do not only point to elements that can lead to grass roots-level change but they also identify the fault lines of society.

While the women in our study endeavoured to remake their worlds in the best way they could, they did not lose sight of the fact that they had a larger story to tell, not only for themselves but for the people of Afghanistan. This aspect was brought home to me in the two sentences that were on the lips of all the women: 'Afghanistan has been destroyed' and 'the people of Afghanistan have been forgotten.' For our research participants the aspect of being forgotten was carried forward to their country of settlement. The women talked about how their basic needs were not met within Canada, as noted above. These women took it upon themselves to tell two intertwined stories: the story of war (Afghanistan) and the story of the war's aftermath (Canada). The most challenging task was to link the two stories – a link that Canada and other Western countries do not recognize, as they have absolved themselves from the responsibility of waging their wars (Cold War and the war on terror) on the soil of Afghanistan. To compound the situation, the West has positioned itself as the saviour and liberator of the people of Afghanistan, the most vocal form of which is gendered. For the West, Afghan women's liberation is measured in terms of whether women can move around without their burqas, which the West considers to be the icon of women's oppression. The West has failed to address substantive issues such as women's education, availability of work, and women's rights in a society whose infrastructure it has helped to destroy. Groundbreaking work in Afghanistan is carried out by initiatives taken by women themselves and also by grass roots-level organizations such as RAWA.

It is to highlight this unarticulated connection between the two countries (Afghanistan and Canada) that the women engage in the act of witnessing their own stories. Our reciprocal engagement must then be to recognize this connection that the women make using the language of everyday life and the language of the wounds. It is at this level that I have presented my argument on witnessing/writing stories of social suffering. To revisit Meena's words:

I have become ill. I have got blood sugar. I am sick because of my stress for my husband. In any case he is my husband. We lived together. He is in India. He is sick as well. He is worried, lots of pressure. I went to my doctor. She wrote a letter that I am sick. I am worried. I long for my husband and I am sad. I gave them [immigration officials] the letter. I have got depression. Doctor said so twice. We have send them the letters. But I do not know why nothing happens.

Meena's husband is sick over there (Afghanistan/India). Meena is sick over here (Canada). The 'sick' bodies/wounds of the husband and the wife connect the two worlds that are otherwise deemed to be separate. Their separation speaks to the cruelty of dividing the world in ways where one world (the West) presents itself as superior and the saviour of the Other, for the purpose of exploitation and control – the colonial narrative (Bannerji 2000; Said 1978).

Witnessing Stories of Social Suffering

Why is the destruction of Afghanistan by the First World not acknowledged despite historical evidence? The historical trajectory is not difficult to grasp. The former Soviet Union attacked and occupied the country; next, the United States embarked on low-intensity warfare (read 'arming local people') to combat its arch-enemy. The two countries turned Afghanistan into an armed camp and destroyed its capacity to govern itself. The inevitable outcome was the production of faction groups that harmed their own people; and in 2001 the Taliban attacked the United States, which led to yet another U.S.-led invasion with deadly ammunition, such as cluster bombs and landmines that continued to kill and maim the civilian population (Goodson 2001). Since the overthrow of the Taliban in 2001, the world has forgotten Afghanistan and its people. This is how Afghan women view their situation in their country of origin as well as that of settlement, a point of view suggested by critical scholars. The promised reconstruction of the country has not occurred. The few projects that have been initiated by world powers are not for the benefit of the local people. Development discourse and practice loom large with the underlying premise that the West has liberated the people of Afghanistan. In the name of liberation, market-oriented projects are introduced for the benefit of foreign-based corporations who fill the coffers of the First World. It is for this reason that the crystal-clear historical reality of Afghanistan is rendered opaque. The oppressive but foreign-produced regime of the Taliban played into the hands of the United States, whose mantra is that it has liberated Afghanistan from the clutches of this regime. The cycle of war and violence set into motion by the former Soviet Union and the United

States and its allies remains unnamed, and with it the long-time suffering of the people of Afghanistan.

The women in our study had experienced suffering in their flesh and blood. They understood what it is like to lose relatives, friends, and neighbours, rendered refugees overnight and maimed as innocent bystanders. They had also witnessed the ongoing destruction of Afghanistan, militarily and through structural violence, the damage of which is not discernable as it tears the fabric of everyday life to bits and pieces. When the women sought asylum in the First World, they encountered indifference and also structural violence. The world did not know or did not want to know these women's long-time suffering.

The women in our study then felt that the onus was on them to tell their stories, but this was a difficult undertaking for two reasons: First, social invisibility translates into social silencing. The women were silenced in the sense that when they told their stories to the few people they had contact with, for example, workers in the welfare agency and in the social service sector, they were dismissed as inconsequential. The women were constantly reminded that they should be grateful that they are in Canada, a supposedly peace-loving country. Canadian social service workers could not picture how a family of five living in a two-bedroom apartment could impact the education of children who have no place to study. One woman related that when she wanted help for her severely depressed husband, no one listened to her until she called the police and said he had a knife. He was promptly hospitalized, a service he had been in need of for several months.

Second, it was difficult for the women to spell out the fact that the First World was responsible for the destruction of Afghanistan, and that in granting refugee status to a handful of people from the several million it had displaced it was only doing its duty, albeit in a small way. In the wake of the powerful West-as-saviour script, there was barely any space for relating this alternative narrative.

People who have been subject to political and structural violence seek other modes of communication to tell their stories of suffering and trauma (Ross 2001). The narrative data from our study revealed the language of everyday life and the language of the body to be salient. Both are powerful mediums of expression and they invariably delineate the broader political context that implicates the system. If the wounds of the women have not healed in the country where they have sought refuge, then we need to look at the fault lines in the host society.

Since the women have taken the initiative to witness their own stories, what is our responsibility as researchers and readers? We cannot overemphasize the point that though we may not have endured such suffering, we do study it. This is the reason why we need to witness with them and not for them, a position that can lead to appropriation of their stories of suffering. It is important to note that the boundary between the two positions is blurred, as I do not think the process of appropriation can be reversed; it can only be minimized through an active process of listening that entails paying attention to alternative means of communication.

I have endeavoured to give central space to the words and worlds of the research participants where on-the-ground reality is linked to the larger political framework they have delineated using the language of everyday life and the language of the body. I want to suggest that it is within a framework of linkages between individual lives and the broader social and political contexts that the act of witnessing can take place. In sum, witnessing stories of suffering must begin in the spaces that the participants have carved and not in the largely textual space created by the experts.

The women in our study took it upon themselves to tell their stories of suffering and pain on their own terms, and this meant using other mediums of expression such as speaking from their wounds. It is in this context that Meena is able to tell a powerful and multi-layered story: she implicates the foreign powers that have systematically destroyed her country, using body language (the language of symptoms and suffering), and linking this language to her native soil: Afghanistan is also a wounded body (bombs, destruction of houses, land filled with blood, land filled with landmines, land where countless number of bodies are buried). Through her wounds, Meena also tells the story of the indifference and structural violence that she encounters in her country of settlement. The wounds on her body speak of her isolation and the loneliness that she experiences on a daily basis. The fact that she has become more sick since migrating to Canada speaks volumes of the link between her body and the political economy. This should prompt us to acknowledge our complicity, as global bystanders/researchers. It is within this space created by the research participants that the act of witnessing can take place, and this is the first step towards bridging the gap between theory and practice. Witnessing stories of social suffering must prompt us to act bottom-up; this means giving up the comfort zone of being mere observers. Nargis put it this way: 'We do not want to tell our stories unless it brought about some results. But we should not let others speak for us. They [the social/welfare workers] do not understand, and maybe our education is higher than that of the welfare worker, but they give themselves the permission to treat us like we are nothing.'

Three themes are salient. First, migrant women (and their families) are entitled to social provision on a scale that would help them build a new life in Canada. This must not take the form of ad hoc measures, but must be systemic and connect with the everyday lives of women. Social entitlement is an issue brought into relief by the women themselves. Second, speaking as wounded storytellers, the women make a connection between here and there, implicating the West in their displacement. Women's transnational connections with kin suggest social and cultural border crossing with its potential to foster interconnections, within and beyond the nation state. It may be that the Afghan women – unrecognized and socially invisible – can suggest an alternative base for civic polity. Third, committed to capturing the local worlds in the context of the global, social scientists can achieve a twofold task. Through reflexive listening, they can recognize research participants as producers of context-specific knowledge, and they can foster a dialogue with policy makers and stakeholders. This is what I have attempted to do in a preliminary way.

ACKNOWLEDGMENTS

The project is funded by the Social Sciences and Humanities Research Council of Canada through the Vancouver Centre of Excellence for Research on Immigration and Integration in the Metropolis (RIIM). For field research, including translation and transcription, I am indebted to Poran Poregbal and to Gulalai Habib. Most of all, I want to thank the Afghan women who opened their hearts and homes to share their experiences with us. I have benefited from the presentations I made at the mini-conference and graduate seminar organized by Sue Wilkinson, Simon Fraser University, and Isabel Dyck, University of British Columbia, respectively.

NOTES

1 The use of body language is significant, as it brings to light the intricate ways in which the body of the national land is linked to the bodies of women. We may note that national narratives are gendered (Yuval-Davis 1997b; Nazmabadi 1998).

2 This is not an across-the-board statement, as there are exceptions (see, for example, Farmer 2003; Scheper-Hughes 1992).

3 My work (Dossa 2004) on Iranian women revealed that women use research settings to advance their goals as well. Note that there is only one Afghan service provider who is hired on a part-time basis.

4 It is not a coincidence that I found myself working with an Afghan and an Iranian research assistant. To begin, Dari and Farsi are kin languages. Anyone who speaks Dari understands Farsi and vice versa. Second, it is not uncommon to have Farsi-speaking health and service providers working with the Afghan community. This is because the Afghan community in metropolitan Vancouver is relatively young.

5 Although one can state that not all women's work is in the gendered ghettos, women who do occupy this niche are used to sustaining the capitalist economy. The majority of the women in this sector are from the non-Western world (Mohanty 2003).

6 The term *The Wounded Storyteller* comes from Arthur Frank's work by the same title (1995). It is the wounds, argues Frank, that gives a person narrative power, effecting a shift from passivity (the biomedical stance) towards activity.

7 My use of ethnographic moment refers to a process that allows us to read the global in the local, and also to explore how the local may impact on the global.

8 I chose to use the fictive name of Meena for the participant; this name carries special significance. Meena, the founder of RAWA (Revolutionary Association of Afghan Women), was assassinated in 1986. Her work continues to this day to the extent that RAWA is known on the international front (Brodsky 2003).

9 These aspects come to light in the documentaries *Daughters of Afghanistan, Return to Kandahar,* and the CBC week-long broadcast from Kabul, 16–20 February 2004.

10 The term *incremental* comes from RAWA's model of change incorporating multiple dimensions: individual, family, community, and society. Small-scale changes are not dismissed.

11 This is my observation from the Iranian women's ESL classes on the North Shore. The classes were held for four hours a week.

PART 3

Communities, Social Capital, Empowerment, and Resilience

10 Advocacy and Social Support: The Multicultural Health Brokers Co-op's Journey towards Equity of Access to Health

LUCENIA ORTIZ AND THE MULTICULTURAL HEALTH BROKERS CO-OP[1]

Yvette[2] and her five children arrived in Edmonton from Rwanda in 2004 after residing in a refugee camp in the Congo. Once their initial settlement needs such as housing, temporary income support, and school for the children were met, it became apparent that Yvette was facing a far more complex situation herself. A single mother with five children under 12 years old, Yvette could not speak English and was suffering from severe mental stress and trauma. Before she came to Canada, her husband was murdered and one of her children was abducted during the civil war. Yvette was referred to a multicultural health broker who helped her find a family doctor, brought her children to the public health centre for their immunizations, introduced her to recreation centres for her children, and connected her with the local Rwandese community. For over a year, the multicultural health broker provided support when Yvette was feeling lonely and helpless. As soon as she was familiar with common bus routes, the multicultural health broker enrolled her in an English as a second language (ESL) class and encouraged her to attend community activities.

Introduction

The relationship between racialization, ethnicity, and gender in creating disparities in health is well documented in the literature (Armstrong 2004; Duffy and Hansen 2005; Zoller 2005; Marmot 2007). Immigrant women's vulnerability to illness has been linked to their inability to access health care and related services due to language and cultural barriers (Kinnon 1999; MacKinnon and Howard 2001; Bhalotra et al. 2007). Beyond these proximal factors, there are structural inequalities that create risk conditions for immigrant women's health. These include lack of or limited employment suitable to the women's international credentials and experience and gender stratification in income and occupation, as well as inadequate social supports for immigrant women experiencing chronic poverty, social isolation, and loss of status (George and Ramkisson 1998; Galabuzi 2006; Stone, Purkayastha, and Berdahl 2006).

Two concepts – *equity* and *access to health* – are crucial to understanding the struggles of immigrant women in reaching their full potential for health and well-being in their new homeland. The concept of *equity*, which is associated with the notion of being just and fair, implies that positive steps must be taken to compensate for various social and natural variations between people such as ethnic minority women, which may arguably confer 'unfair(ness)' (Daniels 1982). A*ccess to health* refers to conditions that enable individuals and population groups to use resources and opportunities to address a need as well as to support and maintain health. To achieve equity of access to health means addressing disparities at the level of personal care, as well as at the level of systems and institutions and societal opportunities.

This chapter focuses on the experience of a group of immigrant women in Edmonton, Alberta, who discovered and nurtured a practice called multicultural health brokering as a model by which immigrant women and their families could access health-promoting and health-supporting resources and increase their life chances for a better life in their new homeland. A collaborative study conducted by the author with the Multicultural Health Brokers Co-op in 2002 explored the multicultural health brokering practice as a community-level response to reduce inequities experienced by ethnic minority individuals and families and to improve their health and well-being in their new homeland (Ortiz 2003). Fifteen multicultural health brokers participated in the study. The research documented the journey of the multicultural health brokers from a group of community volunteers to a formal organization of the Multicultural Health Brokers Co-op. This chapter will highlight excerpts from this research through the words of the multicultural health brokers as they shared their experience, struggles, and insights about their work, and more importantly their vision of an equitable society. We begin with the history of the co-operative and describe how the practice of health brokering has evolved. We then describe the benefits and challenges of operating as a worker's co-op.

The Multicultural Health Brokers: Personal and Collective History

In 1992, a group of immigrant women were recruited from their communities and trained in perinatal health education by the Edmonton Board of Health. The health department was concerned that ethnic minority women were not accessing their prenatal programs. At that time, these immigrant women called themselves 'multicultural childbirth educators'; they delivered perinatal health information to pregnant immigrant women in their own language while blending Western medicine with traditional birthing practices. Their work was funded by Health Canada for three years. Many of these pregnant women were newcomers to this country. As they worked closely with the women, the multicultural childbirth educators became involved in deeper issues of poverty, loss of support, hopelessness, and isolation. They began to connect with service providers and institutions, and advocated with families to obtain the services and resources that families needed. They also looked to the community to provide the social support for which the women longed. Due to this expanded role, and inspired by an article about cultural brokers and cultural brokering, the childbirth educators changed their name to 'multicultural health brokers' to reflect the reality of their work. How this group of immigrant women came to become multicultural health brokers is a remarkable story of resilience and empowerment as women overcame their struggles and shaped their own future in their new homeland.

Immigrating to Canada

The multicultural health brokers' own histories of immigration reflect many stories of newcomers who came to Canada, escaping wars and political upheavals in their home country to seek better lives. The multicultural health brokers who came here as independent immigrants were brought to Canada by their spouses/fiancés or by family members. Most have lived in the country for more than 20 years, including three who arrived as young children. Their children were born and raised in Canada. They came to like Canada for its peaceful and safe environment, for the opportunities that were not available in their home country, and for the amenities of a Western industrialized society. As one multicultural health broker explained, 'It is a safe place to bring the children up, and that was one of the reasons why we live here, and if, you know, the children move to another place for a better future, then we might move; otherwise we are quite happy here.'

The multicultural health brokers who arrived as refugees experienced traumatic events while escaping from their home countries. Some were part of the first wave of Vietnamese refugees who arrived in the United States and Canada in the mid-1970s after the Vietnam War; others arrived in the 1980s when strong anti-Chinese sentiment in Vietnam resulted in the persecution of Chinese merchants and shopkeepers. As one participant said, 'I have one sister and two brothers who came with me, and we escaped; we came in the boat with the people who do fishing, and we paid each of those 13 gold bars, 13 for each of us. My dad said that we got ripped off by those people.'

Although none of the research participants would speak in detail about their lives in the refugee camps, it is well documented that life there was no better than in the boats where many suffered from malnutrition, infectious diseases, and maltreatment at the hands of camp guards (Stephenson 1995). Other political events that brought some of the multicultural health brokers to Canada were the military coup in Chile in 1973, the civil war in Somalia in 1991, and the Bosnian conflict in 1994. The vestiges of these traumatic experiences were still felt by some of the research participants. It has been said that the effects of traumatic experiences are long-lasting and enduring, and it takes a great deal of courage and determination to heal the emotional scars and recapture one's strength to face life again (Stephenson 1995).

Struggling as Newcomers in Canada

Like many newcomers, most of the multicultural health brokers identified the cold weather as the one feature of life in Canada that caused great apprehension for them when they first arrived. All, particularly those who did not have relatives in the new country, spoke of being isolated and lonely. As one participant stated: 'The first year was very lonely for me living in Canada. When I came to Canada, I came to Toronto, Ontario, and I had no friends. I was there in Toronto for about three or four months. After that, we went to Parry Sound. I think it is two- or three-hundred kilometres from Toronto. We were there for roughly a year I think, and that was the loneliest time ever in my life.'

It was not only the unfamiliar physical and social environment to which some of the multicultural health brokers had to adapt, it was also the obvious and glaring change in their life circumstances, particularly their economic status. Another's experience:

... we more suffer poverty [here] than at home ... because back home we were a rich family, and when I moved here, I found myself living in a small house, a small apartment. I never experienced that, or my sister having to work an extra job just to bring money, and then parents later on. We don't want to tell parents that, that they don't have some money, so we still, although my sister's daughters are all grown up, but they still use my parents' money even though they're here, so my parents support us here.

These words echoed the sentiments of many of the multicultural health brokers, particularly those who had to leave their country involuntarily. But the hardest and most painful of all their challenges as immigrants in Canada was coping with the devaluation of their foreign education and work experience. All of them have university degrees. Comparing their foreign education and work experience with their Canadian employment history revealed a marked discrepancy between skills and employment. The occupational history of the foreign-educated multicultural health brokers illustrates the persistent issue of lack of accreditation of foreign credentials, a problem which has not been completely and comprehensively addressed, neither in the public nor private sectors in Canada. It is still the most significant barrier to the occupational mobility of immigrants and refugees (Galabuzi 2001; Kinnon 1999). Table 1 presents the occupational history of the research participants, in their home country and in Canada, prior to their multicultural health brokering work.

To the multicultural health brokers, their occupational history reveals a struggle to survive and adapt to what they perceived to be unreasonable requirements for newcomers finding employment in Canada. As one Co-op member explained:

I kept on applying every time they are advertising and they interviewed me three times, same group of people and then [I] didn't get the job. But you know they did their job and they called up for interview and so one time I asked that one woman who was in the interview panel, 'How come you never hired me?' So they said there was always somebody better than me competing, and also the easy cop-out was that I'm too qualified ... and don't have the Canadian degree. So that was the end of my career.

While there were a few who had been able to find work that matched their educational qualifications, these positions were often the least valued work in the field for which they were qualified. The search for

Table 1
Occupational History of Multicultural Health Brokers

Home Country Education	Home Country Work Experience	Canadian Employment History
Library Science (with post-graduate degree)	Recent graduate before coming to Canada	Retail worker Part-time library assistant Nursing aide Support worker
Statistics	Computer analyst and programmer	Bank employee Volunteer interpreter Parenting educator
Communication Arts	Graphic designer	Support staff in hospital Self-employed in graphic design
Education	High school teacher, math and physics	Day-care worker ESL teacher Group home worker Real estate salesperson Trade worker Electrical technician Sewing machine operator Settlement worker
Nursing	Nurse	Community volunteer
Sociology	Left country after finishing school	Child and family worker Researcher Life skills coach Perinatal educator
Law	Lawyer	Settlement worker

better employment resulted in switching from one job to another. Thus, despite their average length of residence (about 10 years), most had not found stable employment until they became multicultural health brokers in 1992. This is consistent with studies on immigrant employment history, which note that it takes 12 to 15 years of residence before a newcomer can achieve job security and catch up with the earnings of the general Canadian population (Basavarajappa and Jones 1999).

The multicultural health brokers were also expected to fulfill gender role expectations in their culture, and it was often a challenge to balance both work and family responsibilities. For example, as women in their cultural traditions, they were still expected to carry the burden of parenting and managing the household. Another explained:

> It was very hard for me with having five kids under 10 and working full time. From the early morning, we live in the north and I have to drive all the way to work to the computer. So it was very hard to be full-time mom and a full-time worker, and even I was having a big tension in the house because of depression. After a year, I left the work with the computer. I said I couldn't make it, I'll work part-time, and so I work only four months in a bank. After that it was also very hard to do everything by myself and to go out in the new society and to look after the kids and everything on my hands.

It was no accident that the multicultural health brokers were all women. At the time they started to get together as community volunteers, there was a clear recognition that there was inadequate support for immigrant women who were new to Canada, spoke little English, and were socially isolated and unable to navigate the complex web of the formal system. Helping newcomer pregnant mothers was a natural entry point for support when women are at their most vulnerable. Supporting immigrant women who have limited capacities to connect with the formal system was an expression of gender solidarity for the multicultural health brokers, knowing that they themselves have experienced being marginalized because they were women, and, most significantly, women of different racialized groups and ethnicities.

Becoming a Multicultural Health Broker

The dissatisfaction and anguish in their search for suitable employment left a profound impact on the lives of these women in Canada. To them, the demand by employers for Canadian experience represented the inequities of Canadian society, particularly towards immigrants and refugees, who make up the bulk of ethnic minority communities. The employment challenges experienced by the multicultural health brokers exemplify the marginalization of ethnic minorities where a barrier to social and economic mobility is their foreign origin. It was a realization that advancement in Canadian society has less to do with personal abilities and more to do with their racialized and ethnic origins. Furthermore, being an immigrant woman presents another layer of barriers for advancement in a society where there are wide disparities between men and women in all aspects of their lives. Marmot (2007) stresses this point, stating that 'the differential status of men and women in almost every society is perhaps the most pervasive and entrenched inequity' (1156). He identified three key interconnected dimensions of gender disparities where women remain the disadvantaged gender: 'material or the unequal access to and control over property, economic assets and inheritance; psychosocial or the unequal restrictions on physical mobility, reproduction and sexuality; and the political or the unequal participation of women in political institutions' (1156). For the multicultural health brokers, it is this same disillusionment that had spurred them to create opportunities where their inherent talents, skills, and life experiences could be made useful to their communities. In their work, and as women, they decided to take control of their lives, and steered their desired life courses in their new homeland in their own ways.

Many worked as community volunteers before they were introduced into multicultural health brokering. For example, some were translating English health information materials into their own languages, teaching heritage language to second-generation immigrants in their communities, serving on the boards of directors of their cultural associations, and were informally helping people in their communities get connected to programs and services. Their connections with the community provided a natural opportunity for recruiting them to become the first group of multicultural perinatal health educators for the Edmonton Board of Health in 1992. Their compassion and empathy prepared them for cultural brokering work; however, their own life experiences as newcomers were the most compelling reason for their commitment to help others in the community. Two statements:

> Because I personally have experienced this, these difficulties, I don't want anybody else to have to go through that. And so, I will use what I remember in terms of the experience and even the feelings, so that I work in a very authentic way. But then when you're so involved with the people, and often when you work with your heart, people respond with their hearts, and so you have, really, a real relationship emerging.

> It is very rewarding to help people. Especially if you know what it is like to be in their shoes. We were once in the same boat – the war, and refugee camps. I know the immigrant experience, and that makes it easier for me

to understand and help. To best help someone, I need to understand his or her problem.

Some individuals have found suitable and stable employment outside of the Co-op by building on the networks, skills, and solid reputations they developed working as multicultural health brokers. Furthermore, those who are currently working with the Co-op have finally found a place they can call their own. In multicultural health brokering work, cultural background and immigrant experience are regarded as more valuable than Canadian work experience. Multicultural health brokers also enjoy the freedom to make the most of their talent and skills. Two experiences: 'I like the work that I do, it gives me a lot of satisfaction when I've made a difference. I'm valued in the community; I get people telling me that "Oh the radio program is really good." And I can see the improvements in their life, and that's really big for me, because I feel not because my work is very good, but also the feeling that these people appreciate what I'm doing. It's not that I'm looking for a present or anything like that, just I see them happy and they say "Thank you." That's all.'

The feeling of being valued and appreciated can be very important, especially when one has struggled over the years to gain recognition for one's abilities. This validates Wilkinson's (2001) studies of self-esteem as an indicator of health. In his study, pride, dignity, and respect are critical determinants of personal health. According to Wilkinson (2001), these indicators are rooted in structural conditions of equality – not only material wealth, but also social status. This observation supports studies relating to the impact on the personal health of women who work as community health workers. These studies indicate that increased knowledge and skills and improvement of self-esteem are benefits enjoyed by the community health workers (Booker et al. 1997). The most rewarding benefit of all is personal transformation. Booker and colleagues noted that 'the feeling of being capable of helping others is critical to being able to assist others to make decisions about their own health' (458). Roman and colleagues (1999) viewed this as a health promotion opportunity for the community health workers as they gained greater confidence in their capacity to control their own lives.

Multicultural health brokers are members of the cultural group and community they serve; they speak the same language and share their history and experience. They have knowledge of values, beliefs, and health practices of their cultural group, an understanding of traditional and indigenous wellness and healing networks, and have experience navigating health care delivery and supportive systems within communities. Multicultural health brokers enjoy the cultural and linguistic advantage in organizing health promotion and preventive health education activities in their communities. They are also familiar with biomedical culture and Canadian society, which enables them to be trusted by service providers and the institutions they work with. To fulfill their role as cultural and linguistic mediators between families and the formal system, they offer informational, emotional, and social supports in home, communities, and institution settings. In particular, the multicultural health brokers facilitate linguistic access to health education activities by delivering one-on-one and group education in the participants' first language, including translation of health information into different languages. They also act as liaisons for individuals who are culturally unfamiliar with the Canadian health and social service systems. They are knowledgeable in both the health values, beliefs, and practices within their cultural groups or communities and the formal system they have learned to navigate. They therefore serve as effective communicators between immigrant individuals and families and the health care and social service systems to enable clients to meet their health needs and to find relevant resources to achieve healthy outcomes. Multicultural health brokers promote the adoption of positive personal health practices and lifestyles within the cultural traditions of individuals and groups. They are well connected with and enjoy the trust and respect of their communities, capacities that are essential to the delivery of effective health services in communities that are isolated and marginalized from the formal system. They use these capacities to promote increased use of health services, encourage healthy choices, and support the blending of cultural traditions with current standards of preventive care.

The Multicultural Health Brokering Practice

This practice traces its roots in anthropological literature to the works of Wolfe and Geertz (Press 1969; Hopkins et al. 1977; Jezewski 1990). In their studies in Mexico and Indonesia, Wolfe and Geertz found certain individuals who 'straddled between two sub-cultures and acted as cultural translators and go-betweens' (Hopkins et al. 1977:70). The 'cultural broker,' as they have named this person, is an 'insider' (Geertz 1960) and a member of the community (Press 1969).

The notion of cultural brokering in health also predates its modern practice, when spiritual intermediaries attempted to promote an understanding of Western science and medicine with blended native healing (Szasz 1994). By the end of the 1980s, the term 'cultural brokers' gained wider acceptance in health and anthropology. In fact, a cultural broker role has been suggested as part of nursing care in multicultural settings (Jezewski 1993). Jezewski (1990) defines cultural brokering as the 'act of bridging, linking, mediating between groups or persons of differing cultural backgrounds for the purpose of reducing conflict or producing change' (497). In the health arena, it involves 'bridging gaps in cultural meanings or gaps in understanding between health professionals, the patient, his/her community and the broader social system' (1990:80; also Jezewski 1993).

Press (1969) defined the role of the cultural broker based on three concepts articulated in his early studies: ambiguity, innovation, and the marginal person. Ambiguity is a concept wherein the broker acts in a 'clear contextual capacity of the other culture achieving dual competence' (70). This ambiguous role allows the broker to accommodate a number of diverse perspectives that would open the door for negotiation. Innovation means that the broker in the process of bridging may circumvent traditional expectations and create new ways of doing things. This innovative role establishes the broker as a catalyst for change or change processes. Newcomb's concept of the marginal person is someone who is between two cultures and who operates at the borders of these two cultures to achieve a purpose (Press 1969). As such, the broker's relationship with different groups may be fluid, and involves constantly changing friendships and alliances depending on what outcomes are desired. The concepts of ambiguity, innovation, and the marginal person shaped the cultural brokering practice of today. Within the health care setting, the cultural broker is seen as someone who navigates (most often in situations of tension and conflict) within two culture systems: one is the formal health system dominated by Western biomedical beliefs and traditions; the other is all non-Western cultures (Weidman 1982). The notion of parity of cultures implies a symmetrical relationship between cultural brokers and health professionals, and also distinguishes a cultural broker from an outreach worker. While typical outreach workers are agents of the dominant culture they are expected to promote, cultural brokers are purveyors of indigenous knowledge and cultural traditions which may be different but equally important in addressing a health issue (Tripp-Reimer and Brink 1985).

Multicultural health brokering is a holistic and relationship-based practice of building connectedness and brokering support for ethnic minority individuals and communities to achieve equitable access to resources and opportunities for health. It involves providing one-on-one care and support to individuals and families, organizing small groups for education and social support, working with community leaders and organizations to facilitate community actions, promoting culturally competent care among service providers, and advocating for systemic change within institutions and with policy makers. This multidimensional practice assigns a catalytic role for multicultural health brokers to initiate actions that would bring about equity of access to health for marginalized and isolated immigrant women, their families, and their communities.

As the multicultural health brokering practice continued to evolve over time, the multicultural health brokers realized that the empowerment of women will not be complete without the involvement of men in the change process. There are three male multicultural health brokers working in the Co-op who assume the same roles and responsibilities as that of their female counterparts. Although they do not work in the Perinatal Health Program, they provide support within the four dimensions of the multicultural health brokering practice in the other programs of the Multicultural Health Brokers Co-op, such as supporting immigrant seniors, families with children with disabilities, and immigrant youth, and training community leaders. They are motivated by the same commitment to facilitate and enable individuals and families gain access to resources and opportunities.

Cultural Brokering in the Twenty-First Century

In recent years there has been a slow but steady growth of cultural brokering programs in North America, most of them in the United States. This is mainly brought about by the increasing interest in providing culturally competent care and services to culturally, linguistically, ethnically, and 'racially' diverse populations. Cultural competence is defined as the ability to work effectively in a cross-cultural setting (Cross et al. 1989).

In 2004, the National Health Service Corps (NHSC), Bureau of Health Professions (BHPr), funded the National Center for Cultural Competence (NCCC) in Washington, DC, to undertake the Cultural Broker Project. The goal of this collaborative project was to promote and encourage the use of cultural brokering as a key approach to increasing access to, and enhancing the delivery of, culturally competent care to culturally diverse populations, particularly those who are underserved and vulnerable. This project produced a guide called, *Bridging the Cultural Divide in Health Care Settings: The Essential Role of Cultural Broker Programs* (National Center for Cultural Competence 2004). This guide was designed to assist health care organizations in planning, implementing, and sustaining cultural broker programs. Since the release of this guide, many community-based health and social development organizations have implemented cultural broker programs, all of which were aimed at mediating cultural understanding in health care practice, increasing cultural interactions between health care providers and the community, and creating inclusive programs.[3]

Current literature also revealed efforts to encourage health care professionals to assume the role of cultural brokers to meet the needs of growing diverse populations in a variety of service contexts such as nursing care, rehabilitation, and mental health (Jeffreys 2005; Jezewski and Sotnik 2005). The articles suggest that health professionals in any of these settings are in the best position to affect positive change because they work within three key areas of influence in the health care system: clinical practice, workplace settings, and the organization/network. Health care professionals from a dominant culture as cultural brokers present a departure from what has historically been assigned to individuals who come from a minority culture. While this may seem to be an exciting opportunity, it could create a new set of challenges, and perhaps a different set of skills to overcome these challenges will be needed within an institutional context.

The Multicultural Health Brokers Co-operative: Organizational History

The Multicultural Health Brokers Co-operative, perhaps the first of its kind in Canada, was organized in 1998. It marked the formalization of the multicultural health brokers as an organized group that believes in and nurtures the inherent capacities of the immigrant populations. The mandate of the Co-op is to 'support immigrant and refugee individuals and families in attaining optimum health through health education, community development and advocacy support' (Multicultural Health Brokers Co-op 1998:1). The guiding principles of the Co-op are democratic governance, responsiveness, accountability, equity, and social justice. This set of principles reflects a deep and profound understanding of health that encompasses personal health and its collective context. In particular, the Co-op recognizes that ethnic minority populations are inherently disadvantaged in a stratified society like Canada. Health, when viewed from this perspective, dictates that interventions be framed within the principles of addressing inequities and balancing power structures. The Multicultural Health Brokers Co-op lays the formal basis for organizing and consolidating the collective work of the multicultural health brokers.

How the Co-op was formed reveals an ideological orientation to redressing inequities and balancing power relations on the side of the less powerful, in this case that of ethnic minority populations. Responding to a growing demand for multicultural health brokering services in immigrant and refugee communities, the multicultural health brokers were invited to be part of the health care system as employees in 1998. In examining their options, they realized that the nature of their practice required them to work with their communities as well as with institutions – two entities that are not always in congruence with each other. They were also aware that these two entities were unequal, and those with less power, the ethnic minority communities, needed advocates to leverage support for them. If the multicultural health brokers were to be part of the health care system as employees, they feared that a large institution with a corporate structure and less flexibility might limit their ability to advocate for their clients and communities. Thus they decided to form their own organization. One of them recalled: 'We wanted to be in the community. To some degree, not operating out of the system or the institutions or operating even for a while out of a formal office had given us some very strong symbolic value about autonomy and being with the people.'

The need to be in the community so that they could be advocates for and with ethnic minority women was the primary reason for opting not to become institutionalized within the formal health care system. In choosing which form of organization the multicultural health brokers would adopt, they considered several factors. First and foremost was their commitment to democratic and collective processes that allow for diversity and inclusiveness. They chose a co-operative structure because of its egalitarian and democratic foundations. As one member stated:

... because this is a members-owned, members-operated organization, I'm praying that we will never become what other organizations have become, even very, very grassroots organizations, because they chose a different corporate structure where there is a board, there's the executive director, and then the workers, and then the people in the community. Whether it's a public institution or it's a non-profit organization, the danger is it becomes a hierarchical entity where the board is removed from the realities of the people and yet they're making policies, deciding what should happen, right? We see this all the time, where frontline workers are feeling very frustrated because the policies that are made don't reflect the day-to-day reality, and they have very little say over how policy is developed.

So I'm hoping, by consciously choosing to become a worker's co-operative that is flat, where it's democratically all owners and operators and also employees, then we don't have this hierarchy. We are it. All we need to do is stay grounded in people's struggles and their desires and their hopes, right? So it eliminates many of the potential levels of being removed or being, being irrelevant. And so, the structure itself I hope will support our work so we're always, always grounded in the circumstances of the people. And so, the three fundamental unique elements of the Co-op, I hope, will help us: the democratic governance, the accountability to the people rather than the system, which means there will come a time when we might have to choose to let go of certain funding, because it doesn't meet the true need of the people. I hope we'll be decent enough to say, 'Remember, we promised that we're accountable to the people, then therefore we would be willing to let go.'

The second reason for choosing a co-operative structure was the search for an organization whose philosophy resonated with our ideals of equity and social justice. The multicultural health brokers had worked extensively in their communities and were aware of the struggles of ethnic minorities in overcoming barriers to social mobility and advancement.

Co-operatives are organizations that sustain themselves through organizing collective work for a common good. The history of co-operatives is nurtured by the ideals of social emancipation and democracy. From the early 1800s to the present, Fairbarns and colleagues (1990) succinctly summarized the development of co-operatives from a vantage of social and cultural ties that bind memberships together and render the co-operative economically viable. These ties are founded on purely economic interests, but are deepened by a 'shared experience of separateness or discrimination in society, cultural or political awareness' (75). In other words, co-operatives have emerged as a response to social and economic inequities experienced by certain groups in society. The first co-operative, at the turn of the nineteenth century, was a response to the poor working conditions and poverty of factory workers in the newly industrialized England. Fairbarns and colleagues also note that a primary motivation in forming co-operatives has been the political and cultural goals of 'solidifying a minority culture or nationality' (73). Co-operatives began to challenge the dominance of capital in economic endeavours at the time of movements for democratization of society during the mid-eighteenth century. Co-operatives were avenues for the disempowered British working class to gain some control over economic resources and to institute egalitarian forms of distributing power (Oakeshott 1978; Fairbarns et al. 1990; Quarter 1992).

In Canada, the development of co-operatives has been more active in the agricultural sector, as opposed to the British experience in urban industrialized areas. This can be attributed to the lower concentration of urban labour and less polarized social and economic opportunities (Fairbarns et al. 1990). Nevertheless, the growth of farmers' co-operatives was a reaction to the dominance of the economic and political elite in central Canada who was developing policies that impacted rural Canada. The rural sector, represented by farmers across the prairie provinces, desired greater economic and political participation in the country's agricultural development. Agricultural co-operatives were and still are the largest co-operative network in Canada; they earn billions of dollars and have considerable influence in policy making in the agriculture sector (Quarter 1992).

Other forms of small and medium-sized co-operatives are engaged in a wide range of entrepreneurial as well as social development ventures such as consumer or user co-operatives, credit unions, and workers' co-operatives. These form what Quarter (1992) calls the social economy – economic enterprises that are independent of the government, fulfill social objectives, and are 'socially owned.' The concept of social ownership means that members of the co-operatives are owners of their own enterprises. But more than staking a claim to property, social ownership is associated with decentralized and participatory decision-making, greater public accountability, and progressive democratization in the workplace (Quarter 1992).

A workers' co-operative, although one of the least common types of co-operative, is the embodiment of social ownership principles. The workers own the enterprise for which they work. Oakeshott (1978) cites three important features of a workers' co-operative: those who work for the enterprise are not making profits for anyone but themselves, the workforce has no external masters, and there is a more or less democratic regime – one person has one vote. These features articulate basic principles of equity of wealth distribution and democratization in the workplace. Employment is a responsibility of a worker's co-operative; therefore, as a worker's co-operative, the Multicultural Health Brokers Co-op must continuously generate employment for its members.

The multicultural health brokers believed that a crucial role for the Co-op is to promote and nurture the multicultural health brokering practice in the health care system and the social services sector. This role involved consistently doing good work in the community and collaborating effectively with service providers.

The Multicultural Health Brokers' Experience in a Co-operative Organization

Since the Multicultural Health Brokers Co-op was organized in 1998, the multicultural health brokers felt that the organization had provided them with financial support through sustained employment opportunities. It was also a place where they could find emotional support in ways that are more personal than what they said they would experience in other organizations. They valued the warmth and trust among colleagues, especially during difficult moments of working through a complex case. In addition to feeling supported by colleagues, being members of the Co-op had increased their confidence and self-respect. From their experience since the Co-op was organized, the participants felt appreciated by colleagues from other agencies; their credibility had increased and they felt respected even more by health professionals. Two members expressed their thoughts:

I think that as soon as we developed the Co-op, people started to value us, started to recognize us, and treat us with more respect. It's not just like a cultural translator, they realize that we are more than just interpreters.

I think it changed for everybody; it changed for everybody and for all of us. I think that it was great because before we didn't know who we were, we knew that there was something there . . . I think it's great that we have a co-operative today; we could come up with something else, but we came up with the co-operative idea. I think it's important to have a co-operative organization.

Other benefits included training opportunities, access to technical information, and introduction to a network of service agencies. The training opportunities that increased knowledge and skills were benefits that the participants appreciated as being part of an organization. Moreover, they have learned about resources they could access for their clients and communities. These benefits will undoubtedly rebound to the clients' benefit. The multicultural health brokers would say that the organization of the Co-op has improved their work immensely and contributed to their personal growth. One member commented: 'Feeling that you are very formal, established, makes you very strong by yourself, that you are belonging to something and even the working with the other members of the Co-op. I feel very confident that I am belonging [sic], all these people are working from the same background, from the same intention.'

The co-operative model that the Co-op has chosen as an operating structure allows it to live by its principles. It values culture, language, and ethnic heritage of its workers as important assets. Policies and procedures are developed and decided with full participation of the workers as co-owners of the organization. For example, discussions can take time, taking into consideration diverse communication styles and limited English fluency, work hours are flexible to accommodate single moms with children or those who have part-time jobs, or may hire two qualified candidates instead of one and creatively design work arrangements that would fit both their talents and job requirements. The Multicultural Health Brokers Co-op has contributed employment opportunities for immigrant women who have experienced lack of recognition of foreign credentials and were excluded from accessing suitable employment in their new homeland.

Challenges

Although there are many fine examples of successful workers' co-operatives around the world, many of those who have studied co-operatives maintain that workers' co-operatives are the most difficult to sustain (Oakeshott 1978; Quarter 1992). Workers' co-operatives are the least sustainable of all types of co-op for three reasons: first, financing is the co-op's major problem owing to its low capital that comes from the limited funds of the workers themselves; second, the enterprises tend to be labour intensive, as democratic governance requires a large time commitment that is difficult to sustain over time; and third, there may be a lack of managerial skills among the workers (Quarter 1992). The challenges to the Multicultural Health Brokers Co-op resonate with Quarter's observations, and will be discussed in this chapter.

Financial Sustainability

The main concern of the Multicultural Health Brokers Co-op is the sustainability of its funding sources. This threatens members' employment security, and, more importantly, their ability to provide sustained programs and services to their communities. The Co-op's financing comes from service contracts they have negotiated primarily from the local health authorities and social development funding agencies. These service contracts are mostly short-term, covering a period of one to two years. Every year, the Co-op has to develop and negotiate proposals to seek funding for services to ethnic minority clients and communities. As a result, sustainability of the organization is the Co-op's major strategic issue. As the multicultural health brokering practice increases its reach to the community, there will greater demand for services, yet government support has not been consistent. The multicultural health brokers' primary investment in the Co-op is their set of talents and skills rather than monetary capital. Financing of the Co-op depends primarily on public sources that are vulnerable to changes in the political and economic environment.

Fostering Democratic Governance

Democratic governance requires a large time commitment, which is difficult to sustain over a long period. Practising true democracy means equipping members with tools of participation, fostering commitment to participate, and creating relationships that support participation (Hennestad 2000). As one member explained:

> Sometimes we need to make decisions as we are working now; sometimes maybe lack of understanding of the English language, things get twisted or not understood. This happened, because when I had to give an example: 'Gee that's not what I said, that's not what I meant,' and I was right because the multicultural health broker that was sitting beside me, she looked at me, and then I said, 'That's not what I said,' and she said 'Right.' So that just comes up. What I'm saying is I don't know if we're all at the same level there, of understanding, of making decisions.

Another added: 'We have democratic governance in the Co-op and we do decide things together. We need to learn more about decision-making.'

Because of the intensity of their work, it was always difficult to find adequate time for organizational activities. Time is an important resource inherent in the practice. Multicultural health brokers almost operate on a 24-hour work schedule. Since they are known more as members of their own community, they make themselves available anytime. As one member said, 'I wish that all of us would have a full-time job, and then all of us could quit another job, because if you work full time here and part-time there, I don't know how much you could concentrate on doing the work.'

The multicultural health brokers also come from cultures where the concept of participation is not necessarily synonymous with Western-style democracy. The challenge is not that Co-op members have no desire to participate, but that it needs to create participatory processes that are congruent with members' cultural experiences. For example, group discussions may not always be the best forum for inclusive and collective decision-making. Sometimes the effective strategy to generate genuine sentiments could be obtained with one-on-one, individual discussion or written responses. Creating democratic participation within the context of diversity requires an appreciation and understanding of the varying communication styles of different cultures. Language is the most obvious of these differences. Most often when the discussions involved sensitive issues or complex topics, some of the multicultural health brokers were not able to articulate what they really wanted to say because of the difficulty in expressing their views in English. Other areas of cultural differences involved the ability to accept feedback openly, disclosure of personal feelings, and interpreting cues and gestures accurately.

The Multicultural Health Brokers Co-op must be vigilant in sustaining egalitarian relationships in the organization, and must avoid the pitfalls of bureaucratization that most often follow a growing organization. The constant challenge is remaining true to the most essential foundation of co-operatives and democratic governance – the belief that power resides within the members.

Blending Entrepreneurial and Social Objectives

Finally, the Multicultural Health Brokers Co-op must always face the challenge of blending the entrepreneurial objectives of providing employment security and addressing the social objectives of equity of access to health by ethnic minorities. The task of this dual commitment is daunting, and most often the two objectives are not always congruent. The reality of the multicultural health brokers' practice demands that they be sensitive and conscientious in unravelling health issues and all their dimensions, and that they explore holistically all paths to the desired outcomes. This means that responsive interventions can include venues other than the health sector, such as mediating between family members, connecting women to community supports, organizing small groups for practical needs, emotional support, and so on. Unfortunately, these forms of support are not always regarded as having economic value and thus are not translated into remuneration for the multicultural health brokers. In other words, most of this is largely unpaid work that comes from personal commitment to the clients, and is perpetuated by a fragmented and specialized public service system that narrowly defines its services within the strict confines of institutional mandates and/or professional standards. Yet these informal supports within the context of ethnic minorities and other marginalized populations are most critical in promoting and sustaining the health of these individuals and families. Thus, the Multicultural Health Brokers Co-op most often absorbs the cost of unpaid work in providing direct service that should have been supported by public service institutions. This impacts the Co-op through the reallocation of equally important administrative resources to direct services. As a business enterprise, it does not leave the Co-op much room to invest in project development activities, which it needed to sustain the organization in the long term. One member put it succinctly:

It's a reality of the Co-op and it's also a reality each member has to deal with. Because it is a worker's co-operative, we're in it to generate employment for ourselves. There's a great deal of irony in that because there is misfortune in the community, that we have found work ... we often don't all have full-time work and we're working full time but with limited pay; still, we're getting work because of the family's misfortune. And so, there's this delicate balance that on one hand is, there's some degree of self interest, it's generating employment for us; and yet, on the other hand, it's also remembered this is an organization about social justice, right?

We're here to build an organization that is decent and it's here for a greater set of purpose than just get funding and keep going, right? You're always torn between the entrepreneurship of being a member who's a worker, or an organization that generates employment out of a situation of social injustice. And so there is the entrepreneurial piece of it, and yet there is the social objective. Some felt that, not knowing what co-operatives are, thought maybe we were a form of privatization. Others thought, you know, literally, someone said, 'Are you like a communist organization?'

In a study of collective decision-making in a large organization, the above-mentioned problems can lead to degeneration of the co-operative and reversion to the traditional structures of hierarchical organizations, especially if the organization has been taken over by private business organizations (Cornforth et al. 1988). However, another study revealed that the survival rate of workers' co-operatives has been good and that worker participation has increased over time (Cornforth et al. 1988). Quarter (1992) supported this by citing successful workers' co-operatives in micro-businesses. The successful worker co-operatives in this study were those where types of jobs are done by members who have similar skills, and where there is a community-based system with support infrastructure for finance and entrepreneurship. In the experience of the Multicultural Health Brokers Co-op, all the members have similar skills as those of the multicultural health brokers. There is a continuing and progressive demand for their services in the community as shown by the growing number of clients who have accessed their services.

Finally, Cornforth (1992) reiterates that the 'degeneration of a workers' co-operative occurs most clearly when it departs from co-operative principles and thus ceases to be truly co-operative' (120). These principles are open membership and democratic control by members on an equal basis. He proposes safeguards against degeneration that a workers' co-op should adopt. These include: meaningful control over decisions on investment, resource allocation, wages, product/service, technology, and workers' control over aspects of jobs such as conditions of employment, supervision and discipline, work organization, and job content. These safeguards will be important in identifying organizational factors influencing the viability of the Multicultural Health Brokers Co-op as an economic enterprise, to support the multicultural health brokers and as a vehicle for advocating equity and social justice for ethnic minorities. It offers a venue for mutual support among multicultural health brokers while they work at the edges between two cultures. Moreover, the Co-op crystallizes an expression of solidarity when advocating for meaningful changes in promoting the health and well-being of ethnic minorities.

The Multicultural Health Brokers Co-op Today

The Multicultural Health Brokers Co-op has grown from a small group of 13 workers in 1998 to 35 workers serving 18 immigrant and refugee communities in the Edmonton metropolitan region. Each year, the multicultural health brokers serve an average of 1,500 individuals and 500 families. From the Co-op's first years, with its participants carrying on their work from their homes and cars, the Multicultural Health Brokers Co-op is currently renting a house where it is often a hubbub of activity – for example, a group of immigrant parents in one open area actively engage in sharing their bicultural experiences with a multicultural health broker who is providing prenatal education to a young pregnant mom in her own language.

Like all co-operative organizations, the general assembly, composed of all members, is the highest decision-making body in the Multicultural Health Brokers Co-op, which means that the membership is engaged in defining the strategic directions and policies of the organization. The Co-op is governed by a board of directors elected by the members annually. The day-to-day operations are managed by an executive director and supported by a team of program coordinators and administrative staff employed by the Co-op.

The Multicultural Health Brokers Co-op has also ventured into the area of cultural competency training – a venue to share with service providers and practitioners its wealth of knowledge concerning serving and working with culturally diverse families. Since 2002, when it launched its series of cultural competency workshops, the Co-op has delivered training to more than 500 workers in the health and social service sectors.

The Multicultural Health Brokers Co-op is the appropriate organizational vehicle for advancing the multicultural health brokering practice. It is an example of an adaptive strategy that strives to address individual needs for survival while also encompassing broader societal concerns that sustain quality of life. The values of equity, social justice, and democratic governance that underpin the Co-op's work with ethnic minority communities assign a catalytic role to the organization's mandate. As an active agent of social change, this role involves making social inequalities more pronounced and visible, advocating for equitable health policies, and enjoining cross-sectoral participation in reducing economic and social disparities. The Multicultural Health Brokers Co-op stands at the forefront of demonstrating the co-operative organization as an example of inclusive and equitable social structures that can create an impact on individual and community health. The origin of co-operatives is rooted in the concept of reciprocity, a process of gift giving and sharing within a relationship of mutuality. As such, co-operatives are inherently egalitarian in the relationship among members of the organization as well as in sharing benefits from the organization. The Multicultural Health Brokers Co-op is an example of equity in practice; organization members are governed not by traditional and dominant organizational hierarchies but by shared power relations guided by a commitment to collective goals and respect for diversity of capacities and strengths among members. The Co-op strongly believes that real power resides in its membership, thus creating a transformative value system that guides the day-to-day work of the multicultural health brokers. Humility, respect, sacredness, reciprocity, and love are values that underpin the structures and processes of organizational development that are essential to the health and well-being of the Co-op members.

Finally, the practice of multicultural health brokering ushers in a progressive approach to the notion of multiculturalism. It attempts to advance beyond the Canadian mosaic's ideals of tolerance and ac-commodation of cultural differences towards a process of negotiation and mediation of differences. Let me offer a new metaphor, that of a creatively designed Canadian quilt where discernible patterns of co-lours and designs are sewn together into a coherent, functional, and identifiable whole. Multicultural health brokers operate at the borders between cultural patterns and caringly find the right threads to sew the edges together, and in the process create a blended pattern, the product of transformation and change.

NOTES

1 This chapter is based on the collaborative research undertaken by the author with the Multicultural Health Brokers Co-op in 2002–2003. See Ortiz (2003).
2 Names have been changed to preserve the anonymity of the family.
3 For more information on the Cultural Broker Programs, browse the National Centre for Cultural Competence at http://gucchd.georgetown.edu/nccc.

11 Empowering Women through Community Work: Strategies within the Latin American Community in Ottawa

SARA TORRES, ALMA ESTABLE, ANA MERCEDES GUERRA, AND NUBIA CERMEÑO

Introduction

Have Latin American women, and their communities, become empowered through organizing to remove barriers to health and social services? The authors of this chapter have worked for many years assisting Latin American women in Ottawa to achieve equal access to health, which we define in a broad context, one that includes social determinants such as income and social status, social support networks, education and literacy, employment/working conditions, social environments, the physical environment, personal health practices and coping skills, healthy child development, biology and genetic endowment, health services, gender, and culture (Marmot and Wilkinson 1999; Public Health Agency of Canada 2007d; WHO 2003; World Health Organization Commission 2009). Our work questions the assertion that when women organize to remove barriers to health services, women and communities become empowered; but has this actually happened in our community? We wanted to evaluate the organizing strategies we have used to determine how we might improve or change them to best meet the needs of our community. We also wanted to document and celebrate women's contribution to strengthening our community's capacity to enhance our own well-being. As well, we wanted to investigate the complex relationships between empowerment, community capacity, and health. To that end, we undertook a series of interviews and conversations with and among community leaders, asking them to reflect upon the history of our community in Ottawa, the role of women in the community, and the impact of activities, projects, and initiatives that have been directed at increasing women's access to health services.

The issue of lack of access to health services, and the development and maintenance of culturally appropriate informal mechanisms for transmitting information about health within our community, are salient factors for this work (Estable, Torres, and Cermeño 2008; Estable et al. 2009; Torres et al. 2009; Meyer et al. 2009).

This chapter summarizes what we discovered about our community and the strategies we and other women have used to increase women's access to health. We also share our reactions, as community activists and organizers, to what we found, and present some suggestions for the future.

The Latin American Community in Ottawa

It is estimated that approximately 700,000 Latin Americans live in Canada, and that these numbers have been increasing in the last five years (Ginieniewicz and Schugurensky 2006). The Latin American community is drawn from 21 countries and many more cultures. The community is relatively new in Canada (Veronis 2006), with the first wave of newcomers arriving only about 25 to 30 years ago (Estable, Cermeño, and Torres 2005). According to the 2001 Census, 16,650 Spanish-speaking people live in the Ottawa-Hull region, making Spanish the fourth largest non-official language group. The Latin American community in Ottawa is dispersed widely over the city (Estable, Cermeño, and Torres 2005). In contrast to some other minority linguistic communities (such as Chinese, Somali, Arab, Lebanese), there is no Spanish centre offering social, health, or community services to the community (Cermeño, MacLean, and Estable 2004). The most recent data about Spanish-speaking community health needs in Ottawa come from the 'Mujer Sana, Comunidad Sana / Healthy Women, Healthy Communities (MSCS)' project. Results from MSCS's health survey of 212 at-risk Hispanic women revealed that the community is linguistically isolated: only 10 per cent considered themselves to be fluent in English or French, 20 per cent spoke no English, while the remaining 70 per cent spoke English with difficulty. This survey also found that the Latin American community tends to be poor: one-third of respondents lived on a family income of less than $15,000 annually, and another third (33 per cent) earned between $15,000 and $31,000 (Estable, Meyer, and Torres 2003b). Nationally, Latin American Canadians have the fourth-lowest median incomes in the country (just above Haitians, Arabs, and Somalis) (Mohamoud 2007). Linguistic isolation and poverty combined result in difficulties in reaching the Latin American community – particularly as mainstream health promotion and health marketing initiatives are often disseminated only in our two official languages (Estable, Cermeño, and Torres 2004).

The World Health Organization (WHO) recognizes that equal access to health care and eliminating health disparities is a fundamental human right (WHO 1998). Despite Canada's provision of publicly funded health care services, major health disparities persist: 'These health disparities are not randomly distributed; they are differentially distributed among specific populations (e.g., Aboriginal peoples) by gender, educational attainment and income, and other markers of disadvantage or inequality of opportunity' (HDTG 2004:iv). It is well recognized that access to health services is a determinant of population health (PHAC 2007d; WHO 2003), and that 'if health care and public health programs and services do not include a focus on the needs of disadvantaged individuals, populations and communities, there is a risk of increasing rather than reducing health disparities' (HDTG 2004:v). Therefore, marginalized communities such as the Latin American community must be able to rely on the health sector to develop interventions that promote equity within their communities as well as for other disadvantaged individuals, populations, and communities.

In Ontario, the Ministry of Health sets standards for guidelines to improve and maintain population health. 'Equal Access' is the first of three General Standards, with the goal 'To ensure that all Ontarians have access to public health programs,' through 'reduc[ing] educational, social and environmental barriers to accessing mandatory public health programs' (OPHA 2002:1). Barriers can include, but are not limited to: literacy level, language, culture, geography, social factors, education, economic circumstance, and mental and physical ability (OPHA 2002; Ontario Ministry of Health and Long-Term Care (OMHLTC) 1997).

There is considerable evidence that ethnic and racialized minority communities continue to be under-served (OPHA 2002). The needs of Spanish-speaking women are not well understood or documented, making it difficult for service providers to assess and modify programs to remove cultural and linguistic barriers to access (Estable, Cermeño, and Torres 2004). MSCS also confirmed the presence of barriers that make it difficult for community members to maintain and improve their own health. These include having multiple health needs but being reluctant to seek help until it is too late, and lacking accurate and accessible information about health services including health promotion, preventive services, and community health centre availability (Torres, Cermeño, and Smith 2006).

Working with Concepts of Empowerment and Community

Prior to starting this study we had worked extensively with the concept and process of empowerment as part of community development. We understood empowerment as the subjects' 'ability to take collective action on issues of their choosing and to make positive changes in their environments' (Williams 2004:349). We applied an empowerment analysis to our own work as community service providers and researchers. In addition, we had the opportunity of working together in the MSCS project during which we were able to discuss and operationalize many aspects of empowerment.

We therefore entered this study with a well-developed understanding of community empowerment. We knew that removing barriers to accessing health and social services should help empower communities (Justice Institute of British Columbia 2007; Parsons 2001; Reitmanova and Gustafson 2007; Simich, Beiser, and Mawani 2003; Social Planning Council of Ottawa 2004; Weisman 2000), and that empowerment can emerge in various locations, such as within families, neighbourhoods, churches, voluntary organizations, and among networks of friends (Rappaport 1987). We further acknowledged that empowerment is about processes and outcomes that take place at multiple levels – individual, organizational, community, and societal (Nelson and Prilleltensky 2005) – and that empowerment comes about as people learn that they share responsibilities for one another (Rubin and Rubin 2001). For minority women, empowerment has an additional dimension: we have to become transformational leaders (Kelly 2006; Pellicer 2003; Sergiovanni 2007) whose methods are consistent with feminist principles of inclusion, collaboration, and social advocacy (Chin 2007), and we have to transcend barriers of gender, as well as class and ethnicity (Chin 2007; CRIAW 2002, 2006; Hawkesworth 2006).

We also entered this work knowing that our community is about sharing cultural and geographical origins (Nelson and Prilleltensky 2005), about getting people to work together (Rubin and Rubin 2001), and about caring and nurturing (Barnes and Aguilar 2007; NOIVMWC 2005), as well as advocating for social and political change (Staeheli 2003; Williams 2004). Within our Latin American community, we know that women are strengthening the community in addition to maintaining other responsibilities at home, church, or work, and that our community needs leaders committed to building its capacity (Estable, Meyer, and Torres 2006; Coover et al. 1977). We also recognize that our community is disempowered and faces barriers to accessing health and social services.

Recent research about the Latin American community in Canada brings to the forefront other characteristics that affect our work. For example, Ginieniewicz and Schugurensky (2006) note that the community is relatively successful working locally within the ethnocultural community and in Spanish-language or solidarity work, but these skills have not been successfully applied at the level of 'transcultural politics' (between the ethnocultural minority and the majority) or in official languages. These authors use a three-category framework to classify Latin American involvement in civic, political, and community life in Canada: (1) host country politics (community activism within the Latin American community and across immigrant groups); (2) home country politics (solidarity groups supporting various causes in their countries of origin); and, (3) transnational politics (the work of global civil society organizations such as Amnesty International or Greenpeace) (Ginieniewicz and Schugurensky 2006:41). Barriga and Vanzaghi (2006) further point out that the majority of current activities within the Latin American immigrant community are cultural or service-oriented. These may or may not lead to women's empowerment. For immigrant communities to feel empowered, they need both access to mainstream health and social services that respond to their needs *and* the support of ethnospecific community agencies (SPCO 2004) to offer services and lobby on their behalf.

Background

We wanted to do this research because we have worked for many years assisting Latin American women in Ottawa organize to achieve equal access to health and social services and to break down the marginalization that our community experiences in settling in and adapting to Canadian society. We also knew that many other Latin American women and men are working with services and culturally specific projects to strengthen our community's capacity to build a healthier community, but little has been written about it. Conducting this research was a way to document and assess efforts to empower Latin American women and our community.

Methodology

Overall Approach

As we worked collectively to frame our inquiry, the research questions for this study arose from our own practices. We reviewed some of the reports and articles that we ourselves had prepared in the past (Estable, Meyer, and Torres 2003a, 2006; Meyer et al. 2003) and sought new and more up-to-date information, both about Latin American communities in Canada and about women's empowerment (Beteta 2006; Ginienie-wicz and Schugurensky 2006; Justice Institute of British Columbia 2007; Simich, Beiser, and Mawani 2003; Veronis 2006). Our process was in-teractive; we went back to the literature a second time to look for two new concepts that emerged after preliminary analysis of the interviews: leadership and community.

Methods

After considering the available data, timing, and resources at our dis-posal, we decided to undertake a qualitative, interview-based study. We developed an open-ended interview guide in Spanish, pilot-tested it with one informant, transcribed the audiotape, reviewed it in the group, and made some adjustments to the order of the questions. The revised interview guide consisted of nine questions. We translated the interview guide into English for the non-Spanish-speaking informants.

SAMPLE

We identified individuals through our networks, work, and volunteer commitments, and through knowledge of projects, initiatives, and ser-vice locations for Latin American people in the city who we consid-ered – and others referred to as – 'community leaders.' All had been involved in removing access barriers to health and social services and were both known within the Latin American community and knowl-edgeable about the participation of Latin American women in commu-nity organizing. From an original group of 15 individuals, we selected a stratified sample of six community informants, making sure that both women and men were represented, as well as different countries of ori-gin and waves of migration. From a second sample, we identified four participants and selected a woman and a man from mainstream eth-nocultural organizations who could provide an external perspective of

Latin American women's contributions to community empowerment. All the individuals approached agreed to be interviewed and audio-taped.

Data Collection and Analysis

A total of nine interviews of external informants were carried out, each of which took between 45 and 90 minutes. We shared the task of interviewing and transcribing the tapes. Informants reviewed tran-scriptions, and two made a few (minor grammatical) corrections to the transcribed text. Seven of the interviews were in Spanish (quotations in this chapter have been translated by the authors), and two were con-ducted in English. After we completed all informants' interviews, we interviewed ourselves in Spanish (four authors) in a group interview format, to explore and compare our thoughts on the same questions we had asked the nine informants. We took notes and taped the group interview. All authors read the interviews and met at various times to collectively develop the coding framework and analyse node reports. One author applied the coding framework to all interviews using the statistical software NVivo 7. Two authors completed the final analysis and writing, and checked with other authors for validation of findings, interpretation, and accuracy of analysis. All nine informants were pro-vided with the opportunity to comment on the first draft of the chapter.

The stratification of our informants was based on gender, length of residency in Canada, involvement in the Latin American Women's Support Organization (LAZO), other Latin American groups, or other immigrant community organizations, and experience working along-side women in community organizing activities. The literature and our research assumption formed the basis for this breakdown. Table 1 (p. 200) describes our informants:

Findings

In our analysis, we became aware that there were three distinct voices in our data: the voices of nine immigrant Latin American women them-selves (including the authors); the voice of one immigrant Latin Ameri-can man, and the voices of three individuals who are not from Latin America but who know and work with our community. All helped shed light on our questions, albeit from different perspectives. To ac-knowledge these varied viewpoints we categorized the informants in

Table 1
Informants' Selection Criteria and Sample Interviewed

Description	Characteristics	Informants interviewed (N = 9)	Authors (N = 4)
Year/decade of arrival in Ottawa	1970 to 1979	3	2
	1980 to 1989	1	1
	1990 to 1999	2	1
	2000 to 2007	3	
Region of birth	Central America	2	1
	South America	4	3
	The Caribbean	2	
	Other (non-Latin American working with Hispanic community)	1	
Gender	Female	6	4
	Male	3	
Latin American Women Support Organization (LAZO) members		2	4
Works with women's organizations or in mixed-gender organizations	Works with women in community organizing initiatives	9	4
Involvement in organizing of Latin Americans community in Ottawa	Participates in organizing Hispanic community on issues re access to health and social services	7	4

relation to how closely they were living the reality they were describing. In this analysis, Latin American women have the standpoint of 'insiders' (including the authors), while the other two types of informants are relative 'outsiders.'

In our analysis, we sought descriptions of the ways that Latin American women were getting involved in initiatives aimed at removing barriers; we also identified the concepts that informants used to understand and explain that participation, and whether they considered it was making the community stronger and therefore healthier (Blas,

Gilson et al. 2008). These concepts were: empowerment, community, gender roles, leadership, political involvement, disconnection from mainstream society, and investment in the community. The location of communities along these interlinked social determinants and pathways has an impact on the health of communities.

Conceptualizations of Empowerment

Our informants provided many examples of empowerment gained through women's work in their neighbourhood, church, and voluntary organizations. Nelson and Prilleltensky (2005) developed a typology for understanding empowerment as processes and outcomes that take place at multiple levels: individual, organizational, community, and societal. We found this typology useful when we sought to categorize or understand informants' sense of empowerment.

Informants confirmed women's empowerment at the individual and organizational level, but not at the community and societal level. Individual empowerment was described in the context of immigration, spousal relationships, and how it leads to empowerment of others. Many informant 'insiders' indicated that they considered the mentorship they received from those who had immigrated to Ottawa prior to them to be valuable, and that they in turn reciprocated by helping other individuals or the community at large. Organizational empowerment was described in the context of forming community-based organizations, increasing access to programs and services in Spanish, and providing opportunities for women to get together in safe and welcoming environments.

Immigration as Catalyst

Many informants, both insiders and outsiders, believed that immigrant women can feel empowered because Canada offers women individual freedoms that they did not have in their countries of origin. Informant #2, an activist who has worked in women's and community agencies in Canada and in Latin America, explained how Canada's socio-political stability and gender equality provides the opportunity to participate and to grow as women: 'I believe that the fact that where we come from, many of our countries have such turbulent political histories, and that we come from male-dominated societies ('machismo'), as a consequence, in a place like this one, we are able to flourish. Because here we feel that there is more gender equality . . . We are not the objects of violence, as we were in many cases in our countries if we were politically active.'

Informant #5, who has worked with various international and multiethnic immigrant services organization, also believes that immigrant women from all backgrounds, including Latin America, are able to free themselves from male domination when they come to Canada. In his words: 'Personally I think that Canada is great for immigrant women, I see that consistently. Canada is one of the more liberal countries in the world where women have the greatest space ... And I watch the women free themselves.'

Individual Empowerment

At the most personal level, many informants explained how individual empowerment led many women to seek greater equality within their spousal relationships. Both 'insiders' and 'outsiders' had observed women whose increased individual empowerment had led to greater power, independence, and respect in their marriages and personal relationships.

In the words of one 'insider' informant (#2): 'I have heard many women say that their relationship has changed. They have become [equal] partners, and we hope that we will be able to transmit these kinds of values to our children.' Another 'outsider' informant (#1) also recognized that Latin American immigrant women are empowered to overcome the submissive positions in their marriages that they had in their countries of origin. However, he has also observed that women are not always able to negotiate these changes in the balance of power without stress that may lead to separation and divorce: '[Women] find themselves here without that cultural burden of the woman having to be submissive, and therefore at times they take advantage of that situation. Women liberate themselves, but ... sometimes they do it in a violent or abusing way, and that has provoked many divorces that perhaps could have been avoided ... Some of those women regret it afterwards, but it is very difficult to turn back the clock.'

Community Work and Individual Empowerment

Some informants spoke of feeling empowered at the individual level, because their participation within community agencies led them to grow as persons. In turn, they helped other women to do the same. One 'insider' informant (#4), who participated in a health promotion/education program organized by LAZO explains: 'On a personal level, I learned a lot. I was one of the people who took the training as a family visitor; that helped me develop on a personal level, and enabled me to help other women so that they become more aware of the possible signs of cancer, and to recognize the importance of knowing what the resources are.'

Another 'insider' informant (#7), who has been active with her local church and is a member of LAZO and other community groups, speaks of the way her own personal development has helped her to improve the way she works with the rest of the community: 'Thanks to the same help that I received from people ... that type of 'sponsorship' or 'godmothering' is very important ... I have been learning continuously, and carrying all that effort, that assistance, to the community ... I continue to help them, and to help myself.'

Similarly, another 'insider' informant (#3), who has been active with LAZO and who works for a health service provider, expresses her contentment at the work she accomplishes for the community: 'I have been at this job for 10 years and feel very pleased with it ... I like to help the people ... sometimes I do more than what I am supposed to be doing ...'

Community Empowerment

All of our informants had much to share about 'the community'; however, there were nuanced interpretations of what 'the community' actually consists of, and whether or not the community is empowered. As with the concept of individual empowerment described above, we sought examples of ways that our informants described and explained women's participation that were also illustrative of what they understood and how they operationalized the idea of 'community empowerment.'

Service Provision

Almost all our 'insider' informants described how they and other women had become involved in community initiatives that offer services to the Latin American community. Many had set up and participated in non-profit or volunteer community-based organizations. Others had sought employment in 'mainstream' health and social services organizations, or were working with immigrant groups that included Latin

Americans. These informants are aware and concerned about the barriers that Latin American women, and their families, face in accessing services. They describe a need to 'open the doors' for other women from the community as a whole, so they can access all publicly funded health and social programs. They see increased access as directly leading to an empowered community. One informant (#12), who is the co-founder of a seniors' service, describes her experience: 'When we got here, we realized that there was a real absence of organizations that met the needs of the community as such. When we began to get involved, we realized that a whole lot of new initiatives were being born ...'

Another insider informant (#2) recognizes this type of community work as a specialty of women: 'I believe that this community work, that we as women do, is directly oriented to opening the doors for the community, so that they will have access to resources, to services, to programs. This seems to me to be the way that we, as women, direct a great deal of our work towards having an impact for the community.'

Many of the 'outsiders' with whom we spoke, who had also witnessed Latin American women's caring for their own community, describe their contributions to removing barriers to access to health services, and their attempts to empower the community. Informant #10, who has worked with various Canadian and multi-ethnic immigrant women's organizations, explains:

> ... those [Latin American immigrant women] who had been here for a little while have recognized the information gap and have made an attempt to fill that information gap. I'm referring to LAZO, and what it had been doing for the last little while in trying to reach into that community and to provide some health information for the community ... it's not the community [that is] waiting for others to do something for them, but it is the community itself taking the lead role in trying to identify what the issues are and to find the resources to help them to respond to those issues.

Mutual Caring

Many informants provided illustrations of Latin American women's organizing work that are rich in description of emotional content, affection, and mutual caring. They describe warm bonds between people, an openness and friendliness to other Latin Americans, and instances in which members of the community help each other, giving a sense of cohesion. These characteristics create bonds among individuals, and provide an informal and sometimes extended, network of support among Latin American women immigrants. Informant #4 believes that groups like LAZO, which exist because they want to increase access to health services, also offer a collective space for women to gather and share with other women who speak the same language, and who have in common the experiences and challenges of being in another country's culture (see also Vissandjée et al., this volume): 'I think that as Latina women, the interest has been to work so that other women will identify with this, will feel that they have a space where they can remember their culture, where they feel they have a voice, where they can express themselves in their own language.'

Outsider informants who have been working with the Latin American community for a long time also describe how women have cared about other women; and they note that, over time, this has strengthened their capacity to help other women. Informant #1 states: 'Nowadays, I feel that now there is more help within the Latin American community. As soon as one woman knows that something is happening, a group of other women is pulled together; spontaneously and voluntarily they hold out a helping hand to other people, to aid them. At least, for those who really need it, they have received that kind of assistance.'

Family and Neighbourhoods

Both 'insider' and 'outsider' informants mention another dimension of women's involvement: informal participation within the family and neighbourhood, rather than within the context of organizations and groups. They refer to this participation as 'leadership.' As an example, Informant #1 describes Latin American women's leadership role, indicating he has witnessed them as 'women who are very committed to their families, to their children, and also to the environment of the neighbourhood. I have seen women take on leadership. I see them go forward; I see them defending themselves against abuse in relation to workplace wages, to obtain the benefits to which they are entitled.'

As discussed below, it is in this area, among others, informants identified the major challenges to empowerment of women and their communities. In terms of Nelson and Prilleltensky's (2005) typology for understanding empowerment as processes and outcomes that take place at multiple levels, our informants reveal that, regardless of success on a individual or group level, these challenges seem to hinder empowerment at the community and societal level.

Challenges for Women in Empowering Community

The interviews with the informants, and our group discussions as we analysed them, confirm that Latin American women working for empowerment face challenges related to: types and gender of leadership, connection and disconnection with mainstream society, unity and fragmentation within the community, and the availability of resources and support to sustain change.

Women as Community Leaders

It was in relation to community-level leadership that many informants describe the particular challenges that women face as compared to men. Informant #12 indicates that although both women and men are needed to develop community-level empowerment, women continue to face greater challenges that limit their participation, as a consequence of unequal gender roles in the care of the family. She explains: 'We have men who are volunteers, who are always ready to do anything; whereas at times, women find it harder, because of their responsibilities with their families, their household work, and this limits them somewhat ...'

Informant #6, a journalist for a Spanish-language local newspaper, believes that neither men nor women in the Latin American community have been active enough in pushing for change, and that the community lacks the leadership necessary to have an impact, to really advance. In his opinion, Latin American women have participated even less than men; their involvement has only been noticeable recently, and there are few, if any, women who have demonstrated community-wide leadership: '... if the community really hasn't participated [in political and social change activities], women in the community have participated even less in any changes ... only in the last two, three, four years or so we began to see a little bit of movement, a few women beginning to participate in different organizations.'

Another perspective is that of informant #11, who recognizes there is a problem in terms of women's lack of leadership, but attributes this more to a combination of numbers and differing visions of community, rather than only to gender: '... we could really do lobbying [towards a more social justice-based community], we could present an issue, develop a concrete written position, and present it to the politicians. We [the Latin Americans in Ottawa] are very few in number; but we could do that type of work, since we can't have massive demonstrations. It's a question of the type of society we envision, and how we want to get to it.'

Towards Social Justice

Another challenge is with understanding community empowerment as a movement towards social justice. Many 'insiders' who had this vision of participation, spoke about empowerment at a collective level as a socially just community. This conceptualization appears more common among community members who have had a longer history living in Ottawa. For example, several 'insiders' noted that Latin American women's involvement within the community has changed, or even diminished, over time. In the 1970s and 1980s many women were very actively involved in setting up organizations to remove barriers through a social action focus and were less focused on a service delivery approach. However, these organizations gradually disappeared in the 1990s, and many of their leaders moved on, sometimes to focus on goals at a personal level, such as revalidating credentials or seeking professional employment. Informant #11 recalls: 'At one time, there were more organizations ... [such as the Latin American Women's Congress (LAWC), etc.] ... and they studied the process of immigration legislation and policies; we went to lobby politicians on these issues. The Latinas were very organized. Later they became more organized on other things, and they left their work with the LAWC. People went on, they developed their own personal projects and activities.'

This perception is shared by at least one 'outsider' informant, a senior staff member of a large multi-ethnic immigrant services organization, who believes that communities (including the Latin American community) have lost collective power, because the search for individual empowerment has had a negative impact on collective empowerment. In the words of informant #5: 'We have completely, in a sense, given up collective action towards getting, taking possession of our share – our collective share – I am saying that we are not doing enough collectively. And we are not doing enough particularly together as a group.'

Connection/Disconnection

Many of our informants, both 'insiders' and 'outsiders,' noted that while the Latin American community has been growing and increasing internal capacity, it remains disconnected from mainstream Canadian society. This keeps women, and the community as a whole, from advancing.

Many informants emphasize that Latin American women need an 'affective' community, but as immigrants facing language, ethnic, and racialized barriers, they do not easily form part of the majority/mainstream 'affective' community. This means that Latin American women working in their communities face a double burden: they/we have to build, support, and nurture the development of a local Latin American minority community, while simultaneously assisting individuals and the community as a whole to break through, join, and have access to all dimensions of the 'mainstream' community, including the 'affective' dimensions of friendship, neighbourliness, and social solidarity.

One 'insider' informant (#13), who has been involved with both the Latin American and mainstream communities, is seeking different approaches to establish links with mainstream society. In her opinion, activities such as the annual Latin festivals should not be seen as a 'thing' that belongs to people who come from different (minority) cultures, but rather as a thing that belongs to people in this (majority) culture as well. She suggests that Latin American women and men leaders can be ambassadors within the mainstream community, but: 'ambassadors actually of who we are, not who we were there [in countries of origin], and how is the family there. No. How we are, here and now. Because by telling them who we are here, and what we do here, there is a better degree of interaction; and we, as immigrants, will feel we are a part of where we live.'

An 'insider' informant (#8) who has worked both with the Latin American and mainstream communities acknowledges that the Latin American community has not made a dent on mainstream community: 'but as a community ... that lives here, there is very little impact ...'

The absence of Latin American leaders from the mainstream public sphere has been noticed by leaders from other minority community groups. Although the Latin American community has set up, over the years, various groups that provide services, do training, or undertake small projects, neither Latin American women nor men are particularly visible in the public fora, lobbying to let politicians know about the socio-economic problems that the community faces, and advocating for changes that will benefit the community's members. In the words of informant #5: 'You know, you are not out there pushing. So, the casual observer will think that there are no problems ... because that's the way things work here, if you are not saying that I have a problem, it's because there isn't one. If you are keeping quiet, it is because everything is okay' [chuckles].

One 'insider' (#9), who has been involved with both the Latin American and mainstream communities, believes that the disconnect stems from the lack of lead organizations that can lobby and speak on behalf of the community: 'That's the challenge: since we don't have those vanguard organizations that represent the community, and that the community feels represented by ...'

Unity and Fragmentation

For many informants, the main challenge to linking with mainstream society is that the Latin American community in Ottawa is itself not yet united. Informant #6 believes that this lack of unity keeps the community from being visible within the mainstream. In order to lobby politicians and advocate for better health and other services, the community must be united: 'What it is in reality is a lack of unity: a lack of a physical, mental, ideological unity among the Latinos; we need to work together so that we can impress politicians, have an impact on the organizations that offer those services.'

One 'insider' (#7) thinks that Latin American women face challenges in making their issues more visible within the mainstream community because the community is very diverse, composed of people originating from diverse Latin American regions, nations, and cultures. Several 'insiders' believe that Latin American women are working to create a new cultural vision that, recognizing our heterogeneity, focuses on what we have in common (a collective identity). Only then will we be able to ascertain how this vision matches up with the mainstream community.

Discussion

As mentioned at the beginning of this chapter, we started this study knowing that the Latin American community in Ottawa is disempowered by the barriers that impede access to health and social services. Our approach was also informed by the knowledge that empowerment of individuals and communities is a goal of health promotion and of efforts to reduce health disparities (Raphael 2009; Rose and Hatzenbuehler 2009; WHO 2009). We knew that to promote empowerment, service providers must be able to assist the women and their communities to break through language barriers, to access information, to meet material needs, and to establish social networks to break their social isolation (Justice Institute of British Columbia 2007; Reitmanova and Gustafson 2007; Simich, Beiser, and Mawani 2003).

Our study helped us to operationalize Nelson and Prilleltensky's (2005) typology for understanding empowerment as processes and outcomes that take place at multiple levels: individual, organizational, community, and societal. Our results have shown that the strategies that were used contributed to the empowerment of Latin American women at the individual and organizational levels, but not at the community and societal levels.

We also found evidence of Staeheli's (2003) two ways of conceptualizing community in our study: 'community as a space in which values and norms can be nurtured and in which affective bonds of trust and mutuality are fostered ...' (218) [and] '... community as a strategy to create political and material spaces for caring, empowerment, and justice' (815). However, this does not necessarily mean that these are dichotomous ways of 'building community'; for the Latin American women who most actively work on women's health issues in Ottawa, these two spaces are complementary and mutually reinforcing (Hardy-Fanta 1997). The lack of political influence of our work cannot be attributed solely to the fact that women activists devote considerable time and energy to the important dimensions of family, caring, friendship, nurturing, and neighbourhood building. Rather, it is as much, or more so, a consequence of the double burden imposed on women in this and other societies (Escobar 2006); the small number of Latin Americans in Ottawa and Canada in comparison to other 'minority' groups; the language barrier (Tossutti 2003); the diversity and divisions within the Latin American community; the decrease in funding from state programs (Luther and Prempeh 2003); and the racism and sexism of the mainstream society (Escobar 2006:171; Hawkesworth 2006:184; Young 2002:26). In addition, Latin American women have to learn to survive the urban isolation associated with Ottawa's long, bitter winters.

Latin American women in Ottawa are feeling increasingly empowered at the individual and organizational levels because we are organizing around both the removal of barriers and a vision of 'nurturing, affective' community. However, we experience disempowerment at the community and societal levels because we lack the strategies to combine the 'caring' with 'political and material empowerment and justice.' The results are consistent with the position of Ginieniewicz and Schugurensky (2006), and of del Pozo (2006), who write about Latin Americans' lack of capacity to 'act in a united fashion through organizations that will permit them to have a role in public life, that will bring the authorities to consult with them more frequently' (Cruz Herrera 2005, as cited in del Pozo 2006:52; translation ours). Our study confirms that we lack collective capacity to bring our issues front and centre among decision-makers in the health and social services field, and within other realms of the society. Our findings also coincide with those of Barriga and Vanzaghi (2006), who point out that the dismantling of Canadian-Latin American solidarity groups, which were the central concern of many Latin American activists in the 1970s and 1980s, led to a subsequent shifting of energies to local service organizations, and a reduction in social activism. In part, this change resulted from shifting political conditions in Latin American countries. Moreover, the refocusing of energies was a consequence of entrenched gender roles and limitations to women's individual empowerment and leadership in traditional solidarity groups.

To some extent, this is also evident in Ottawa, where Latin American women who were once very active in Latin American solidarity groups have in the last decade moved on to take a leadership role in service-oriented and cultural organizations, as well as women-oriented organizations such as LAZO. Our findings, however, suggest that leadership within gender-mixed, service-oriented organizations may not always be formally recognized unless women play along with a liberal style male leadership (Suyemoto and Ballou 2007).

For instance, some informants working in such organizations did not necessarily recognize women's contribution to the strengthening of the community. This means that just because men and women work side by side, it does not mean that men will necessarily embrace women's equality or encourage women's leadership. Similarly, just because women help other women does not mean that they advocate a critical gender analysis.

The paucity of literature on feminist leadership (Chin 2007:4) embodying feminist principles of inclusion, collaboration, and social advocacy represents another challenge in empowering women leaders to be collaborative and nurturing consensus builders while advocating for policies (Lott 2007:28) to remove barriers to accessing health and social services.

What does this mean for us, as Latin American women trying to work for empowerment of women and our community? We are keenly aware that, as well as 'engendering health' we have to transcend the barriers of sexism, racism, and class division within our own community, and between our community and mainstream society, and that these issues require more analysis, especially at the collective and community levels. We are convinced that we need to strengthen a vision of community that involves social justice by working on issues that strengthen community unity, that build gender equality and equality for ethnic/racialized minorities, and that develop leadership. Furthermore, by lobbying and pushing for change that links us both to other immigrant groups facing similar issues, and to mainstream social change organizations, we can collectively promote political action. Community empowerment must therefore be about collective action, not only or particularly for women, but also for the 'whole community,' acting together to gain power, remove barriers, build healthier communities, and thus be able to participate fully in Canadian society.

12 The Global Ottawa AIDS Link (GOAL): The Story of an 'Un-Project'

CAROL AMARATUNGA, LAURA M. BISAILLON, ALLISON FARBER, LUCIE KALINDA, SUJATHA LIYANAGE, FÉLICITÉ MURANGIRA, AND MELISSA ROWE

Introduction

In Lewis Carroll's 1865 fantasy novel, *Alice's Adventures in Wonderland*, the protagonist navigates an imaginary world where language is often nonsensical; for instance, the characters refer to the famous tea party as an 'unbirthday' party. Similarly, the Global Ottawa AIDS Link (GOAL) was an 'unproject' for its first three years of life, insofar as it lacked conventional research funding while still finding ways to organize numerous HIV-education activities and slowly build a dedicated constituency of volunteers, community leaders, academics, and students.

In this chapter we describe the evolution of this community-based research initiative, the purpose of which was to address issues of gender, diversity, and migration in the context of HIV and AIDS, specifically among African and Caribbean communities in Ottawa, Canada. The chapter is arranged into three sections: the social epidemiology of HIV/AIDS, both globally and locally; an overview of the GOAL initiative, including its development, achievements, and next steps; and a discussion of the potential for community-based research methodology as a tool to mobilize communities to address complex issues such as gender, diversity, and migration, while simultaneously breaking the silence and stigma around HIV/AIDS.

The Social Epidemiology of HIV/AIDS

HIV and AIDS-related illnesses have killed more than 25 million people since 1981, and the death toll was expected to reach 45 million by 2010, making it one of the most destructive epidemics in recorded history

(United Nations Children's Fund (UNICEF) 2007; Joint United Nations Programme on HIV/AIDS (UNAIDS) 2007; World Health Organization (WHO) 2007). Put another way, the most recent estimates of the number of people living with HIV/AIDS (PHAs) is roughly the same as the population of Canada, at between 30 and 36 million people (UNAIDS 2007; WHO 2007).

Globally, the rate of HIV infection is believed to have peaked in the late 1990s and to have subsequently stabilized. Where rates are in decline, it is attributed to increased prevention efforts, improved surveillance methods, and changes in behaviour (Public Health Agency of Canada (PHAC) 2007a; UNAIDS 2006a, 2007; WHO 2007). Nevertheless, at this time rates of infection are still increasing in a number of countries, and HIV/AIDS remains a leading cause of death worldwide, especially in those regions where HIV is considered endemic. Sub-Saharan Africa remains the global epicentre of the AIDS epidemic, with an estimated adult prevalence rate (i.e., percentage of population) of 7.4 per cent; the Caribbean is considered the second most affected area in the world at 2.3 per cent prevalence. This translates into an estimated 450,000 PHAs in the Caribbean, where AIDS is the leading cause of death among adults aged 15 to 44 years (UNAIDS 2007; WHO 2007). In these regions, the extent and nature of the disease – as well as government and civil society response – varies considerably from country to country.

In Canada, the Public Health Agency estimates that approximately 58,000 Canadians are HIV positive, and 3,400 Canadians are infected annually, with the greatest number of new infections occurring in the provinces of Ontario, Québec, British Columbia, and Alberta. Ninety-five per cent of reported HIV+ tests and AIDS diagnoses in Canada occur in these jurisdictions, although HIV has been reported in every jurisdiction in Canada since approximately 2003 (PHAC 2007a). In Ontario, approximately 1,200 people test positive for HIV each year (Ontario Ministry of Health and Long-Term Care (OMHLTC) 2007b). Between 1985 and 2006, there were 26,579 positive HIV infections recorded across Ontario (PHAC 2006a). Ontario has consistently had the highest number of positive HIV tests in Canada, with its capital and most populous city of Toronto accounting for approximately 66 per cent of all positive HIV tests. By comparison, the city of Ottawa accounted for approximately 11 per cent of all positive tests nationally over the same 20 years (Remis et al. 2010). Nevertheless, Ottawa's incidence rates of HIV, both in general and among specific subgroups, are second only to Toronto in the province, and are among the high-

Figure 1. Crude Incidence Rates of AIDS, City of Ottawa and Ontario, 1994–2006

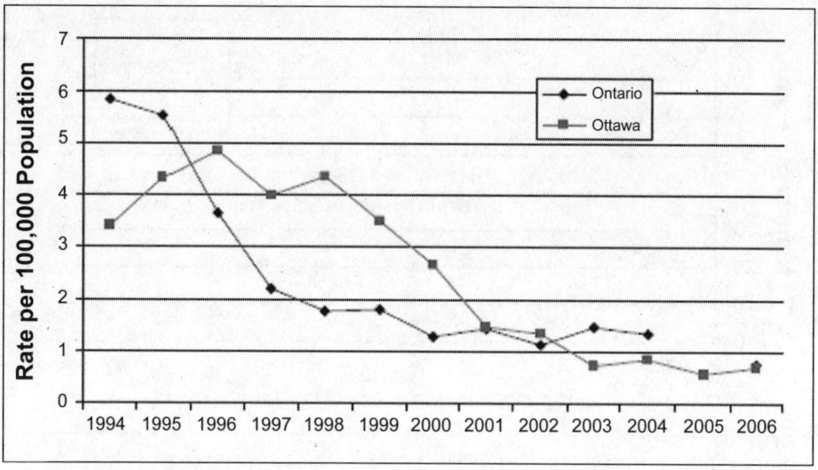

Source: Ottawa Public Health (OPH) 2007.

est across Canada (PHAC 2007a; Remis et al. 2010; Remis and Merid 2004a). Moreover, while the incidence of HIV has declined steadily in Ottawa since 1994, there has been a modest upturn in recent times reported by Ottawa Public Health (OPH) (see Figure 1).

For prevention and treatment efforts to be successful, it is crucial to understand who, how, and why individuals are infected and affected by HIV/AIDS. In Canada, there has been a dramatic increase in infection rates among people originating from regions of the world where HIV is endemic, such as Africa and the Caribbean. In 1998, the proportion of overall positive test results in Canada attributed to the HIV-endemic category was 2.9 per cent; by 2005, this had increased to 7.7 per cent (PHAC 2007a). The same year, Ontarians born in African or Caribbean countries accounted for 14 per cent of PHAs and 20 per cent of new diagnoses, and the proportion continues to increase, as it did by 34 per cent between 2000 and 2005 (OMHLTC 2007b; (Remis et al. 2010). The prevalence rate in Ontario among individuals from HIV-endemic countries is now about 20-fold higher than for the general population (Remis and Merid 2004a,b).

This increase has been particularly notable in Ottawa, an increasingly diverse city and a destination of choice for newcomers from both

Figure 2. HIV Cases by Risk Factor, City of Ottawa, 1990–2003

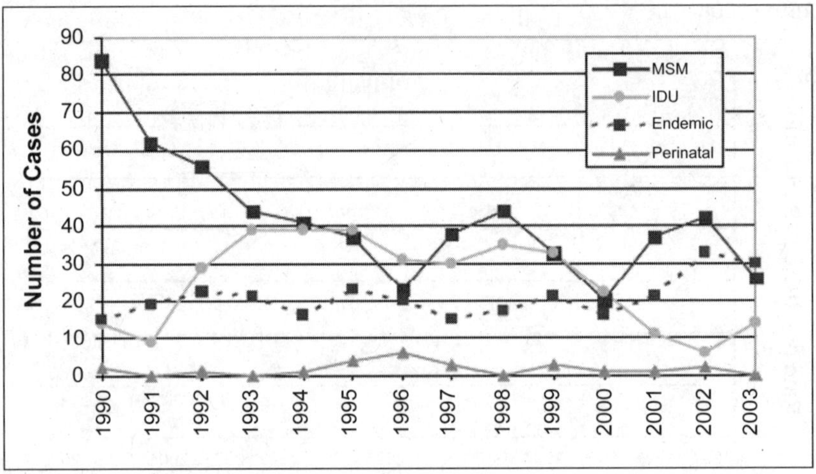

Source: Ottawa Public Health (OPH) 2007.

English- and French-speaking countries. While in 1985 there were no identified cases of HIV among persons from HIV endemic countries, by 2001 this group represented 26 per cent of all HIV cases in Ottawa (Interagency Coalition on AIDS and Development (ICAD) (2006a), and the second-largest group of new infections (Anne Wright and Associates 2003). Figure 2 shows that by 2003, for the first time, the prevalence of HIV/AIDS among African and Caribbean communities in Ottawa ranked even higher than for men who have sex with men (MSM) and injection drug users (IDU) (OPH 2007; Remis and Merid 2004b).

A particularly disturbing aspect of this trend is the number of persons with HIV who do not know they are infected because they have not been tested (UNAIDS 2007). It is estimated that roughly one-third (27 per cent) of Canadians with HIV are unaware of their seropositive status (PHAC 2007a), but among people from endemic countries living in Ottawa, the estimate increases to more than 40 per cent (Anne Wright and Associates 2003).

In addition to ethnocultural populations, the other group for whom the Canadian government has developed a 'population-specific approach' for HIV is women (Government of Canada 2004), reflecting the fact that HIV is increasingly becoming a 'women's disease' (Zimmer and Thurston 1998). The proportion of women diagnosed with HIV has increased dramatically in Canada – from 1.8 per cent in 1985 to almost 28 per cent in 2006 of all new infections (PHAC 2007c). Young women aged 15 to 29 and female immigrants from HIV-endemic countries are among those most at risk of acquiring the virus (Remis and Merid 2004a), the latter group recently accounting for 52 per cent of all HIV+ tests among people from HIV-endemic countries (PHAC 2007c). In Ottawa, approximately 66 per cent of women who tested positive for HIV between 2001 and 2003 were born in an HIV-endemic country (OPH 2006). Internationally, too, women and girls account for the majority of new infections (Csete 2004), and more women than ever before are living with HIV (UNAIDS 2006). In sub-Saharan Africa, for instance, there are 14 HIV+ adult women for every 10 HIV+ adult men, and across all age groups, 60 per cent of all PHAs are women. In the Caribbean, as in some other regions, the ratio of HIV+ women to men is almost 1:1 (UNAIDS 2007; WHO 2007).

Why the disparity in infection rates? Physiologically, women are more vulnerable to HIV infection and are at greater risk of the negative impacts of HIV and AIDS than men (WHO 2007). Since they are generally infected at an earlier age than men (UNAIDS 2007b), women are at greater risk of either a diminished life span or greater number of years of ill health and disability. For HIV+ women who are pregnant, not only are their own health and lives at risk, but also their children's, particularly if anti-retroviral medication is not taken throughout at least two trimesters of pregnancy. Moreover, as with many other diseases and health conditions, vulnerability to HIV is related to a wide variety of social and systemic factors (McKeown, Reid, and Orr 2004; PHAC 2007a). HIV spreads along fault lines of society, fuelled by societal and structural factors such as poverty, disorder, racism and sexism (ICAD 2002). The pandemic disproportionately focuses on vulnerable individuals and communities who are at the same time coping with wider health and socio-economic issues.

National and international reports demonstrate that gender inequalities are at the heart of these disproportionate rates (Remis and Merid 2004a; UNAIDS 2006a,b). Globally, women are disadvantaged by the dominant social and cultural norms that characterize power relations between men and women, as well as between health care providers and clients (ICAD 2002, 2006). Women often have less access to prevention, care, treatment, and support. It is no accident that the largest gender gap in HIV infection rates is recorded between 15- to 24-year-olds. A considerable body of opinion purports that women and girls have more limited access to health information, including sexual and reproductive health information (Baksh-Soodeen and Amaratunga 2002; WHO 2007; PHAC 2007a; Government of Canada 2004).

As a consequence of these gendered dimensions of HIV/AIDS, women often lack the requisite resources and power (whether economic, social, or personal) to protect themselves, either by obtaining needed information and services, negotiating safer sex, or by leaving high-risk relationships (ICAD 2002). Women and girls are also more likely to have to assume the role of caregiver to others who are HIV+ or sick with AIDS; in some regions, girls are more likely than boys to be taken out of school to care for family members and to save on costs. Furthermore, women are more likely to experience stigma and discrimination related to HIV/AIDS, as they are often blamed for bringing the disease and subsequent shame into the family, regardless of how the disease was contracted. The stigmatization can also be subtle, such as with the commonly accepted HIV terminology of 'mother-to-child transmission' (MTCT), which is seen by many as blaming the woman for 'vertical transmission' from mother to child instead of emphasizing the structural forces and societal barriers that made her infection possible in the first place.

Gender, however, does not by itself account for the fact that female immigrants from racialized communities in particular remain the most at risk to HIV infection (Apanovich, McCarthy, and Salovey 2003; Fortin 2005; Ploem 2002). In *Silent Voices of the HIV/AIDS Epidemic* (Tharao, Massaquoi, and Teclom 2006), it is reported that African and Caribbean women bear the greatest burden of HIV/AIDS stigmatization in Canada. The 2001 report of the Ontario HIV-Endemic Task Force noted that Canada has a poor record of addressing issues related to HIV/AIDS in our racialized and ethnocultural communities. Moreover, recent studies have demonstrated that many African and Caribbean Canadians are uncomfortable with and even avoid health and social services due to language and cultural barriers and subtle racism (Amaratunga, Sranton, and Clow 2002; Spitzer 2004). It is beginning to be recognized that 'gender and migration, and more particularly the dynamic imbrications between them, are determinants of health' (Vissandjée et al. 2007:221). Inequalities in health relate to the determinants of health, and particularly to the interactions between gender and migration (Dunn and Dyck 2000; Evans, Barrer, and Marmor 1994). Adding gender, migration, and systemic racism to the existing list of social determinants of health may begin to address the existing knowledge gap in immigrant health research in Canada.

Additional scholarship and research is needed to systematically examine the health of newcomers through a 'gendered' lens (Vissandjée et al. 2007:221). Epidemiological and community-based research that are both culturally appropriate and gender-sensitive are potentially powerful tools for this work. With these approaches, the Global Ottawa AIDS Link team recognized that public health policy and programming could be made much more responsive to the health and social service needs of Canada's racialized communities, and at the same time be more effective in helping to control the spread of HIV in Canada.

Around the world, women and girls are blamed for bringing diseases and shame into the family, regardless of how the diseases were contracted (UNAIDS 2007b; WHO 2007; UNAIDS 2006b); these attitudes are found in Canada as well. For instance, the Global Ottawa AIDS Link (GOAL) project has found that women and girls, especially those from racialized immigrant, refugee, and First Nations communities, are likely to experience such HIV/AIDS-related stigma and discrimination. In the next section, we will give an example of a community-based research initiative that is working to accomplish these ambitious goals.

The Global Ottawa AIDS Link (GOAL) Initiative

The GOAL project is an action research initiative of community leaders and volunteers, service providers, clinicians, students, and academics who have been working diligently since 2003 to support more effective responses to HIV/AIDS, particularly within Ottawa's African and Caribbean communities. In the founding year, strategic plans were released by both the Ottawa Carleton Council on AIDS (OCCA) and the *Healthy Sexuality and Risk Reduction Program of the* City of Ottawa's Public Health department (OPH). Both documents outlined increasing rates of infection among people from HIV-endemic countries, and the lack of a culturally appropriate response from the local service system. At that point in time, there was only one local program that specifically targeted its HIV interventions to the needs of Ottawa's African and Caribbean communities: the Ethnocultural HIV Peer Education program (EHPEP) of Somerset West Community Health Centre.

Both the OCCA and OPH documents called for a community development approach to develop strategies that would meet the specific needs of Ottawa's ethnocultural communities. Discussion began about the need to support the EHPEP, develop other services like it, and undertake research to support such service planning. As a result, OPH took the lead in developing a task force with representatives of social services and Ottawa's African and Caribbean communities to address service development. At the same time, a small group of OCCA members, staff from Somerset West Community Health Centre, and researchers from the Women's Health Research Unit (WHRU) at the University of Ottawa began to discuss research possibilities and the formation of a network. Ever mindful of both the global and local dimensions of HIV/ AIDS, the group named itself the Global Ottawa AIDS Link (GOAL).

Over the course of the next few years, GOAL sharpened its focus and slowly expanded its core group, reaching out to dynamic, progressive, feminist leaders from Ottawa's diverse African and Caribbean communities, HIV service providers, as well as other academic researchers and graduate students. These women and men continue to function as bridge-people among the various stakeholder groups; GOAL provides a platform for various groups and individuals to join together in dialogue on HIV, exploring opportunities for collaboration and resource sharing.

In the process of these discussions, and with support from OCCA, GOAL, and OPH, a leadership coalition on HIV issues emerged from within local African and Caribbean communities. From its inception, GOAL members were committed to supporting Ottawa's African and Caribbean communities and HIV service providers to mobilize to develop culturally appropriate and effective responses to HIV/AIDS. Community meetings were held in 2004 to assess needs and brainstorm ideas, and, from the organizing group, the African Caribbean Health Network of Ottawa (ACHNO) was formed. ACHNO has gone on to stimulate public dialogue on HIV/AIDS, provide leadership in program planning, and develop strong links with its provincial counterpart the African Caribbean Council on HIV/AIDS in Ontario (ACCHO). GOAL members were honoured to have been involved in the founding of ACHNO, and the two Ottawa-based groups now work closely together, the former focusing primarily on research and the latter on service development in relation to HIV/AIDS. A GOAL representative continues to serve on ACHNO's Research Committee.

Inspired by the work of social activists such as Ivan Illich (1999), Saul Alinsky (1989), and Paulo Freire (1973, 1974), GOAL engages members of these communities in dialogue and praxis (i.e., reflective action) in relation not only to the more obvious health and social issues related to

HIV and AIDS, but also underlying considerations of gender, diversity, migration, social justice, power structures, and social conventions. The GOAL initiative's three objectives are as follows:

1 To generate and disseminate new knowledge about how gender, diversity, and migration affect the experience of HIV/AIDS within ethnocultural communities;
2 To build capacity and expertise in culturally competent community-based research on HIV/AIDS through applied research, training, and mentoring of graduate students and community members;
3 To create a community of practice in which community leaders from Ottawa's African and Caribbean communities engage researchers, policy makers, and service providers in Canada and in Africa to share knowledge and experience about promising practices in the design and delivery of culturally competent HIV interventions.

GOAL members also committed early on to the use of community-based research as the most appropriate methodology for achieving these objectives. Inspired by and building upon Paulo Freire's 1974 work, *Pedagogy of the Oppressed*, the GOAL team embraced community-based research as its modus operandi. The belief is that sustainable and effective solutions emerge when those most affected are responsible for developing them, and that community leadership is critical to this sense of ownership. Community-based research has transformative capacity through its emphasis on community involvement, skills development, open dialogue, action research, and capacity building (University of Washington 2007; University of Victoria 2007). These qualities are the very spirit and ethos of the GOAL initiative.

Despite having identified its goals and objectives and its methodology, GOAL remained an orphan project (an 'unproject') for the first three years while its members searched for research project funding. Early activities were fuelled primarily by the personal capital of the core members, in the sense that they committed considerable time and energy to meeting regularly, creating plans and proposals, and developing relationships of mutual trust, without any external resources for coordination or support.

The GOAL Project has enjoyed numerous successes in a short time, and with limited finances. From the beginning, GOAL tried to stimulate public dialogue, and to break the silence on the complex issues of gender, diversity, and migration in relation to HIV/AIDS. GOAL team members chaired community meetings, engaged citizens from a variety of sectors, and mobilized the participation of women, men, and youth in public forums on HIV/AIDS. With an action plan and a variety of communication and outreach materials, GOAL team members continue to work collaboratively and across numerous disciplines to generate new knowledge, build expertise in community-based research methods, and collaborate with community and international partners. A number of GOAL's achievements are presented below.

In June 2004, the GOAL Project was identified as a pilot project for the academic non-governmental organization (ACANGO) initiative sponsored by the Centre for Global Health, Faculty of Medicine, and the Institute of Population Health, University of Ottawa. ACANGO's purpose was to develop partnerships for research, training, and social action in global health (Robinson et al. 2007). Through ACANGO, potential partners for GOAL from Thailand and Sri Lanka were identified; follow-up meetings articulated several areas of common interest and research activity in HIV/AIDS and sexual health. These meetings generated ongoing interest and discussion in professional and academic training and exchange for faculty and students, as well as the need to raise awareness for the inclusion of gender and HIV/AIDS curriculum development for graduate programs (Baksh-Soodeen et al. 2002)

Another early success was Bangkok or Bust, an initiative to send a team of graduate students and youth, academics, and community members to the 15th International AIDS Conference in Bangkok, Thailand, in July 2004. With resources from an international twinning project, another team attended the 16th International AIDS Conference in Toronto in August 2006, along with two colleagues from Rwanda. After both of these conferences, GOAL team members conducted workshops with AIDS service organizations (ASOs) in Ottawa to report on promising practices and disseminate resource materials collected at the conference. This lead to an invitation for core GOAL team members to visit the National University of Rwanda and to deliver workshops on Gender and HIV/AIDS as well as project management for community based research. .

With time, GOAL attracted modest funding from several funding organizations supporting HIV/AIDS research, education, and/or capacity building. These included the Canadian Institutes for Health Research (CIHR), the Public Health Agency Canada (PHAC), and the Canadian International Development Agency (CIDA). The latter funds one of GOAL's most significant initiatives, the above-mentioned twin-ning linkage with the Ligue Universitaire Contre le Sida (LUCS), a research unit at the National University of Rwanda in Butare, south-eastern Rwanda. In typical 'unproject' fashion, the GOAL Project team designed a reverse overseas development assistance project in which promising practices in HIV prevention education from a southern HIV-endemic country are shared and exchanged with Canadian coun-terparts. In this instance, GOAL (represented by the Women's Health Research Unit at the University of Ottawa), Somerset West Community Health Centre, and LUCS share information, materials, and expertise, and collaborate to develop opportunities for training, organizational development, and joint publications. The overarching goal is to help each organization reduce the impact of HIV/AIDS in its respective community.

This international exchange was built first upon professional re-lationships of trust; two key GOAL members are from Rwanda and helped establish the partnership, after which followed a proposal and funding. The project has reached several milestones, including visits by team members to each country. The LUCS twinning linkage is nascent, and the early exchange visits have been mutually beneficial, strength-ening the collaboration among partners, developing knowledge and expertise, and providing opportunities for developing creative solu-tions to local challenges. These include culturally relevant and appro-priate interventions and education programs suitable for both African and Ottawa contexts. The Rwandan-Canadian collaboration on com-munity theatre has been a particularly successful and creative outcome of reciprocal knowledge flow between the two countries.

An Arts-Based HIV/AIDS Prevention: Best-Practices Workshop was held in Ottawa in November 2007, and was an international gather-ing featuring speakers from Canada, the United States, and Rwanda. The workshop featured a range of imaginative presentations on body mapping, radio drama, community theatre, poetry, visual arts, hip-hop, photography, and forum theatre. A presentation was also made by Operation Hair Spray, an innovative program offered by Ottawa Pub-lic Health that involves hairdressers as peer educators. International presenters included forum theatre specialist Dr Paulin Basinga from the National University of Rwanda; radio serial drama specialist and founder of Vermont's Population Media Center, Mr William Ryerson; and the Rwandan ambassador to Canada and former Rwandan minis-ter of justice, Her Excellency Mrs Edda Mukabagwiza.

This workshop, designed, organized, and facilitated by community leaders, was widely attended by university-based HIV/AIDS researchers, members of Ottawa ASOs, graduate and undergraduate students from Ottawa's universities, members from local youth groups, actors from popular theatre groups, and representatives from Toronto's ACCHO. The workshop demonstrated not only the range of creative vehicles that can advance culturally competent modes of HIV prevention education, but also the importance of collaboration and community-led initiatives for citizen engagement.

A final example of GOAL's achievements was its success in obtaining research development funding from the community-based HIV/AIDS program of Canadian Institutes of Health Research (CIHR). While this support has yet to translate into operational funding for a larger research project, it provided the necessary resources for GOAL to extend its reach to the broader African and Caribbean communities of Ottawa, and to involve them in a series of consultations to develop a framework for community-based research on HIV/AIDS in their communities. In other words, it allowed GOAL to put into action another stage of its plan for using community-based research as a tool for community mobilization regarding HIV/AIDS. The process and outcome of these consultations are presented in the next section.

Community-Based Research in Action

As mentioned earlier, GOAL aims to use community-based research as an instrument for social change and social justice in Ottawa, stimulating a 'micro social movement' among Ottawa's African and Caribbean communities. Team members chose community-based research methodology in part because of the methodology's values of collaboration, empowerment, and social justice. However, the methods are also well suited to the early stage of development these communities were at in terms of speaking out about the problem of HIV/AIDS and the lack of appropriate HIV services in their communities, and taking action for change.

Until the 1990s the African and Caribbean communities in Ottawa, indeed in Canada, had played limited roles in formal, systems-level efforts for HIV/AIDS prevention and programming. This resulted in minimal involvement of these communities in health promotion, fuelled by a lack of evidence on which to base programs and services (Tharao, Massaquoi, and Teclom 2006). The emergence of groups such as ACCHO (then called the HIV-Endemic Task Force (HETF) in Ontario) and Women's Health in Women's Hands, a community health centre specifically for women of colour in Toronto helped spur the development of other community-driven HIV/AIDS initiatives for ethnocultural groups. This surge of activity augurs well for the advancement of better population health practice and culturally competent service delivery in Canada. Regrettably, many of these excellent initiatives remain under-resourced and under-promoted, which means that the progressive work of many grass-roots, community-based organizations does not gain full recognition. At the end of the day, unrecognized work remains unrecognized.

GOAL's own research development process needed to demonstrate respect for these early calls for change, as well as for those not yet able to come forward; to demonstrate support to amplify 'voices,' as well as acknowledge the plurality of perspectives. Community-based research methods are well suited to such efforts, in that they integrate mechanisms for community ownership (through the use of reference groups or co-direction of the research project, for example) for cooperative decision-making and collective action.

In this case, the project developed directly from the initial community meetings in 2005, when African and Caribbean community members themselves started speaking out about the issue. After hiring several research assistants from these communities to plan and coordinate the process, GOAL embarked on a series of community 'brainstorming sessions' in late 2005 and early 2006. Both English and French sessions were held, as were sessions specifically inviting youth and service providers. While each group raised specific concerns, there were common themes in people's experiences of HIV/AIDS, whether as someone living with the disease, as a friend or family member, or as a concerned member of a community of increased risk.

A key message that emerged from community dialogues highlighted that it is crucial to recognize the diversity of new Canadian populations in terms of language, education, culture and ethnicity, history and politics, and migration experience. Even the term *community* implies a homogeneity of perspectives and experiences that may not be accurate. Community leaders realized that it is important to sort fact from fiction. It was suggested that many immigrants to Canada assume 'they have left HIV behind' and that it is not a health issue here. Research has now determined that the majority of HIV infections among people of African descent actually occur in Canada (i.e., almost 60 per cent of infections in 2002), thus dispelling the myth that HIV and AIDS are being imported by immigrants (Remis and Fikre-Merid 2006).

Research indicates that reproductive health, human sexuality, and HIV/AIDS are often taboo topics for African and Caribbean and other ethnocultural communities in Canada (ACCHO 2006; Falconer 2005; ICAD 2006 b; Lawson et al. 2006). This general reserve about public dialogue on sexuality is related to the power of myth (e.g., regarding transmission and 'cleansing') and stigma that was referred to time and again at the GOAL sessions.

Recent research among African and Caribbean communities in Canada also reveals that there is reticence at speaking openly about one's sero-status due to fear of blame and shame (Tharao, Massaquoi, and Teclom 2006). Participants at the GOAL sessions spoke of discrimination both from outside and within their communities, of reluctance to having their community labelled by 'mainstream' Euro-Canadian society as 'the source for HIV/AIDS,' and the risk of being entirely excluded from their own community if one is suspected of being HIV+. Though not unique to the African and Caribbean communities, there is also a persistent, moralistic association between HIV/AIDS and 'deviant' lifestyles and 'immoral' behaviour. Many people in HIV-affected communities describe religious institutions as an important source of support, one that they fear losing if they speak up about HIV in their community (Tharao, Massaquoi, and Teclom 2006).

Problems of ignorance, fear, and taboo contribute to the cumulative challenges HIV affected communities face in relation to stigma, systemic discrimination, and linguistic and cultural barriers. Apart from underscoring the need for prevention education, the appropriate responses for HIV-related services are not quite so clear. While it was generally acknowledged that it was vital to have more people of colour among the staff of health and social service agencies, many participants also attested to the fact that most African and Caribbean people would likely *not* want to talk to someone from their own community about sexual health and HIV for fear of disclosure beyond the confines of the medical encounter. Service providers spoke of people never returning for follow-up services after testing HIV-positive, some of them moving to a larger city where they could remain relatively anonymous.

Several participants underscored the societal barriers of racism and discrimination for people of colour, whether recent or established migrants or those whose families had lived in Canada for generations. For newcomers, however, these problems are compounded by language

barriers, cultural differences, and the myriad and pressing needs to ar-
range for an income, housing, schooling, and childcare. Social norms
dictate that many of these settlement affairs are within the woman's
realm, and several women attending the GOAL sessions reported jug-
gling so many responsibilities that little time was left to dedicate to
health issues such as HIV/AIDS. Since women generally access health
care for their families, it was suggested that women, in addition to
youth, ought to be identified as priority groups for education and prevention interventions. This would seem particularly important, given
the feedback from the community awareness sessions, that like Canadian women in general, married immigrant women from African and Caribbean communities did not see themselves at risk for HIV infection.

The range of systemic and socio-economic factors that affect both
the transmission and experience of HIV among African and Caribbean
communities also affects how and why HIV-related services may be
underutilized by these groups. Reports from ACCHO's 2001 community forum entitled 'For Us, By Us, About Us' highlight key factors of
vulnerability of racialized immigrant and refugee populations in Canada, many of which were mentioned at the GOAL sessions and are described above. These include: silence and denial about HIV and AIDS;
lack of community mobilization around health issues; lack of research
funding; absence of prevention and treatment services tailored to African and Caribbean communities; and stigmatizing behaviours towards
individuals who may be HIV positive. Also common to the lived experiences of people living with HIV and AIDS (PHAs) in these communities are underemployment and unemployment, social exclusion and
isolation, depression, and fear of disclosure.

As suggested at the GOAL sessions and in ACCHO's (2001) research,
PHAs from racialized communities may need additional supports such
as housing, immigration, mental health, and psychosocial support,
which may in turn affect the type and quality of help they seek and/
or receive (ACCHO 2001, 2002). PHAs report discrimination from mis-
informed or insensitive health care providers with limited HIV/AIDS
care experience, especially for those patients or clients from an HIV-
endemic country (ICAD 2002a). Taken together, ACCHO's research and
the feedback from the GOAL sessions underscored the importance of
inclusive, culturally appropriate prevention and treatment programs.
The GOAL researchers concluded that multidisciplinary approaches
and programs must be designed and implemented by and for African
and Caribbean communities in Canada. Public health programs should

be routinely and regularly reviewed and revised to identify more effective ways to serve the needs of ethnocultural communities. As the GOAL 'unproject' demonstrated, community-based research methods can be a valuable tool for social change and social justice.

Conclusion

In this chapter, we have outlined how global HIV/AIDS trends are mirrored in Canada. The Global Ottawa AIDS Link or GOAL project specifically engaged citizens and practitioners in Ottawa, where people originally from HIV-endemic regions such as Africa and the Caribbean are at significantly higher risk for HIV infection than the general population. A range of cultural and socio-economic factors – including gender, culture and ethnicity, migration experience, and immigration status – can increase vulnerability, particularly for women. The GOAL project corroborated research which demonstrates that these factors prevent some migrants with HIV/AIDS from accessing health and social service, treatment, and prevention programs (Tharao, Massaquoi, and Teclom 2006). Misunderstanding and misinformation can also profoundly affect the quality of the service that newcomers to Canada receive.

There is growing awareness that HIV/AIDS is not solely a health problem, but an issue of gender, diversity, and power. Planning efforts to reduce HIV transmission therefore need to focus on the interplay among the social determinants of health for population subgroups at highest risk, and need to include women, men, and youth from Canada's diverse ethnocultural communities. To successfully address the HIV and AIDS pandemic, a gendered and human rights perspective must be mainstreamed into a broad-based, multi-sectoral policy and program response (Baksh-Soodeen and Amaratunga 2002). As demonstrated by the GOAL 'unproject,' these policy and program areas can be designed in consultation and in partnership with HIV and AIDS affected communities.

Community-based research initiatives such as GOAL, which represent the heart and spirit of the community, can be particularly effective and powerful tools for community resiliency and recovery. The GOAL response focused upon and listened to the voices of people most directly affected by HIV/AIDS. The researchers were able, with limited resources, to forge positive, collaborative partnerships to mobilize community action for social change. The process provided a platform for citizen advocates to meet with health care service providers and planners and to better understand each other's needs and priorities.

As discussed in this chapter, the GOAL initiative demonstrated that the creation of trust among partners from diverse sectors and communities can have powerful outcomes. The academic partners served as technicians and scribes and the project provided a 'real world' platform for community members to identify and express their voice. In this model, research is viewed, not as an end in itself, but as a tool and a process. The project supported the generation of new knowledge, community mobilization, advocacy, and, ultimately, policy change. The role of facilitating knowledge exchange with policy audiences is thus another critical role for academic partners.

Service providers, too, played an important role in the GOAL model, since they were among the first to express the gaps in HIV-related services to Ottawa's ethnocultural communities, and to commit to a community development approach. Their willingness and courage to admit to the limitations of services helped to stimulate a public health dialogue. Their practical support (in terms of funding, coordination, and planning) continues to help the leadership within local African and Caribbean communities to mobilize and coalesce around the issue of HIV/AIDS, and to organize to address the problem.

It is the community leaders, however, who are the real champions of the GOAL initiative. Their involvement from the outset helped establish credibility for the 'unproject'; their insights and passion stimulated 'buy-in' from the broader communities, strengthened research capacity, and provided valuable cross-cultural perspectives. While a concrete objective of GOAL was to develop culturally appropriate tools for HIV/AIDS prevention education, the larger goal is to bridge gaps in policy and service delivery and to address the inequities inherent in the health system. Community mobilization and empowerment are essential prerequisites for social change and social justice. The successes achieved by the GOAL 'unproject' in Ottawa belong to the African and Caribbean communities and their leadership.

In addition to the specific outcomes mentioned in this chapter, there have also been indirect benefits, including a greater appreciation of community-based research as a method to inform local health service planning. There has been an increasing openness among African and Caribbean communities in Ottawa to talk about HIV/AIDS and stigma. One example comes from the 2007 creation of a peer support group for HIV-positive women from African and Caribbean communities in cooperation with Somerset West Community Health Centre. This support group represents an important step forward to co-develop resources with socially excluded and under-funded communities in Ottawa. Although good progress has been made, additional research is required to explain the complex interplay among the social determinants of health and ethnocultural communities. In recent years, prevention education for African and Caribbean communities in Ontario has made huge strides, largely as a result of the early efforts of ACCHO community researchers and the academic partners at the University of Toronto. The battle against ignorance and stigma towards HIV/AIDS in Canada, however, is far from over. The GOAL initiative demonstrated that sometimes modest, community-based initiatives can have a significant impact. Such projects rely on the qualities of trust and respect that are the foundation of interpersonal relationships. Team members have shared commitment, vision, and moral ownership of the process and outcomes. It is often the personal testimonials, anecdotal evidence, stories, and commitment of community and academic research partners that are particularly effective in communicating a sense of social urgency. Academic and community researchers do not always work well together. But when they find common ground they can work together effectively. They can also be a powerful, persuasive force to influence decision-makers to make greater investments in prevention and treatment programs.

As HIV/AIDS gains an ever-pervasive foothold in Canada, it will be imperative that researchers, service providers, and community members work together to push the boundaries of public health practice and policy. As Archimedes once said, 'If you give me a lever, I can move the world.' The GOAL 'unproject' experience is testimony that community-based research is a powerful tool to engage and mobilize communities to find their voice, speak up, and identify solutions from within. It is hoped that this story will inspire and empower other HIV and AIDS affected communities in Canada to have courage, to mobilize, and to take action!

ACKNOWLEDGMENTS

The authors gratefully acknowledge the contributions of Heather Smith Fowler, Sarah Crowe, and Patricia Thille to this chapter.

13 At the Intersection of Migration, Gender, and Health: Accounting for Social Capital

BILKIS VISSANDJÉE, STEPHANIE ANN CLAIRE
ALEXANDER, ALISHA NICOLE APALE, AND MADINE
VANDERPLAAT

Introduction

In the introduction to his book *Social Capital* (2003), Field summarizes his central thesis by stating quite simply that 'relationships matter' (1). A similarly pithy and oft-cited phrase distilling the core idea behind the concept of social capital additionally suggests that 'it's not what you know, but who you know' that matters for health and well-being (Field 2003:2; Putnam 2007; Vissandjée, Wieringa, and Apale 2009). Considering such descriptions, notions conveyed by the term *social capital* are not novel. In fact, the importance of relationships and the obvious value of 'whom one knows' reflect common knowledge and make intuitive sense to most people.

The concept of social capital has been taken up by numerous fields of research. Recently, considering the challenges faced by newcomers and their capacity to mobilize resources for health 'at entry to the host society,' social capital has been invoked as one of the most important protecting factors (Bruegel 2005; Llácer et al. 2007; Putnam 2007; Vissandjée, Wieringa, and Apale 2009; Wakefield and Poland 2005).

In this chapter, we focus on accounts in the literature regarding the complexities associated with the resources – namely, social capital resources and related support systems – that women use as they undergo the experience of progressive integration in a host country. We ask how the specific conditions that migrant women face might shape their experiences of access to various types of support during the migratory process. We also examine the ways in which social capital has been addressed as a potential resource and source of support for well-being and health, along with a sense of autonomy. Finally, we discuss how social capital combined with the discourse of empowerment might inform policies and practices designed to address the health of women experiencing migration.

Though the situation is evolving, it is well documented that most research focusing on gender and health has historically equated gender with biological sex rather than defining this 'complex' determinant shaping women and men's social world in a differential manner. Gender refers to the differences and commonalities between women and men that are set by convention and other social, economic, political, and cultural forces (Johnson, Greaves, and Repta 2007). Here gender is taken in its definition as a social construct that cuts across identities held by women and men and influences socially constructed roles and relationships (Greaves and Barr 2000; Health Canada 2003; Johnson, Greaves, and Repta 2007; Hankivsky and Cormier 2009). A more comprehensive understanding of gender and the way it shapes access to social capital is required in order to gain a complete appreciation of the role social capital plays in the health of migrant women. In the context of the current discussion, gender is considered above and beyond sex as a determinant of health, shaping the way migrant women and men acquire social capital to maintain and improve their health and wellbeing.

An overview of literature focusing on the ways in which social capital has been understood in the public health literature is presented with a critical assessment of the relevance of social capital for women migrants' health. Suggestions are provided for a more systematic integration of the analysis and application of social capital with migration experiences as gendered determinants of migrant women's health.

Social Capital: Diversity of Use

The prominence that social capital has been enjoying in academic and social-policy circles can be largely attributed to the contributions of a number of seminal authors, such as Bourdieu, Coleman, and Putnam, who, working within the fields of sociology and political science, have conceptualized social capital in distinct ways (Anucha et al. 2006; Bourdieu 1980; Coleman 1988; Della Giusta and Kambhampati 2006; Field, 2003; Moore et al. 2005; Putnam 1995). In this regard, Della Giusta and Kambhampati (2006) summarize some points of convergence stating that while Bourdieu (1986) argues that 'one can acquire social capital through purposeful actions and can transform it into conventional economic gains' (822), Coleman (1988) suggests that social capital concerns aspects of social structure, such as obligations and norms, which facilitate the actions of women and men within a specific structure. Putnam (1995), on the other hand, has highlighted that social capital involves social organization; for instance, the ability to establish forms of trust and working networks that should, in turn, facilitate action in society at the community level.

Social capital's wide appeal and diversity of application has also meant that researchers from a broad range of disciplines, including sociology, economics, political science, socio-politics, history, health sciences, public health, and feminist studies have endeavoured to incorporate it into their work (Field 2003; Fine 2001; Kinitz 2004; Makinko and Starfield 2001). While this diversity has resulted in a rich body of knowledge, social capital still lacks an unequivocal definition.

Moore Lappe and Du Bois (1997) have made reference to the elasticity of the term, while more recently Fassin (2003) has argued that, despite its popularity, the relevance of social capital to public health has been called into question. Scholars such as Wakefield and Poland (2005), Franklin (2005), Salaff and Greve (2004), Mackian (2002), Drevdahl et al. (2001), Adler and Kwon (2000), and Kawachi et al. (1997) have also critically questioned its assumed positive impact on an expected 'proper' integration of migrants, while definitions of what adequate integration may be remains generally unclear. Further, Frank (2003) suggests that it is precisely the versatility of the concept that makes it 'run the risk of being rendered meaningless by becoming everything to everyone' (3). Such debates and discussions surrounding the operational usefulness of the concept thus persist, particularly as it pertains to social inequalities in health (Campbell and Gillies 2001; Fassin 2003; Lochner, Kawachi, and Kennedy 1999; Moore et al. 2005; Muntaner and Lynch 1999; Stephens 2008). Nonetheless, the myriad ways in which the concept is used clearly illustrate its potential fruitfulness.

For the purpose of this chapter, the debate around the complexities of social capital and gender issues have led to definitions, including social capital as a resource supporting health, well-being, and empowerment for vulnerable groups, or, alternatively, as sites and sources of control, isolation, and manipulation (Vissandjée, Wieringa, and Apale 2009). Social capital may not always benefit migrants; however, it potentially profits those already living in the host country (Kawar 2004; Sassen 2000).

Social Capital as a Resource

Social capital is generally understood as being manifest through a diversity of not only accessed – but also perceived to be accessible – social resources as reciprocated through social networks and relations; its value resides in the capacity as much as the perceived capacity to mobilize it (Campbell and McLean 2003; Edwards 2005; Policy Research Initiative (PRI) 2005; Putnam 2007). The complexities associated with structural changes and individual abilities in the mobilization of social capital have been eloquently discussed by Mohindra and Haddad (2005) in their application of Amartya Sen's *capability approach* to women's health. They suggest that such a perspective clearly highlights the difference between *functionings* and *capabilities* for a woman and a man trying to achieve good health. *Functionings* are the things one *is* or *does*, which include being in good health, having a social network, and being socially integrated in accordance with societal expectations. A *capability* represents *freedom* or the 'real opportunities of individuals to lead the lives that they value' (357). Two men, two women, or a woman and a man may thus have access to the same quantity of a resource, but their *functionings* (for instance, level of good health and well-being) may differ because of their individual *capabilities*, that is, their *real opportunities* to live a 'healthy' life (Mohindra and Haddad 2005; Sen and Östlin 2008).

One might then argue that increasing these *capabilities* may lead to improved and more equitable *functionings* with regard to mobilizing and using social capital for health and well-being. The classic example involves increasing access to resources through social networks, such as assistance in finding an appropriate job or housing, support in starting an educational program, or navigating the health care or legal system more comfortably (PRI 2005; Putnam 2007; Vissandjée et al. 2007).

Such an analysis leads to the argument that the experience of progressive integration by migrant women and men needs to be understood in terms of several intersecting elements. These include the category of migration (for instance, chosen, forced, with or without family), the availability of social resources, and the opportunity to use social resources depending on length of stay in the new society. All these factors affect a woman's or a man's *functionings*, and, consequently, also shape a productive and successful integration (Bruegel 2005; Laurie and Petchesky 2008).

Current Literature Considering Social Capital at the Intersection of Migration and Gender

The Canadian Policy Research Initiative has identified the process of integration by newcomers to Canada as one of the priority policy areas that is most ripe for a social capital approach (Frank 2003). Described as critical resources for recent immigrants, particularly as a specific 'way of fulfilling the ideal of social justice and equity' (4), at least two types of social capital have been considered as critical for the process of progressive integration of migrants. First, *horizontal* or *bonding* social capital reflects ties within groups of women and men, including ties with family members, neighbours, close friends, and colleagues. Horizontal social capital has also been defined as *bridging* social capital, and refers to social interactions among women, men, and communities of different ethnic, occupational, and economic backgrounds (Coutts et al. 2007). Second, *vertical* social capital, also called *linking* social capital, stems from hierarchical power and status-based relations (Coutts et al. 2007; Kunz 2003). Scant literature exists regarding the effects of these forms of social capital on the progressive integration experience of newcomers; further reflection on this issue is certainly needed, since the experience is unique to each woman, man, family, and group.

Previous work points out that the notion of social capital has not sufficiently addressed the intersectional dimensions of the various social determinants of health involved (Bilge 2005; Morrow, Hankivsky, and Varcoe 2004; Vissandjée et al. 2004; Hankivsky and Cormier 2009). Llàcer and colleagues (2007) argue that research ought to consider the 'determinants in origin, transit and destination' (ii6) of migration. These include 'distal and contextual' determinants of health, such as socio-economic conditions, status, sex, gender, and the associated indicators, as well as 'proximal and individual' determinants, such as evolving health behaviours (Hyman et al. 2006; Kunz 2005; Vissandjée and Hyman 2011).

Indeed, being an immigrant 'does not simply refer to a legal status but encompasses a set of complex realities and experiences' (Vissandjée et al. 2004:3). Siegmann and Thieme (2007), Salaff and Greve (2004), Della Giusta and Kambhampati (2006), Bruegel (2005), and Hyman et al. (2006) add that integration processes lead to inequality of access to social networks and that they are gendered processes rooted in social capital mobilization capacities, which need to be better understood and measured. Siegmann and Thieme (2007) argue that a 'growing feminist literature on the social capital debate has shared the criticism of the naïve equation of social networks as promoting growth as well as reducing poverty and vulnerability' (7) of women and men.

A number of other studies point out that women migrants are particularly disadvantaged in terms of their access to social capital, and that they are more vulnerable than men to suffering inequality and various forms of discrimination (Anucha et al. 2006; Kawar 2004; Premji, Messing, and Lippel 2008). Kawar (2004) and Gravel and colleagues (2008) show that women migrants with adequate training and skills tend to be caught more frequently in irregular or exploitive employment situations, and that their work generally involves fewer responsibilities with no opportunity for career advancement. Similarly, Hawthorne (2006) has found that age tends to be more of an impediment to finding work for women migrants than for their male counterparts, and Anucha and colleagues (2006) report that the creation of social capital is more difficult for immigrant women than men, since women are more likely to be cut off from their social network and because child rearing impacts the size of women's networks differently than men's. VanderPlaat and Barrett (2006) also argue that research is needed that recognizes how the centrality of caregiving and kinship work affects women's immigration experiences, including their participation in formal and informal social networks.

Women migrants, who are often dependents or family-class migrants, also deal with inequalities with respect to full participation in the life of the host country. This is the case primarily due to structural variations in access to social, economic, political, and cultural resources (Abel 2006; Galabuzi and Labonté 2002). These resources are often linked to inequalities and oppression related to ethnic background, gender, and immigrant status (Abel 2006; Galabuzi and Labonté 2002). Consequently, immigrant women frequently do not belong to the mainstream community and do not have access to the appropriate networks of social relationships, values, norms, and behavioural patterns that contribute to a healthy life (Abel 2006). These findings are especially relevant today, as globalization entails a much larger flow of female migrants than in previous decades (Della Giusta and Kambhampati 2006).

Considering how important social capital is for the experience of migration, the intersection of social determinants of health such as ethnic background, pre-migration experience, and gender roles has elicited little discussion. Furthermore, Anucha and colleagues (2006) suggest that the dearth of literature that 'directly addresses the experiences of immigrant women particularly within the context of settlement' (13) is a major challenge for public health. Social and structural environments need to be better understood with regard to their contributions to the 'mobilization of social capital' by migrant women and men towards a 'successful' integration into a new host society. As gender determines the probability of emigrating, combining individual factors, family factors, and social factors, it is suggested that *empowerment* for health involves being able to achieve a certain level of equality in personal relationships as well as in the social and political spheres (Dyck and Dossa 2007; Llacér et al. 2007; Mohindra and Haddad 2005).

The objective of the next section is to share results from a targeted literature review meant to identify how social capital may have been specifically conceptualized and addressed as a resource for women migrants in the public health literature. A larger keyword search, including such terms as *social capital, gender/women,* and *migration/ethnicity* resulted in very few articles that considered the intersection of any of these terms with health (see Tables 1 and 2 below).

Table 1
Keywords Used

- Social capital
- Gender
- Men, male
- Women, female
- Migration
- Ethnicity, ethnic affiliation
- Culture
- Health, perceptions of

Table 2
No. of Articles Discussing Social Capital

1 or more of the keywords; n = 79	2 or more of the keywords; n = 27	Intersection of 3 or more of the keywords; n = 15

Out of the 15 papers, three emerged from our literature search that dealt specifically with the intersection of three or more of our concept categories (social capital, gender/men/women, migration/ethnicity/culture, and health). The articles examine how access to social capital during the migratory process is shaped by being a female or male migrant and how social capital resources are addressed as a source of support for good health. The term *gender* was often used as a proxy for male and female sex rather than being understood as a social construction that shapes women migrants' acquisition of social capital and their subsequent health.

Ooka and Wellman (2003) used survey data to examine the job searches of three generations of women and men from five ethnic groups in Toronto. They analysed which factors influence the use of intra-ethnic and inter-ethnic ties (elements of social capital) when women and men conduct job searches. Their study did not explicitly concern the social construct of gender, but the authors discussed the differential in men's and women's use of networks to find employment. They suggested that the more ethnically heterogeneous an immigrant's networks, the more likely they are to use inter-ethnic ties to find employment and that men and women do not differ in this respect. However, the way in which inter- and intra-ethnic ties and job searches are themselves gendered is left unexplored.

While Bezanson and Carter's (2006) report based on Canada's 2004 General Social Survey does not directly address migrant health, it focuses on issues associated with social capital using a gendered lens. The authors argue that the gender biases inherent in social capital must be addressed if it is to be used as a tool for social policy development in Canada. It is not that women experience a social capital deficit relative to men. It is more likely that the gendered nature of their formal and informal ties may lead to gendered forms of social capital. The subsequent investment of this social capital reaps differing returns (Farmer 2003). Context matters. The authors concede, however, that inherent in surveys are underlying assumptions about the nature of certain networks, and that since the questions and answer options are predetermined some subtleties cannot be captured. Nonetheless, their overview provides the basis for a discussion of policies, as it highlights the way networking and access to resources are gendered.

While the studies by Ooka and Wellman (2003) and Bezanson and Carter (2006) allowed for a somewhat quantitative analysis of differences between men and women in terms of the development of social capital and health achievement, they left unexamined nuances and details regarding the gendered experience of migration. Pilkington (2002) also argues that the use of quantitative measures for examining gender and social capital may not be very useful, particularly since social capital is multi-dimensional and gender is a social experience not easily captured in individually administered survey forms. Moreover, when differences are found between men and women migrants regarding social capital and health, the reasons for these differences are often not addressed, nor are potential solutions to the inequalities discussed.

In the following section, we consider these papers and outline the way in which social capital can be addressed in future public health research so as to be cognizant of gender-sensitive migration experiences.

Llácer and colleagues (2007) make a strong argument for integrating a gender perspective into epidemiology and into considerations of migrant women's health. The authors address the gendered nature of social capital in their discussion of the way social networks, social support and services, employment opportunities, and ethnic density in neighbourhoods in the host country differentially impact men's and women's experiences of migration and health. They highlight migrant women's increased vulnerability to situations of violence, and point to some significant gaps in our knowledge of the differential adverse health effects that poverty, unemployment, health behaviour, use of services, and discrimination can have on men and women migrants.

Arguing for the importance of the social construct of gender, the authors suggest that a gender perspective on the migration process involves recognizing that men and women 'operate in a historically configured relationship of subordination which influences all aspects of their lives, rendering them differentially vulnerable' (Llácer et al. 2007:ii4).

Supporting previous research (Lippel 1998; Messing 1999), the authors argue that such inequities between women and men arise from 'unequal social and economic valuation of productive work (gainful employment) and reproductive work (unpaid work, such as household tasks and care-giving)' (Llácer et al. 2007:ii4).

Salaff and Greve (2004) consider the way dual-career couples from the People's Republic of China (PRC) organize care for their children and rebuild their professional careers after immigration to Canada. Through qualitative interviews with migrants, they directly address the problems Chinese immigrant women face in rebuilding their professional careers, given their loss of social capital upon migration to Canada. The authors demonstrate that the acquisition of social capital among Chinese migrants is gendered, women sharing more losses than their husbands in a context where dual-career couples simultaneously face demands from work and for family reorganization (Salaff and Greve 2004).

Salaff and Greve (2004) confirm, as other studies have done previously, that women are more likely to interrupt their schooling and careers for family responsibilities proceeding with a 'staggered approach' (151) that may run counter to the demands of expected professional career development. Furthermore, the authors indicate that while men's social support and networks allow them to combine work and community effectively, women's social networks bring together work and family. Although these social networks may allow women to find work, they do not help them attain better or more suitable employment. The inability to find or manage employment and family responsibilities in a new country can be a considerable burden, particularly for women, and may constitute a significant source of stress.

The third study, conducted by Della Giusta and Kambhampati (2006), focuses on women migrants in the United Kingdom. The objective of this study was to better understand the role that social networks (micro-level social capital) and local institutions (macro-level social capital) play in shaping women's integration and settlement in a host society. The authors consider that women's acquisition of social capital in the host country is particularly important because geographical mobility may destabilize community and family life, and, consequently, increase the incidence of mental illness among women while lowering the level of trust among individuals.

For example, the authors mention the experience of transnational motherhood. In these situations 'women who leave their families behind are less able to settle and integrate in the host communities' (Della Giusta and Kambhampati 2006:821). However, the logistics of bringing these children with them to the host society and the required childcare can become overwhelming to the mothers. The result is decreased well-being among women migrants. The authors hypothesize that one of the main factors determining the ability of women migrants to feel settled in the UK and in their new neighbourhood is the type of social capital they can access.

Della Giusta and Kambhampati's (2006) findings suggest that the more settled women migrants are in their new environment, the more likely they are to be satisfied with their new lives. In particular, the authors argue that it is critical to consider micro-level social capital through social links with the new host community and links to their own immigrant community. These links in turn allow for a stronger capacity to build macro-social sustainable capital such as adequate housing and access to resources, including immigration services.

Such findings certainly have implications for immigration policy if they are to be 'socially' sensitive and aim to build on the inherent 'capital' that the new migrants bring along as they arrive and settle in a new society. In this regard, the responsibilities given to institutions, both formal (government, social services, voluntary sector) and informal (various social networks) may need to be revisited in view of accounting more systematically for the diverse 'types' of 'capital' that women and men newcomers bring along.

Implications for Public Health

As noted earlier, different fields of research have conceptualized social capital in ways that are quite distinct (Anucha et al. 2006; Field 2003; Moore et al. 2005). The wide appeal and diversity of application of the concept have also meant that it risks 'becoming everything to everyone' (Frank 2003:3) irrespective of the gendered nature of the concept. While there is little consensus as to what social capital specifically consists of, or how gender affects experiences of migration, there is some consensus regarding the need for health strategies and 'successful' integration to take into account the social resources that newcomers can mobilize.

A discourse of empowerment may provide a useful framework within which to construct a research and program agenda focusing on migrant women, social capital formation, and public health. The concept of empowerment admittedly has as many definitions as does that of social capital (See Torres et al., this volume, for further exploration), but some of the key features provide promising direction for public health policy, programming, and practice. For example, a majority of formulations of the idea of empowerment recognize that the process must start from the perspective of everyday life (Gittell, Ortega-Bustamente, and Steffy 2000; VanderPlaat and Barrett 2006). As noted earlier, we know that employment and the workplace may not be particularly empowering spaces for migrant women in terms of social-capital formation; however, we have not explored where such spaces *do* exist. As Lister (2005) points out, women, especially marginalized women, tend to live in the interstices of the public and the private. VanderPlaat and Barrett (2006) argue for the importance of recognizing the potential that these women's spaces hold for empowerment and informal network formation.

Furthermore, when considered in the context of social capital formation, empowerment may be more useful when formulated as a collective
rather than an individualistic activity (Raven et al. 2003; VanderPlaat,
Samson, and Raven 2001). The implications for social capital formation
are best articulated in the community development and community
health literature (Allen and Dillman 1994; Besser 1998; Flora 1998; Gittell and Thompson 2001; James, Schulz, and van Olphen 2001; Kawachi 2001; Portes and Mooney 2002). In terms of this discussion, what
is important is whether we are aiming for a discourse of social capital
and health that addresses individual as opposed to collective empowerment and agency (Bruegal 2005). The answer has significant implications for how programs and practices are formulated.

A better understanding of women's spaces and the role of collective
agency also demand referring to 'communicative space' as essential
(VanderPlaat 1998; Dyck and Dossa 2007). As Bruegel (2005) argues:
'The development of social capital requires resources of time and space,
the existence of safe, accessible public space, and the social and physical
means of on-going, repeated communication' (6). These spaces need to
be consistent with the everyday reality of migrant women's lives (Lister
2005; Molyneux 2002; VanderPlaat and Barrett 2006).

In the end, discussions regarding issues of empowerment as it interacts with gender-sensitive mobilization of social capital need to be
anchored in the experiences and trajectory of immigration. As the demographic landscapes of host countries are transformed, a crossed understanding of empowerment, social capital, and gender issues needs
to be pursued in research, practice, and policies while being sensitive
to the cultural variations of meanings and experiences of integration in
a new society.

PART 4

Conclusion

14 Engendering Migrant Health: Final Reflections

DENISE L. SPITZER

Introduction

The authors in this text have examined a diverse range of foreign-born residents in Canada, from Latina immigrants in Ottawa, Afghan refugee women in Vancouver, and South American women living a liminal existence in Toronto as non-status immigrants, to Sudanese fathers in Calgary and gay and lesbian immigrants in Vancouver. By complicating the topic of immigrant and refugee health, they have helped to illuminate the multiple and dynamic forces that may negatively influence both perceptions of health status and incidences of certain acute and chronic conditions that can be read as loss of the healthy immigrant effect.

Migrant Health Redux

Downward mobility and diminished possession of and access to resources reflect emergent and shifting forms of social stratification that are the by-products of global capitalism. Currently, over one-third of economic immigrants to Canada report a decline in socio-economic status, citing the lack of recognition of foreign credentials and work experience as prominent reasons for their exclusion from suitable employment (Salaff, Greve, and Ping 2002; Schellenberg and Maheux 2007). The devaluation of skills and work experience gained outside Canada highlights the demarcation lines of social and economic exclusion and launches newcomers on a downward spiral characterized by underemployment and poor wages. Immigrants' declining circumstances are evidenced by the disproportionately high rates of unemployment and underemployment (Zietsma 2007), and statistics that show that 65 per cent of immigrants fall into low income within their first decade in Canada regardless of educational attainment (Picot, Hou, and Coulombe 2007). Notably, financial return on foreign experience has declined to zero in the last decade (Picot and Hou 2009).

Movement towards poverty, with its attendant impacts on health and well-being, also leads to a growing disparity between expectations, ambitions, hopes, dreams – and lived reality. Over 35 per cent of economic immigrants serving as principal applicants on their immigration files presumably possessed attributes deemed to align with the needs of the labour market. Consequently, they anticipated that they would attain financial and professional success; however, life in Canada has fallen short of their expectations (Schellenberg and Maheux 2007).

Imbued with racist underpinnings, country of origin, ethnicity, religion, and phenotype figure prominently in structuring the opportunities offered newcomers in Canada (Grant 2005; Teelucksingh and Galabuzi 2005a), potentially resulting in disappointment, anger, frustration, bitterness, and stress (Grant 2005). For many, these experiences are embedded in 'everyday racism … the integration of racism into everyday situations … that activate[s] underlying power relations' (Essed 1991:50) and reinforce social exclusion.

Complicating their attempts to navigate the shifting terrain of life in Canada are changes to gender roles in particular as they intersect with expectations of productive and reproductive labour. Resultantly, individual and collective identities are challenged under the process of migration and its aftermath, requiring renegotiation as certain roles and values that underpin identity are lost or altered, potentially leading to increased mental health problems and violence. In some circumstances these confrontations and renegotiations may open new sources of meaning and support; for instance, some women may find more economic independence in Canada. Concomitantly, unwanted identities can also be inscribed on migrant bodies – potentially constraining their ability to take action on their lives as they wish they could (Spitzer 2008).

The health implications of this phenomenon can be viewed as the body's response to the social environment. Poverty and the dynamics of downward mobility; the loss of identities, social networks, and stability; the lack of meaningful, steady, and remunerative employment; exposure to racism, sexism, homophobia, and/or Islamophobia; and lack of control in the workplace – taken together with frustrated

ambitions, unfulfilled dreams, and the pressures of gendered role expectations – may induce chronic stress that can lead to negative health
outcomes precipitated by a cascade of effects involving the nervous
and endocrine systems (Hyman 2007b; Krieger, Chen, and Selby 2001;
Lightman 2008; Siegrist and Marmot 2004; Spitzer 2005).

Importantly, transitioning to poverty and/or to poor health status
is neither uniform nor universal. Social location, the configuration of
intersecting identifiers including gender, ethnicity, religion, sexuality, dis/ability, and migration status, among others, can structure the
pathways and direction of one's socio-economic mobility. Furthermore,
newcomer status as immigrant or family member thereof, refugee or
refugee claimant, migrant worker, or non-status immigrant, shapes access to governmental programs and to both formal and social citizenship that can likewise constrain or facilitate upward mobility.

In our efforts to operationalize intersectionality and highlight diversity of locations and experiences, authors in this volume have helped
to illuminate the hetereogeneity of individuals, communities, and
contexts that are subsumed under the category of 'immigrant,' and to
challenge the dominant discourse that often constructs a singular immigrant experience marked by lack and vulnerability. This text, however, provides several concrete examples of healthful interventions which
build on individual and communal strengths and resources, and which
further enhance collective and personal social capital and the ability to
give and receive social support. Significantly, social capital, the availability of social support, and a place (physical or metaphoric) to connect are vital to sustaining community members and have the potential
to mitigate deleterious effects for individuals and communities.

Whither Migrant Health?

Moving towards more equitable health for foreign-born Canadians and
their descendents requires a critical approach to notions of health and
well-being, the realm of policy, and to supporting individual and communal strengths.

First, both qualitative and quantitative research indicates that social
determinants of health influence the health and well-being of migrants
more significantly than biogenetic factors (Dunn and Dyck 2000).
Whether expressed in terms of identifiable conditions or through symptoms that elude biomedical categorization, these health outcomes often
emerge from or are exacerbated by interactions between individuals

and the social environment they inhabit. As a result, narrowly focused biomedical analyses fail to grasp the complexity of migrant health issues and limit interventions primarily to the biomedical realm.

Realigning attention towards the body and its response to the environment provides a more holistic platform with which to regard migrant health and launch more efficacious interventions and policies. Governmental response need also reflect the embrace of this approach, requiring departmental and jurisdictional cross-border cooperation instead of the current fractured policy environment where policy makers are often confined to singular policy silos. Indeed, the current policy making context belies Canada's commitment towards population health that requires joint policy action. For instance, while raising minimum wage may be more beneficial to foreign-born Canadians than biomedical services, there does not appear to be a forum for bringing diverse policy interests together to produce policy changes that reflect what we know about issues such as social determinants of health.

A more nuanced approach is also needed to ensure that policies and programs are appropriately targeted and have minimal untoward effects. The heterogeneity of individuals, communities, histories, and identities contained under rubrics such as immigrant, refugee, migrant, refugee claimant, and undocumented worker complicate the implementation of programs and policies. In addition, consequences of inclusion under a particular category intersects with gender, ethnicity, religion, sexuality, and so on to produce a disparate array of presentations and responses to policy interdictions. Attention to social location, migration status, bodily response, and lived experience along with policies and practices that attend to the heterogeneity and lived experiences of newcomers to Canada are essential. In addition, we need to consider ongoing changes to the discursive construction of immigrants and refugees and its impact, not only on public opinion and consequently political action, but also on self-regard of cultural communities and individuals. While social determinants of health are of major significance to migrant health, better access to health services is also important to the development of an equitable, engendered migrant health.

Conclusion

To advance this approach, further research is required to learn more about the application of intersectional analysis to policy-relevant research on migrant health that will, among other effects, account for the dynamic and flexible application of identities that are part of quotidian existence.

More research is also needed with those who fall outside of the major immigration categories such as undocumented immigrants, refugee claimants, and family members of principal applicants. Further examinations are needed into the impact of policies on the diversity of individuals under each category, and into the dominant discursive constructions that sustain the images of those who fall under the assigned category that can also facilitate or constrain newcomers' ability to maintain or attain good health status.

Immigration contributes significantly to Canada. We rely on immigration to sustain our population and our economy; thus, even in the most utilitarian sense, good migrant health benefits us all.

I opened this text by posing the question: 'Is migrating to Canada bad for your health?' As a society, Canadians must ask ourselves: 'Must it be?'

References

Abel, T. 2006. Cultural capital in health promotion. In *Health and modernity: The role of theory in health promotion,* ed. D.V. McQueen, I. Kickbusch, L. Potvin, J.M. Pelikan, L. Balbo, and T. Abel. New York: Springer.

Abella, I., and H. Troper. 1982. *None is too many: Canada and the Jews of Europe 1933–1948.* Toronto: Lester and Orpen Dennys.

Abella, R.S. 1984. *Égalité en matière d'emploi. Rapport de la Commission sur l'égalité en matière d'emploi.* Ottawa: Approvisionnements et Services Canada.

ACCESS Alliance. 2005. *Racialised groups and health status.* http://accessalliance.ca/index.php [accessed 26 September 2007].

Adler, P.S., and S.W. Kwon. 2000. Social capital: The good, the bad and the ugly. In *Knowledge and social capital: Foundations and applications,* ed. E. Lesser. Boston: Butterworth-Heinemann.

African and Caribbean Council on HIV/AIDS in Ontario (ACCHO). 2001. African and Caribbean Council on HIV/AIDS in Ontario.

– 2002. *Report on phase two of community consultation.* Toronto: African and Caribbean Council on HIV/AIDS in Ontario.

– 2006. *AIDS 2006 African/Black Diaspora stream: Bringing the hidden epidemic to an international audience.* Toronto: African and Caribbean Council on HIV/AIDS in Ontario.

Agardh, E., A. Ahlbom, T. Andersson, S. Efendic, V. Grill, J. Hallqvist, A. Norman, and C. Östenson. 2003. Work stress and low sense of coherence is associated with Type 2 diabetes in middle-aged Swedish women. *Diabetes Care* 26:719–24.

Ahearn, F. 2000, ed. *Psychosocial wellness of refugees: Issues in qualitative and quantitative research.* Vol. 7 of *Studies in forced migration.* New York: Berghahn Books.

Ahmad F., A. Shik, R. Vanza, A.M. Cheung, U. George, and D.E. Stewart. 2004. Voices of South Asian women: Immigration and mental health. *Women and Health* 40(4):113–30.

Alcock, P., and L. Christensen. 1995. In and against the state: community-based organisations in Britain and Denmark in the 1990s. *Community Development Journal* 30:110–20.

Alcuitas, H., L. Alcuitas-Imperial, C. Diocson, and J. Ordinario. 1997. *Trapped: 'Holding on to the knife's edge': Economic violence against Filipino migrant/immigrant women.* Vancouver: Philippine Women's Centre of BC.

Ali, A., N. Massaquoi, and M. Brown. 2003. *Women's health in women's hands community health centre: Racial discrimination as a health risk for female youth: Implications for policy and healthcare delivery in Canada.* Toronto: Canadian Race Relations Foundation.

Ali, J.S. 2002. Mental health of Canada's immigrants. *Health Reports* 13(suppl.):1–12.

Ali, J.S., S. McDermott, and R.G. Gravel. 2004. Recent research on immigrant health from statistics Canada's population surveys. *Canadian Journal of Public Health* 95(3):I9–13.

Alinsky, S. 1989. *Rules for radicals: A pragmatic primer for realistic radicals.* New York: Vintage Books.

Allen, J.C., and D.A. Dillman. 1994. *Against all odds: Rural community in the information age.* Boulder, CO: Westview Press.

Altman, D. (2004). Gay/lesbian movements. *International Encyclopedia of the Social and Behavioral Sciences* (pp. 5895–9). www.sciencedirect.com/science/referenceworks/ [accessed 2 May 2009].

Amaratunga, C., J. Stanton, and B. Clow, eds. 2002. *Race, ethnicity and women's health.* Halifax: Atlantic Centre of Excellence for Women's Health.

American College of Physicians. 2004. Racial and ethnic disparities in health care: A position paper of the American College of Physicians. *Annals of Internal Medicine* 141:226–8.

Amnesty International. 2006. Sexual minorities and the law: A world survey [updated 2006]. www.ai-lgbt.org [accessed 2 May 2009].

Anderson, J., and S. Reimer Kirkham. 1998. Constructing nation: The gendering and racializing of the Canadian health care system. In *Painting the maple: Essays on race, gender, and the construction of Canada,* 242–61. Ed. V. Strong-Boag, S. Grace, A. Eisenberg, and J. Anderson. Vancouver: University of British Columbia Press.

Anderson, L.M., S.C. Scrimshaw, M.T. Fullilove, J.E. Fielding, J. Normand, and Task Force on Community Preventive Services. 2003. Culturally competent healthcare systems: A systematic review. *American Journal of Preventive Medicine* 24:68–79.

Anderson, P. 2004. Survival on the margins: Summary of a research project on the undocumented in Munich. *Journal of International Migration and Integration* 5(1):53–76.

Andrew, C., L. Cardinal, M. Kérisit, H. Dallaire, F. Boudreau, D. Farmer, L. Bouchard, D. Lemire, D. Adam, D. Culligan, A. Rochon-Ford, and Institute for Clinical Evaluative Studies. 1997. *Les conditions de possibilité des services de santé et des services sociaux en français en Ontario: Un enjeu pour les femmes.* Toronto: La Table féministe Francophone de concertation provinciale de l'Ontario.

Anne Wright and Associates, Inc. 2003. *From sprint to marathon: A strategic plan for getting in shape for a new era of HIV/AIDS in Ottawa.* Prepared for the Ottawa-Carleton Council on AIDS. Ottawa: Ottawa-Carleton Council on AIDS.

Anucha, U., N.S. Dlamini, M.C. Yan, and L. Smylie. 2006. *Social capital and the welfare of immigrant women: A multi-level study of four ethnic communities in Windsor.* Ottawa: Status of Women Canada.

Apanovitch, A.M., D. McCarthy, and P. Salovey. 2003. Using message framing to motivate HIV testing among low-income, ethnic minority women. *American Psychological Association* 22(1):60–7.

Archer, B. 1999. The end of gay (and the death of heterosexuality). Toronto: Doubleday Canada.

Armstrong, P. 1996. The feminization of the labour force: Harmonizing down in a global economy. In *Rethinking restructuring: Gender and change in Canada,* 29–54. Ed. I. Bakker. Toronto: University of Toronto Press.

– 2004. Health, social policy, social economies and the voluntary sector. In *The Social Determinants of Health: Canadian Perspectives,* 341–4. Ed. D. Raphael. Toronto: Canadian Scholar's Press.

Armstrong, P., and H. Armstrong. 2001. *Thinking it through: Women, work and caring in the new millennium.* Halifax: Maritime Centre of Excellence for Women's Health.

Aroian, K. 1993. Health risks and problems encountered by illegal immigrants. *Issues in Mental Health Nursing* 14:379–97.

Ashcraft, C. 2000. Naming knowledge: A language for reconstructing domestic violence and systemic gender inequity. *Women and Language* 23:3–10.

Astbury J. 2001. *Gender disparities in mental health.* World Health Organization Ministerial Round Tables.

Audy, R. 1994. Collaboration between police and social service practitioners: Failure or success? *Social Worker* 62:133–6.

Austin, C., and D. Este. 2001. The working experiences of underemployed immigrant and refugee men: Implications for social work practice. *Canadian Social Work Review* 18(1):213–29.

Aycan, Z., and J.W. Berry. 1996. Impact of employment-related experiences on immigrants' well-being and adaptation to Canada. *Canadian Journal of Behavioral Science* 28(3):240–51.

Baksh-Soodeen, R. (series editor), C. Amaratunga, J. Gahagan, S. Bentley (Canadian eds.), and T. Johnson (contributing ed.). 2002. *Gender mainstreaming in HIV/AIDS: Taking a multisectoral approach.* London: Commonwealth Secretariat and the Maritime Centre of Excellence for Women's Health.

Bannerji, H. 2000. *The dark side of the nation: Essays on multiculturalism, nationalism and gender.* Toronto, Canada: Canadian Scholars' Press.

– 2004. Immigrant women: Labour in the North American continent. In *Globalization*, 87–92. Ed. M. Bhattacharya. New Delhi: Tulika Books.

Bannerman, M., P. Hoa, and R. Male. 2003. *South Riverdale Community Health Centre's exploration of services for non-insured people of East Toronto.* Toronto: South Riverdale Community Health Centre.

Barnes, D.M., and R. Aguilar. 2007. Community social support for Cuban refugees in Texas. *Qualitative Health Research* 17 (February):225–37. http://qhr.sagepub.com [accessed 4 July 2007].

Barriga, M., and G. Vanzaghi. 2006. Mujeres inmigrantes latinoamericanas: identidad, participación y familia. In *Ruptures, continuities and re-learning. The political participation of Latin Americans in Canada*, 101–10. Ed. Jorge Ginieniewicz and Daniel Schugurensky. Toronto: Ontario Institute for Studies in Education/University of Toronto (OISE/UT).

Basavarajappa, K.G., and F. Jones. 1999. Visible minority income differences. In *Immigrant Canada: Demographic, Economic and Social Challenges*, 230–60. Ed. S. Halli and L. Driedger. Toronto: University of Toronto Press.

Basran, G., and Zong, L. 1998. Devaluation of foreign credentials as perceived by visible minority professional immigrants. *Canadian Ethnic Studies* 30(3):6–23.

Bassolé, A., H. Hamboyan, M. Kérisit, N. Plante, and M. Young. 2004. *L'impact du conflit armé sur l'intégration des femmes immigrantes et des réfugiées Francophones en Ontario.* Rapport présenté au Mouvement ontarien des femmes immigrantes Francophones (MOFIF). Ottawa.

Bauder, H. 2003. 'Brain abuse,' or the devaluation of immigrant labour in Canada. *Antipode* 35(4): 699–717.

Baukje, M., and S. Wachholtz. 1999. A complex web: Access to justice for abused immigrant women in New Brunswick. *Canadian Women's Studies* 19:175–81.

Beaulieu, M., M. Kérisit, P. Michaud, and D. Lemire. 2000. La santé communautaire en français: Analyse de quatre modèles au sein des communautés Francophones et acadiennes. http://www.fcfa.ca [accessed 10 October 2007].

Behar, R. 1996. *The vulnerable observer: Anthropology that breaks your heart*. Boston: Beacon Press.

Beiser, M. 1990. Migration: Opportunity or mental health risk. *Triangle* 29(2/3):83-90.

– 1999. *Strangers at the gate: The 'Boat People's' first ten years in Canada*. Toronto: University of Toronto Press.

– 2005. The health of immigrants and refugees in Canada. *Canadian Journal of Public Health* 96(2):S30–44.

– 2006. Longitudinal research to promote effective refugee resettlement. *Transcultural Psychiatry* 43:56–71.

Beiser, M., M. Cargo, and M.A. Woodbury. 1994. A comparison of psychiatric disorder in different cultures: Depressive typologies in Southeast Asian refugees and resident Canadians. *International Journal of Methods in Psychiatric Research* 4:157–79.

Beiser M., and F. Hou. 2001. Language acquisition, unemployment and depressive disorder among Southeast Asian refugees: A 10-year study. *Social Science and Medicine* 53(10):1321–34.

Beiser, M., and I. Hyman. 1997. Southeast Asian Refugees in Canada. In *Ethnicity, Immigration and Psychopathology*, ed. I. Al-Issa and M. Tousignant. New York: Plenum Publishing.

Beiser, M., L. Simich, and N. Pandalangat. 2003. Community in distress: Mental health needs and help-seeking in the Tamil community in Toronto. *International Migration* 41(5):233–45.

Beiser, M., and K.A. Wickrama. 2004. Trauma, time and mental health: A study of temporal reintegration and depressive disorder among Southeast Asian refugees. *Psychological Medicine* 34(5):899–910.

Berinstein, C., J. McDonald, P. Nyers, C. Wright, and S. Sahar Zerehi. 2006. Access Not Fear: Non-Status Immigrants and City Services Preliminary Report. (February) Toronto. http://www.socsci.mcmaster.ca/polisci/emplibrary/Access%20Not%20Fear%20Report%20(Feb%202006).pdf [accessed 3 May 2009].

Berk, M., and C. Schur. 2001. The effect of fear on access to care among undocumented Latino immigrants. *Journal of Immigrant Health* 3:151–6.

Besser, T.L. 1998. The significance of community to business social responsibility. *Rural Sociology* 63(3):412–31.

Beteta, H.C. 2006. What is missing in measures of women's empowerment? *Journal of Human Development* 7(2):221–41.

Bezanson, K., and E. Carter. 2006. *Public policy and social reproduction: Gendering social capital*. Ottawa: Status of Women Canada.

Bhandari, S., S. Horvath, and R. To. 2006. Choices and voices of immigrant men: Reflections on social integration. *Canadian Ethnic Studies 38*(1):140–8.

Bhalotra S., M.B.M. Ruwe, G.K. Strickler, A.M. Ryan, and C.L. Hurley. 2007. Disparities in utilization of coronary artery disease treatment by gender, race and ethnicity: Opportunities for prevention. *Journal of the National Black Nurses Association* 18(1):36–49.

Bhugra, D., C. Harding, and R. Lippett. 2004. Pathways into care and satisfaction with primary care for black patients in South London. *Journal of Mental Health* (UK) 13(2):171–83.

Bilge, S. 2005. *Between a rock and a hard place: Minority women's citizenship in Canada, its intersecting inequalities, and what an intersectional theorizing can offer*, 71–6. Proceedings of the symposium: Muslim Women's Equality Rights in the Justice System: Gender, Religion and Pluralism. Toronto: Canadian Council of Muslim Women.

Blas, E., L. Gilson, M. Kelly, R. Labonté, J. Lapitan, C. Muntaner, P. Östlin, J. Popay, R. Sadana, G. Sen, T. Schrecker, and Z. Vaghri. 2008. Addressing social determinants of health inequities: What can the state and civil society do? *Lancet* 372:1684–9.

Booker, V., J. Robinson, B. Kay, L. Najera, and G. Stewart. 1997. Changes in empowerment: Effects of participation in a lay health promotion program. *Health Education and Behavior* 24(4):452–65.

Both, P. 2003. *South Sudan: Forgotten tragedy.* Bloomington, IN: Author House.

Bouchard, C. 2003. Nurturing dads. In *On fathers ground: A portrait of projects to support and promote fathering*, 5–9. Ed. C. Bolte, A. Devault, M. St-Denis, and J. Gaudet. Montreal: Canadian Institute of Child Health.

Bourdieu, P. 1980. Le capital social. *Actes de la Recherche en Sciences Sociales* 31:2–3.

– 1986. Forms of capital. In *Handbook of Theory and Research for the Sociology of Education*, 241-60. Ed. J.R. Richardson. Westport, CT: Greenwood Press.

Boudreau, F., and D. Farmer. 1997. *Profil épidémiologique des francophones de l'Ontario au niveau de la santé et du mieux-être : Les faits sallants revisités et comparés*. Toronto: Table féministe francophone de concertation provinciale.

Bowen, S. 2001. Language barriers in access to health care. Ottawa: Health Canada. http://www.hc-sc.gc.ca/hppb/healthcare/equity/index.html [accessed 10 October 2007].

Boyd M., and E. Grieco. 2003. *Migration fundamentals – women and migration: Incorporating gender into international migration theory*. Migration Information Source. http://www.migrationinformation.org/Feature/display.cfm?ID =106 [accessed 3 April 2005].

Boyd, M., and D. Pikkov. 2005. *Gendering migration, livelihood and entitlements:*

Migrant women in Canada and the United States. (Occasional Paper 6). Geneva: United Nations Research Institute for Social Development.

Brodsky, A. 2003. *With all our strength: The revolutionary association of the women of Afghanistan.* New York: Routledge.

Brondolo, E., R. Rieppi, K.P. Kelly, and W. Gerin. 2003. Perceived racism and blood pressure: A review of the literature and conceptual and methodological critique. *Annals of Behavioral Medicine* 25(1):55–65.

Brooker, A.-S., and J. Eakin. 2001. Gender, class, work-related stress and health: Toward a power-centred approach. *Journal of Community and Applied Social Psychology* 11:97–109.

Brotman, S., B. Ryan, Y. Jalbert, and B. Rowe. 2002. The impact of coming out on health and health care access: The experiences of gay, lesbian, bisexual and Two-Spirit people. *Journal of Health and Social Policy* 15(1):1–29.

Browne, A., V. Smye, and C. Varcoe. 2007. Postcolonial-feminist theoretical perspectives and women's health. In *Women's health in Canada. Critical perspectives on theory and policy,* 124–42. Ed. M. Morrow, O. Hankivsky, and C. Varcoe, Toronto: University of Toronto Press.

Browne, A., C. Varcoe, V. Smye, S. Reimer-Kirkham, M.J. Lynam, and S. Wong. 2009. Cultural safety and the challenges of translating critically oriented knowledge in practice. *Nursing Philosophy* 10:167–79.

Bruegel, I. 2005. Social capital and feminist critique. In *Women and social capital.* Ed. J. Franklin. Families and Social Capital ESRC Research Group Working Paper No. 12. London South Bank University.

Brunet, L., and M.-L. Garceau. 2004. *Faire autant avec si peu ... Bilan et profil des services français en matière de violence contre les femmes.* Ottawa: Action ontarienne contre la violence faite aux femmes.

Bui, H.N., and M. Morash. 1999. Domestic violence in the Vietnamese immigrant community: An exploratory study. *Violence Against Women* 5(7):769–95.

Cabrera, N., C. Tamis-LeMonda, R. Bradley, S. Hofferth, S., and M. Lamb. 2000. Fatherhood in the twenty-first century. *Child Development* 71(1):127–36.

Cameron, H. 2005. *Barriers and issues in access to French-language health services in BC / Obstacles et problèmes relatifs à l'accès en français aux soins de santé en Colombie Britannique.* Société Santé en Français. Vancouver: Provincial Health Authority.

Cameron, M. 2005. Two-spirited Aboriginal people: Continuing cultural appropriation by non-Aboriginal society. *Canadian Woman Studies* 24(2/3):123.

Campbell, C., and P. Gillies. 2001. Conceptualizing 'social capital' for health promotion in small local communities: A micro-qualitative study. *Journal of Community and Applied Social Psychology* 11:329–46.

Campbell, C. and C. McLean. 2003. Social capital, local community participation and the construction of Pakistani identities in England: Implications for health inequalities policies. *Journal of Health Psychology* 8(2):247–62.

Campbell, J., A.S. Jones, J. Dienemann, J. Kub, J. Schollenberger, P. O'Campo. 2002. Intimate partner violence and physical health consequences. *Archives of Internal Medicine* 162:1157–63.

Canadian Centre for Justice Statistics. 2003. *Family violence in Canada: A statistical profile 2003*. Ed. H. Johnson and K. AuCoin. Cat. no. 85-224-XIE. Ottawa: Statistics Canada.

– 2005. *Family violence in Canada: A statistical profile 2005*. Ed. K. AuCoin.. Cat. no. 85-224-XIE. Ottawa: Statistics Canada.

Canadian Council for Refugees (CCR). 1998. Best settlement practices: Settlement services for immigrants and refugees in Canada. Ottawa: Canadian Council for Refugees.

– 2004. *More than a nightmare: Delays in refugee family reunification*. Montreal: Canadian Council for Refugees. http://www.web.ca/ccr [accessed 8 August 2007].

Canadian Council on Multicultural Health. 1989. Proceedings of the Canadian Council on Multicultural Health. In First Nations Conference. Toronto: Canadian Council on Multicultural Health.

Canadian Race Relations Foundation. http://www.crr.ca/ [accessed 8 August 2007].

Canadian Research Institute for the Advancement of Women (CRIAW). 2002. *Women's experience of racism: How race and gender interact*. http://www.criaw-icref.ca/indexFrame_e.htm [accessed 4 July 2007].

– 2006. *Intersectional feminist frameworks (IFFs): An emerging vision*. http://www.criaw-icref.ca/indexFrame_e.htm [accessed 7 July 2007].

Canadian Task Force on Mental Health Issues Affecting Immigrants and Refugees. 1988. *After the door has opened: Mental health issues affecting immigrants and refugees*. Ottawa: Minister of Supply and Services Canada.

Caragata, L. 1999. The privileged public: Who is permitted citizenship? *Community Development Journal* 34:270–86.

Cardinal, Linda. 2001. *Chroniques d'une vie politique mouvementée. L'Ontario Francophone de 1986 à 1996*. Ottawa: Le Nordir.

Carty, L., and D. Brand. 1993. 'Visible minority' women: A creation of the Canadian state. In *Returning the gaze: Essays on racism, feminism and politics*, 169–81. Ed. H. Bannerji. Toronto: Sister Vision Press.

Castles, S. 2002. Migration and community formation under conditions of globalization. *International Migration Review* 36(4):1143–68.

Catholic Immigration Centre (CIC). n.d. *Last stop Canada: Promoting creative dialogue*. Ottawa: Catholic Immigration Centre.

Caulford, P., and Y. Vali. 2006. Providing health care to medically uninsured immigrants and refugees. *Canadian Medical Association Journal* 174:1253–4.

Cermeño, N., L. MacLean, and A. Estable. 2004. Expected impact of spending cuts on population groups. In *Public Forum*. Presentation given to the Health and Social Services Advisory Committee. Ottawa: Health and Social Services Advisory Committee.

Chauvin, P., and I. Parizot. 2006. Enquete européenne sur l'acces aux soins des personnes en situation irreguliere: Données de l'Observatoire European de Médecins du Monde, Rapport final. Equipe de recherches sur les determinants sociaux de la sante et du recours auz soins, UMRS 707 (INSERM), Universite Peirre et Marie Curie, Paris.

Chard, J., J. Badets, and L. Howatson-Leo. 2000. *Women in Canada: A gender-based statistical analysis*, 189–217. Ottawa: Statistics Canada.

Chavez, L. 1992. *Shadowed lives: Undocumented immigrants in American society*. Fort Worth, TX: Holt, Rinehart and Winston.

Chen, J., E. Ng, and R. Wilkins. 1996. The health of Canada's immigrants in 1994–95. *Health Reports* 7(4):33–45.

Chen, J., R. Wilkins, and E. Ng. 1996. Health expectancy by immigrant status, 1986 and 1991. *Health Reports* 8(3):29–38.

Chin, J.L. 2007. Overview: *Women and leadership – transforming visions and diverse voices*, 1–17. Ed. J. L. Chin, B. Lott, J. K. Rice, and J. Sanchez-Hucles. Malden, MA: Blackwell Publishing.

Christensen, C.P. 2001. Immigrant minorities in Canada. In *Canadian social welfare*, 180–209. 4th ed. Ed. J.C. Turner and F.J. Turner. Toronto: Pearson Education Canada.

Chui, T. 2003. *Longitudinal Survey of Immigrants to Canada: Process, Progress and Prospects*. Ottawa: Statistics Canada.

Churchill, W. 1967. *Homosexual behavior among males: A cross-cultural and cross-species investigation*. New York: Hawthorn Books.

Citizenship and Immigration Canada (CIC). 2005. *Annual report to Parliament on immigration, 2005*: Sec. 6, Gender-based analysis of the impact of Immigration and Refugee Protection Act. www.cic.gc.ca/english/resources/publications/annual-report2005/section6.asp [accessed 26 January 2008].

– 2006a. *Plan stratégique pour favoriser l'immigration au sein des communautés Francophones en situation minoritaire*. Ottawa: http://www.cic.gc.ca/english/resources/publications/settlement/plan-minorities.asp [accessed 8 April 2007].

– 2006b. *Consultations on the settlement and language training services needs of newcomers*. In support of the Canada-Ontario Immigration Agreement. Ottawa: CIC.

– 2007. *Annual report to Parliament on immigration: Facts and figures.* Ottawa: CIC. www.cic.gc.ca/english/resources/publications/annual-report2007/section6.asp [accessed 2 May 2009].

– 2008a. *Facts and figures: Immigration overview: Permanent and temporary residents.* Ottawa: CIC.

– 2008b. *Sponsoring your family.* www.cic.gc.ca/english/immigrate/sponsor/index.asp [accessed 3 October 2008].

– 2009a. Medical exam requirements for permanent residents. http://www.cic.gc.ca/english/resources/publications/welcome/wel-06e.asp [accessed 26 May 2009].

– 2009b. Welcome to Canada: What you should know – health services. http://www.cic.gc.ca/english/information/medical/medexams-perm.asp [accessed 26 May 2009].

– 2010. *Annual report to Parliament on immigration 2010.* Section 2: Managing permanent and temporary immigration. Ottawa: CIC. http://www.cic.gc.ca/english/resources/publications/annual-report2010/section2.asp [accessed 3 February 2011].

City of Calgary 2003. *Facts about Calgary immigrants.* Calgary, AB: City of Calgary, Community Strategies, Policy and Planning Division.

– 2007. *Facts about Calgary immigrants.* Calgary, AB: Community and Neighbourhood Services, Social Policy and Planning Division.

Clark, D., R. Shimoni, and D. Este. 2000. *Supporting immigrant and refugee families: A training manual for human services workers.* Calgary, AB: Calgary Immigrant Aid Society.

Coderre, C. 1995. Femmes et santé, en français, s'il vous plaît. *Reflets* 12(1):38–71.

Cohen, R. 2001. The new immigrants: A contemporary profile. In *From immigration to integration: The Canadian Jewish experience: A millennium edition,* chap. 14. http://www.bnaibrith.ca/institute/millennium/millennium14.html [accessed 31 March 2008].

Coker, E. 2004. 'Traveling pains': Embodied metaphors of suffering among southern Sudanese refugees in Cairo. *Culture, Medicine and Psychiatry* 28:15–39.

Coleman J. 1988. Social capital in the creation of human capital. *American Journal of Sociology* 94:S95–120.

Coleman, R. 2003. Gender equality in the Genuine Progress Index. In *Made to measure: Women, gender and equity,* 43–54. Ed. C. Amaratunga. Halifax: Maritime Centre of Excellence for Women's Health.

Connell, R.W. 1994. The state, gender and sexual politics: Theory and appraisal. In *Power/gender: Social relations in theory and practice,* 136–73. Ed. H.L. Radtke and H.J. Stam. Thousand Oaks, CA: Sage.

Cooley, J.K. 1999. *Unholy wars. Afghanistan: American and international terrorism.* London: Pluto Press.

Cooper, P.J. 2000. Canadian refugee services: The challenges of network operation. *Refuge* 18:14–26.

Coover, V., E. Deacon, C. Esser, and C. Moore. 1977. *Resource manual for a living revolution.* Philadelphia: New Society Publishers.

Cornforth, C. 1992. Co-operatives. In *Concise encyclopaedia of participation and co-management.* Ed. G. Szell. New York: Walter de Gruyter Inc.

Cornforth, C., A. Thomas, A. Lewis, and R. Spear. 1988. *Developing successful worker co-operatives.* London: Sage.

Côté, A., M. Kérisit, and M-L. Côté. 2001. *Sponsorship . . . for better or for worse: The impact of sponsorship on the equality rights of immigrant women.* Ottawa: Status of Women Canada.

Coutts, A., P.R. Pinto, B. Cave, and I. Kawachi. 2007. *Social capital indicators in the UK: A research project for the commission for racial equality.* London: Ben Cave Associates.

Canadian Research Institute for the Advancement of Women (CRIAW). 2006. *Intersectional feminist frameworks: An emerging vision.* Ottawa: CRIAW.

Coghlan, B., R. Brennan, P. Ngoy, D. Daffara, B. Otto, M. Clements, and T. Stewart. 2006. *Mortality in the Democratic Republic of Congo: A national survey.* *Lancet* 367(9504):44–51.

Crompton, L. (2003). *Homosexuality and civilization.* Cambridge, MA: Harvard University Press.

Cross, T., B. Bazron, K. Dennis, and M. Isaacs. 1989. *Towards a culturally competent system of care.* Vol. 1. Washington, DC: National Technical Assistance Center for Children's Mental Health, Georgetown University Child Development Center, and NWICWA.

Csete, J. 2004. Bangkok 2004. Not as simple as ABC: Making real progress on women's rights and AIDS. *HIV AIDS Policy Review* 9:68–71.

Csordas, T. 1994. Introduction: The body as representation and being-in-the-world. In *Embodiment and Experience: The Existential Ground of Culture and Self,* 1–24. Ed. T. Csordas. Cambridge, UK: Cambridge University Press.

– 1999. Embodiment and cultural phenomenology. In *Perspectives on embodiment: The intersections of nature and culture,* 143–64. Ed. G. Weiss and H.F. Haber. London: Routledge Press.

– 2002. *Body/Meaning/Healing.* Houndmills, UK: Palgrave Macmillan.

Culbertson, F.M. 1997. Depression and gender. An international review. *American Psychologist* 52(1):25–31.

Daley, A. (2006). Lesbian and gay health issues: OUTside of Canada's health policy. *Critical Social Policy* 26(4):794–816.

Daniels, N. 1982. Equity of access to health care. *Health and Society* 60(1):51–81.

Danso, R. 2001. From 'there' to 'here': An investigation of the initial settlement experiences of Ethiopian and Somali refugees in Toronto. *GeoJournal* 55:3–14.

Das, V. 2001. Sufferings, theodicies, disciplinary practices, appropriations. *International Social Science Journal* 49(4):563–72.

Das, V., and A. Kleinman. 2001. Introduction. In *Remaking a world: Violence, social suffering, and recovery*, 1-30. Ed. V. Das, A. Kleinman, M. Lock, M. Ramphele, and P. Reynolds. Berkeley: University of California Press.

Das Gupta, T. 1994. Political economy of gender, race and class: Looking at South Asian immigrant women in Canada. *Canadian Ethnic Studies* 26 (1):59–73.

– 1996. *Racism and paid work*. Toronto: Garamond Press.

Davis, D. 1983. *Blood and nerves: An ethnographic focus on menopause*. St John's: Institute of Social and Economic Research, Memorial University of Newfoundland.

– 1997. Blood and nerves revisited: Menopause and privatization of the body in a Newfoundland postindustrial fishery. *Medical Anthropology Quarterly* 11(1):3–20.

Deetz, S., and D.K. Mumby. 1990. Power, discourse, and the workplace: Reclaiming the critical tradition. In *Communication Yearbook/13*, 18–47. Ed. J.A. Anderson. Thousand Oaks, CA: Sage.

DeLaet, D. 1999. Introduction: The Invisibility of Women in Scholarship on International Migration. In *Gender and Immigration*, 1–17. Ed. G. Kelson and D. DeLaet. New York: New York University Press.

Della Giusta, M., and U. Kambhampati. 2006. Women migrant workers in the UK: Social capital, well-being and integration. *Journal of International Development* 18:819–33.

del Pozo, J. 2006. La participación política de los latinoamericanos en la provincia de Quebec: El caso de los chilenos. In *Ruptures, continuities and relearning. The political participation of Latin Americans in Canada*, 101–10. Ed. Jorge Ginieniewicz and Daniel Schugurensky. Toronto: Ontario Institute for Studies in Education/University of Toronto (OISE/UT).

De Maio, F., and E. Kemp. 2010. The deterioration of health status among immigrants to Canada. *Global Public Health* 5(5):462–78.

Denzin N., and Y. Lincoln. 2000. Introduction: Entering the field of qualitative research. In *Handbook of Qualitative Research*, 1–17. Ed. N. Denzin and Y. Lincoln. Thousand Oaks, CA: Sage.

DesMeules, M., J. Gold, A. Kazanjian, D. Manuel, J. Payne, B. Vissandjée, S. McDermott, and Y. Mao. 2004. New approaches to immigrant health assessment. *Canadian Journal of Public Health* 95(3):I22–6.

Diallo, L., and G. Lafrenière. 2007. Intervenir auprès des survivants de guerre, de torture et de violence organisée. *Reflets* 13:41–77.

Diamond, M. (1993). Homosexuality and bisexuality in different populations. *Archives of Sexual Behavior* 22(4):291–310

Di Leonardo, M. 1993. The female world of cards and holidays: Women, families and the world of kinship. In *Gender in Cross-Cultural Perspective*, 379–89. Ed. C. Brettel and C. Sargent. Englewood Cliffs, NJ: Prentice Hall.

Din-Dzietham, R., W. Nembhard, R. Collins, and S. Davis. 2004. Perceived stress following race-based discrimination at work is associated with hypertension in African-Americans. The Metro Atlanta Heart Disease Study, 1999–2001. *Social Science and Medicine* 58:449–61.

Dobbins, J., and J. Skillings. (2000). Racism as a clinical syndrome. *American Journal of Orthopsychiatry* 70(11): 14–27.

Dobrowolsky, A., and E. Tastsoglou. 2006. Crossing boundaries and making connections. In *Women, Migration and Citizenship: Making Local, National and Transnational Connections*, 2–35. Ed. E. Tastoglou and A. Dobrowolsky. Aldershot, UK: Ashgate Palgrave.

Dodgson, J., and R. Struthers. 2005. Indigenous women's voices: Marginalization and health. *Journal of Trancultural Nursing* 16(4):339–46.

Donner, L., T. Horne, W. Thurston, and Prairie Women's Health Centre of Excellence. 2001. *Population health data through a gender lens: A gender analysis of Toward a Healthy Future: Second Report on the Health of Canadians and selected other population health documents.* Ottawa: Federal/Provincial/Territorial Status of Women Forum, Health Canada.

Dossa, P. 1988. Women's space and time: An anthropological perspective on Ismaili immigrant women in Calgary and Vancouver. *Canadian Ethnic Studies* 20(1):45–65.

– 2003. The body remembers: A migratory tale of social suffering and witnessing. *International Journal of Mental Health* 32(3):50–73.

– 2004. *Politics and poetics of migration: Narratives of Iranian women from the diaspora.* Toronto: Canadian Scholars' Press.

Douglass, A., and T. Vogler, eds. 2003. *Witness and Memory: The Discourse of Trauma.* New York and London: Routledge Press.

Doyal, L. 1995. *What makes women sick? Gender and the political economy of health.* London and Houndsmills, UK: Macmillan Press.

– 2002. Putting gender into health and globalization debates: New perspectives and old challenges. *Third World Quarterly* 23(2):233–50.

Dressler, W. 1991. *Stress and adaptation in the context of culture: Depression in a southern black community.* Albany: State University of New York Press.

Dressler, W., M.C. Balieiro, and J. Dos Santos. 1998. Culture, socioeconomic status, and physical and mental health in Brazil. *Medical Anthropology Quarterly* 12(4):424–46.

Dressler, W., G. Grell, and F. Viteri. 1995. Intracultural diversity and the sociocultural correlates of blood pressure: A Jamaican example. *Medical Anthropology Quarterly* 9(3):291–313.

Drevdahl, D., S. Kneipp, M. Canales, and K. Dorcy. 2001. Reinvesting in social justice: A capital idea for public health nursing. *Advanced Nursing Sciences* 24(2):19–31.

Dua, E. 2000. 'The Hindu women's question': Canadian nation building and the social construction of gender for South Asian-Canadian women. In *Anti-Racist Feminism*, 55–72. Ed. A. Calliste and G. Sefa Dei. Halifax: Fernwood Publishing.

Duffy, M., and K. Hansen. 2005. *One hundred years of buying care: Gender, race, immigration and market care work in the twentieth century.* Dissertation, Brandeis University, Waltham, MA.

Dunn, J., and I. Dyck. 2000. Social determinants of health in Canada's immigrant population: Results from the National Population Health Survey. *Social Science and Medicine* 51:1573–93.

Duster, T. 2003. Buried alive: The concept of race in science. In *Genetic nature/culture: Anthropology and science beyond the two-culture divide*, 258–77. Ed. A. Goodman, D. Heath, and S. Lindee. Berkeley: University of California Press.

Dyck, I. 1995. Putting chronic illness 'in place': Women immigrants' accounts of their health care. *Geoforum* 26:247–60.

– 1998. Methodologies on the line: Constructing meanings about 'cultural difference' in health care research. In *Painting the maple: Essays on race, gender and the construction of Canada*, 19–36. Ed. V. Strong-Boag, S. Grace, A. Eisenberg, and J. Anderson. Vancouver: University of British Columbia Press.

– 2004. *Immigration, place and health: South Asian women's accounts of health, illness and everyday life.* Research on immigration and integration in the metropolis (RIIM). Working Paper Series No. 04-05. Vancouver: Research on Immigration and Integration in the Metropolis (RIIM).

Dyck, I., and P. Dossa. 2007. Place, health, and home: Gender and migration in the constitution of healthy space. *Health and Space* 13:691–701.

Edwards, R. 2005. *Social capital: A Sloan work and family encyclopedia entry.* Families and Social Capital ESRC Research Group, South Bank University. http://www.bc.edu/bc_org/avp/wfnetwork/rft/wfpedia/wfpSCent.html [accessed 7 July 2005].

Eichler, M. 2001. Moving forward: Measuring gender bias and more. In *Gender-based analysis in public health research, policy and practice: Documentation of the International Workshop in Berlin*, 11–21. Berlin: Berlin Centre for Public

Health, European Women's Health Network, and German Society for Social Medicine.

Elabor-Idenmudia, P. 2000. Challenges confronting African immigrant women in the Canadian workforce. In *Anti-racist feminism: Critical race and gender studies*, 91–110. Ed. A. Calliste and G. Sefa Dei. Halifax, NS: Fernwood Publishing.

Eliasson, M., and C. Lundy 1999. Organizing to stop violence against women in Canada and Sweden. In *Women's organizing and public policy in Canada and Sweden*, 280–309. Ed. L. Briskin and M. Eliasson. Montreal and Kingston: McGill-Queen's University Press.

Escobar, Mónica. 2006. Nation and gender views from Chilean-Canadian women in post exile. In *Ruptures, continuities and re-learning: The political participation of Latin Americans in Canada*, 164–76. Ed. Jorge Ginieniewicz and Daniel Schugurensky. Toronto: Ontario Institute for Studies in Education/ University of Toronto (OISE/UT).

Espiritu Y.L. 1999. Gender and labor in Asian immigrant families. In *Gender and U.S. immigration: Contemporary trends*. Ed. P. Hondagneu-Sotelo. Berkeley: University of California Press.

Essed, P. 1991. *Understanding everyday racism: An interdisciplinary theory*. Newbury Park, CA: Sage.

Estable, A., N. Cermeño, and S. Torres. 2005. *Providing effective culturally sensitive public health services at a relatively low cost*. Paper presented at Our Diverse Cities Symposium. Ottawa, 23 February.

Estable, A., M. Meyer, and S. Torres. 2003a. *Building community capacity and equitable access to cancer screening for ethnoracial minority women*. Research report prepared for the Ontario Women's Health Council. Ottawa: Ontario Women's Health Council.

– 2003b. *Combining health promotion and participatory research methods: Reaching out to isolated immigrant women to increase health information and knowledge*. Poster presented at Fostering Research Connections, University of Ottawa Applied Health and Social Research Network Inaugural Symposium. Ottawa, 18 November.

– 2004. *Lessons learned in participatory evaluation of a community-based project with multiple partners*. Paper presented at Community of Enquiry Symposium, Toronto, 10 July.

– 2006. Challenges of participatory evaluation within a community-Based health promotion partnership: Mujer Sana, Comunidad Sana-Healthy women, healthy communities. *Canadian Journal of Program Evaluation* 21(2):25–57.

Estable, A., S. Torres, and N. Cermeño. 2008. *Experiences of Latinas with the Canadian health care system: A qualitative study*. Poster presented at Public

Health Without Borders, APHA 136th Annual Meeting and Expo. San Diego, CA, 25–29 October.

Estable, A., S. Torres, N. Cermeño, and M. Meyer. 2009. *Addressing barriers to health services through community-based lay health promotion: Experiences of Latinas in the MSCS project*. Paper presented at the Canadian Public Health Association 2009 Annual Conference, Public Health in Canada: Strengthening Connections. Winnipeg, MB, 7–10 June.

Evans, R., M. Barrer, and T. Marmor, eds. 1994. *Why are some people healthy and others not? The determinants of health population*. New York: Aldine de Gruyter.

Fadiman, A. 1997. *The spirit catches you and you fall down*. New York: Noonday Press.

Fairbarns, K., C.S. Axworthy, M. Fulton, L.K. Hammond, and D. Laycock. 1990. Co-operative institutions: Five disciplinary perspectives. In *Co-operative organizations and Canadian society: Popular institutions and the dilemmas of change*, ed. M. Fulton. Toronto: University of Toronto Press.

Fairclough, N. 1992. A social theory of discourse. In *Discourse and Social Change*, 62–99. Cambridge: Polity Press.

Falconer, D.A. 2005. *Springboard of a national HIV/AIDS strategy for Black Canadian, African and Caribbean communities project: Environmental scan report*. Prepared for the Interagency Coalition on AIDS and Development (ICAD). Ottawa: ICAD.

Farmanova-Haynes E., A. Bose, and B. Vissandjée. 2006. Impact of immigration and settlement on women's mental health, mental illness, substance use and addiction. In *Ad hoc working group on women, mental health, mental illness and addictions. Women, mental health and mental illness and addiction in Canada: An overview*. Canadian Women's Health Network. http://www.cwhn.ca [accessed 8 August 2007].

Farmer, P. 1999. *Infections and inequalities: The modern plagues*. Berkeley: University of California Press.

– 2003. *Pathologies of power: Health, human rights, and the new war on the poor*. Berkeley: University of California Press.

Fassin, D. 2003. Le capital social, de la sociologie à l'épidémiologie: Analyse critique d'une migration transdiciplinaire (full text in English on www.e2med.com/resp). *Revue d'Epidémiologie et de Santé Publique* 51:403–13.

– 2005. Social illegitimacy as a foundation of health inequality: How the political treatment of immigrants illuminates a French paradox. In *Unhealthy Health Policy: A critical anthropological examination*, 203–14. Ed. A. Castro and M. Singer. Walnut Creek, CA: Altamira.

Fédération des communautés Francophones et acadiennes du Canada (FCFA).

2001. Pour un meilleur accès à des services de santé en français. http://www.fcfa.ca [accessed 8 April 2007].

Featherstone, B. 2003. Taking fathers seriously. *British Journal of Social Work* 33(2):239–54.

Fenta, H., I. Hyman, and S. Noh. 2004. Determinants of depression among Ethiopian immigrants and refugees in Toronto. *Journal of Nervous and Mental Disease* 192(5):363–72.

Field, J. 2003. *Social capital.* London: Routledge.

Fine, B. 2001. *Social capital versus social theory: Political economy and social science at the turn of the Millennium.* London: Routledge.

Finkler, K. 1994. Sacred healing and biomedicine compared. *Medical Anthropology Quarterly* 8(2):178–97.

Fisher, E.B., W. Auslander, L. Sussman, N. Owens, and J. Jackson-Thomson. 1991. Community organization and heath promotion in minority neighborhoods. *Ethnicity and Disease* 293:252–72.

Flora, J.L. 1998. Social capital and communities of place. *Rural Sociology* 63(4):481–506.

Floch, William. 2003. *Official languages and diversity in Canada.* Conference proceedings on Canadian and French perspectives on diversity. http://www.pch.gc.ca/pc-ch/pubs/diversity2003/index_e.cfm [accessed 15 October 2007].

Forgues, E., and R. Landry. 2006. *Defining francophones in minority situations: An analysis of various statistical definitions and their implications.* A study for the Joint Commission on Health Care Research for Francophones in Minority Situations. http://www.cnfs.ca [accessed 6 October 2007].

Fortin, M-C. 2005. *Le déséquilibre du pouvoir dans les relations de sexe et la qualité de vie: Le cas des femmes immigrantes séropositives de Québec et de Montréal.* PhD diss., Université de Laval.

Fortin, S. 2002. Social ties and settlement processes: French and North African migrants in Montreal. *Canadian Ethnic Studies* 34(3):76–98.

Fowler, N. 1998. Providing primary health care to immigrants and refugees: The North Hamilton experience. *CMAJ.* 159(4):388–91.

Francour, R.T., and R.J. Noonan, eds. 2004. *Continuum complete international encyclopedia of sexuality.* www.kinseyinstitute.org/ [accessed 6 October 2008].

Frank, A. 1995. *The wounded story-teller.* Chicago: University of Chicago Press.

Frank, J. 2003. Making social capital work for public policy. Policy Research Initiative. *Horizons* 6(3):3–6.

Franklin, J. 2005. *Women and social capital.* London: London South Bank University.

Franks, F., and S. Faux. 1990. Depression, stress, mastery, and social resources in four ethnocultural women's groups. *Research Nursing Health* 13(5):283–92.

Fraser, N. 1989. *Unruly practices: Power, discourse and gender in contemporary social theory.* Minneapolis: University of Minnesota Press.

Freire, P. 1973. *Education for critical consciousness.* New York: Seabury Press.

– 1974. *Pedagogy of the oppressed.* New York: Seabury Press.

Freund, P. 2006. Socially constructed embodiment: Neurohormonal connections as resources for theorizing about health inequalities. *Social Theory and Health* 4:85–108.

Frigon, S., and M. Kérisit, eds. 2000. *Du corps des femmes: Contrôles, surveillances et résistances.* Ottawa: Les presses de l'Université d'Ottawa.

Gagnon, A. 2002. *Responsiveness of the Canadian health care system towards newcomers.* Commission on the Future of health Care in Canada. Discussion paper no. 40.

Gagnon, A., G. Doughtery, R. Platt, O. Wahoush, A. George, E. Stanger, J. Oxman-Martinez, J.-P. Saucier, L. Merry, and D. Stewart. 2007. Refugee and refugee-claimant women and infants post-birth: Migration histories as a predictor of Canadian health system response to needs. *Canadian Journal of Public Health* 98(4):287–91.

Galabuzi, G.E. 2001. *Canada's creeping economic apartheid.* Toronto: Centre for Social Justice.

Galabuzi, G.E. 2005. *Canada's economic apartheid: The social exclusion of racialized groups in the new century.* Toronto: Canadian Scholars' Press.

– 2006. *Canada's creeping economic apartheid.* Toronto: Canadian Scholar's Press.

Galabuzi. G.E., and R. Labonte. 2002. *Social inclusion as a determinant of health.* Summary document based on presentations prepared for the Social Determinants of Health across the Life-Span Conference, Toronto, 2002. http://www.phac-aspc.gc.ca/ph-sp/phdd/overview_implications/03_inclusion.html [accessed 21 September 2007].

Garceau, M-L. 1996a. Bénévolat des femmes vieillissantes à l'aube de l'an 2000. *Reflets* 2(2):58–81.

– 1996b. La pauvreté des Franco-Ontariennes de 45 à 64 ans du Nord-Est de L'Ontario. In *Changing lives: Women in Northern Ontario*, 224–31. Ed. M. Kechnie and M. Reitsma-Street. Toronto and Oxford: Dundurn Press.

Garcia-Moreno, C., H.A.F.M. Jansen, M. Ellsberg, L. Heise, and C. Watts. 2006. Prevalence of intimate partner violence: Findings from the WHO multi-country study on women's health and domestic violence. *The Lancet* 368:1260–9.

Gates, G.J. 2006. *Same-sex couples and the gay, lesbian and bisexual population: New estimates from the American Community Survey.* Los Angeles: Williams Institute, UCLA School of Law.

Gee, G. 2002. A multilevel analysis of the relationship between institutional and individual racial discrimination and health status. Miscellaneous. *American Journal of Public Health. Women of Color* 92(4):615–23.

Gee, G.C., A. Ryan, D.J. Laflamme, and J. Holt. 2006. Self-reported discrimination and mental health status among African descendants, Mexican Americans, and other Latinos in the New Hampshire REACH 2010 Initiative: The added dimension of immigration. *American Journal of Public Health* 96(10):1821–8.

Geertz, C. 1960. The Javanese Kijaji: The changing role of a cultural broker. *Comparative Studies in Sociology and History* 2:228–49.

George, U., and S. Ramkisson. 1998. 'Race, gender and class.' Interlocking oppressions in the lives of South Asian women in Canada. *Affilia* 13(1):102–19.

Gilbert, A., M. Kérisit, C. Dallaire, C. Coderre, and J. Harvey. 2005. Les discours sur la santé des organismes franco-ontariens: Du rapport Dubois à la cause Montfort. *Reflets* 11:20–48.

Ginieniewicz, J., and D. Schugurensky. 2006. The Latin American migration to Canada: Eight outlooks. In *Ruptures, continuities and re-learning. The political participation of Latin Americans in Canada*, 2–16. Ed. J. Ginieniewicz and D. Schugurensky. Toronto: Ontario Institute for Studies in Education/ University of Toronto (OISE/UT).

Gittell, M., I. Ortega-Bustamente, and T. Steffy. 2000. Social capital and social change: Women's community activism. *Urbain Affairs Review* 36:123–47.

Gittell, R., and J.P. Thompson. 2001. Making social capital work: Social capital and community economic development. In *Social capital and poor communities*, 115–35. Ed. S. Saegert, J.P. Thompson, and M.R. Warren. New York: Russell Sage Foundation.

Gjerdingen, D., P. McGovern, M. Bekker, U. Lundberg, and T. Willemsen. 2000. Women's work roles and their impact on health, well-being, and career: Comparisons between the United States, Sweden, and the Netherlands. *Women and Health* 31(4):1–20.

Goldman D.P., J.P. Smith, and N. Sood. 2005. Legal status and health insurance among immigrants. *Health Affairs* 24:1640–53.

Goodson, L. 2001. *Afghanistan's endless war: State failure, regional politics, and the rise of the Taliban.* Seattle: University of Washington Press.

Government of Canada. 2004. *The federal initiative to Address HIV/AIDS in Canada: Strengthening action in the Canadian response to HIV/AIDS.* Ottawa: Minister of Public Works and Government Services Canada.

– 2006. *The human face of mental health and mental illnesses in Canada.* Ottawa: Minister of Public Works.

Government of Canada, Department of Justice. 2001. Immigration and Refugee Protection Act (2001, c. 27). http://www.canlii.org/ca/sta/i-2.5/whole .html [accessed 3 September 2007].

Graham, J.M., and W.E. Thurston. 2005. Overcoming adversity: Resilience and coping mechanisms developed by recent immigrant women living in the inner city of Calgary, Alberta. *Women's Health and Urban Life* 4:63–80.

Grant, P. 2005. *The devaluation of immigrants' foreign credentials: The psychological impact of this barrier to integration into Canadian society.* Edmonton, AB: PCERII.

Grant, P., and S. Nadin. 2007. The credentialing problems of foreign-trained personnel from Asia and Africa intending to make their home in Canada: A social psychological perspective. *Journal of International Migration and Integration* 8:141–62.

Gravel, S., J.-M. Brodeur, B. Vissandjée, F. Champagne, and K. Lippel. 2008. Incompréhension par les travailleurs immigrants victimes de lésions professionnelles de leurs difficultés d'accès à l'indemnisation. *Migrations et Santé* 131:12–37.

Graves, J. 2001. *The Emperor's new clothes: Biological theories of race at the millennium.* New Brunswick, NJ: Rutgers University Press.

Greaves, L., and V.J. Barr. 2000. *Filtered policy: Women and tobacco in Canada.* Vancouver: BC Centre of Excellence for Women's Health (BCCEWH).

Green, A., and D. Green. 2004. The goals of Canada's immigration policy: A historical perspective. *Canadian Journal of Urban Research* 13(1):102–39.

Grenon, É., M. Kérisit, and F. Magunira. 2008. *La réunification des femmes immigrantes et réfugiées avec leurs enfants.* Ottawa: Mouvement Ontarien des femmes immigrantes francophones.

Griffen, J., R. Fuhrer, S. Stansfield, and M. Marmot. 2002. The importance of low control at work and home on depression and anxiety: Do these effects vary by gender and social class? *Social Science and Medicine* 54:783–98.

Grosfuguel, R. 2004. Race and ethnicity or racialized ethnicities? Identities within global coloniality. *Ethnicities* 4(3):315–36.

Grove, N.J., and A.B. Zwi. 2006. Our health and theirs: Forced migration, othering, and public health. *Social Science and Medicine* 62(8):1931–42.

Gunewardena, N., and A. Kingsolver. 2007. Introduction. In *The gender of globalization: Women navigating cultural and economic marginalities,* 3–22. Ed. N. Gunewardena and A. Kingsolver. Sante Fe, NM: School for Advanced Research.

Guruge, S., G. Donner, and L. Morrison. 2000. The impact of Canadian health care reform on recent women immigrants and refugees. In *Care and consequences: The impact of health care reform*, 222–42. Ed. D. Gustafson. Halifax: Fernwood Publishing.

Gushulak, B., and D. MacPherson. 2000. Health issues associated with the smuggling and trafficking of migrants. *Journal of Immigrant Health* 2:67–78.

Gushulak, B., and L. Williams. 2004. National immigration health policy: Existing policy, changing needs and future directions. *Canadian Journal of Public Health* 94(3):127–9.

Halpin, S., and Allen, M. 2004. Changes in psychosocial well-being during stages of gay identity development. *Journal of Homosexuality* 47(2):109–26.

Hankins, C., T. Tran, L. Hum, C. Laberge, N. Lapointe, D. Lepine, M. Montpetit, and M.V. O'Shaughnessy. 1998. Socioeconomic geographical links to human immunodeficiency virus seroprevalence among childbearing women in Montreal, 1989–1993. *International Journal of Epidemiology* 27(4):691–7.

Hankivsky, O. 2005. Gender mainstreaming vs. diversity mainstreaming: A preliminary examination of the role and transformative potential of feminist theory. *Canadian Journal of Political Science* 38(4):977–1001.

– 2007. Gender-based analysis and health policy: The need to rethink outdated strategies. In *Women's health in Canada: Critical perspectives on theory and policy*, 143–68. Ed. M. Morrow, O. Hankivsky, and C. Varcoe. Toronto: University of Toronto Press.

Hankivsky, O., R. Cormier, and J. Chou DeMerich. 2009. *Intersectionality: Moving women's health research and policy forward*. Draft primer for Women's Health Research Network Intersectionality Workshop (April 17–18, 2008). Vancouver: Institute for Critical Studies in Gender and Health.

Hardy-Fanta, C. 1997. Latina women and political consciousness, La chispa que prende. In *Women's studies in the academy, origins and impact 2004*, 493–504. Ed. R. Rosen. New Jersey: Pearson Prentice Hall.

Harper, G. W., and M. Schneider. 2003. Oppression and discrimination among lesbian, gay, bisexual, and transgendered people and communities: A challenge for community psychology. *American Journal of Community Psychology* 31(3/4):243–52.

Harrell, S. 2000. A multidimensional conceptualization of racism-related stress: Implications for the well-being of people of color. *American Journal of Orthopsychiatry* 70(11):42–57.

Harris, M.B., J. Nightengale, and N. Owen. 1995. Health care professionals' experiences, knowledge, and attitudes concerning homosexuality. *Journal of Gay and Lesbian Social Services* 2(2):91–107.

Harris, R., M. Tobias, M. Jeffreys, K. Waldegrave, S. Karlesen, and J. Nazroo.

2006. Effects of self-reported racial discrimination and deprivation on Maori health and inequalities in New Zealand: Cross-sectional study. *The Lancet* 367(9527):2005–9.

Hawkesworth, M. 2006. *Feminist inquiry: From political conviction to methodological innovation.* New Brunswick, NJ: Rutgers University Press.

Hawkins, R., and W. Stackhouse. 2004. U.S.A. adults: Homoerotic, homosexual and bisexual behaviors. In *Continuum complete international encyclopedia of sexuality.* Ed. R.T. Francour and R.J. Noonan. http://www.kinseyinstitute .org/ [accessed 7 May 2009].

Hawthorne, L. 2006. *Labour market outcomes for migrant professionals: Canada and Australia compared – executive summary.* Melbourne: University of Melbourne.

Health Canada. n.d. *Language barriers in access to health care.* Health Canada. http://www.hc-sc.gc.ca/hcs-sss/pubs/acces/2001-lang-acces/gen_e.html [accessed 7 July 2007].

– 1994. Strategies for population health: Investing in the health of Canadians. Public Health Agency of Canada. http://www.phac-aspc.gc.ca/phsp/ phdd/determinants/determinants.html#culturePHAC [accessed 8 August 2007].

– 1996. Canadian Research on Immigration and Health. http://dsp-psd .pwgsc.gc.ca/Collection/H21-149-1999E.pdf [Accessed 4 March 2007].

– 2002. *A report on mental illnesses in Canada.* Ottawa: Health Canada.

– 2003. *Exploring concepts of gender and health.* Ottawa: Women's Health Bureau, Health Canada.

Health Disparities Task Group of the Federal/Provincial/Territorial Advisory Committee on Population Health and Health Security. 2004, December. Reducing health disparities – Roles of the health sector. Discussion paper. Public Health Agency of Canada(PHAC). http://www.phac-aspc.gc.ca/ph-sp/ disparities/ddp_e.html [accessed 7 July 2007].

Heiley, J. 2001. Beyond the formulaic: Process and practice in South Asian NGOs. In *Participation: The New Tyranny?*, 89–101. Ed. B. Cooke and U. Kothari. London-New York: Zed Books.

Heise, L. 1993. Violence against women: The hidden health burden. *World Health Statistics Quarterly* 46:78–85.

Heise, L., A. Raikes, C.H. Watts, and A.B. Zwi. 1994. Violence against women: A neglected public health issue in less developed countries. *Social Science and Medicine* 39:1165–79.

Helly, D. 2004. Are Muslims discriminated against in Canada since September 2001? *Canadian Ethnic Studies* 36:24–47.

Helman, C. 1990. *Culture, health and illness.* 2d ed. Oxford: Butterworth-Heinemann.

Hennestad, B.W. 2000. Implementing participative management: Transition issues from the field. *Journal of Applied Behavioral Science* 36(3):314–36.

Herek, G.M. 2004. Beyond 'homophobia': Thinking about sexual prejudice and stigma in the twenty-first century. *Sexuality Research and Social Policy* 1(2):6–24.

Highes, D. 2004. Disclosure of sexual preferences and lesbian, gay and bisexual practitioners. *British Medical Journal* 328:1211–12.

Hill-Collins, P. (1990) 2000. *Black feminist thought: knowledge, consciousness, and the politics of empowerment*. New York: Routledge.

HIV-Endemic Task Force (HETF). 2001. Summary report of the community forum *For us, by us, about us: An opportunity for African and Caribbean communities to address the issue of HIV/AIDS-related stigma and denial*. http://www.phs.utoronto.ca/ohemu/doc/CF-%20Sum-Rep-june28.pdf [accessed 25 November 2007].

Hopkins, N., M. Ekpo, J. Heileman, M. Michtom, A. Osterweil, R.T. Sieber, and G. Smith. 1977. Brokers and symbols in American urban life. *Anthropological Quarterly* 50(2):65–75.

Horne, T., L. Donner, and W.E. Thurston. 1999. *Invisible women: Gender and health planning in Manitoba and Saskatchewan and Models for Progress*. Winnipeg, MB: Prairie Women's Health Centre of Excellence.

Horowitz, J.L., and M.D. Newcomb. 2001. A multidimensional approach to homosexual identity. *Journal of Homosexuality* 42(2):1–19.

Hsieh, H.F., and S.E. Shannon. 2005. Three approaches to qualitative content analysis. *Qualitative Health Research* 15(9):1277–88.

Huang, F.Y., and S. Akhtar. 2005. Immigrant sex: The transport of affection and sensuality across cultures. *American Journal of Psychoanalysis* 65(2):179–88.

Hughes, D. 2004. Disclosure of sexual preferences and lesbian, gay and bisexual practitioners. *British Medical Journal* 328:1211–12.

Hulewat, P. (1996). Resettlement: A cultural and psychological crisis. *Social Work* 41(2):129–35.

Hyman, I. 2001. Immigration and Health, In *Working paper 01-05, 47–57*. Ottawa: Health Canada.

– 2002. Immigrant and visible minority women. In *Ontario women's health status report, Women's Health Council*. Ed. D.E. Stewart, A. Cheung, L. Ferris, I. Hyman, M. Cohen, and I.J. Williams. http://www.womenshealthcouncil.on.ca [accessed 13 February 2007].

– 2004. Setting the stage: Reviewing current knowledge on the health of Canadian immigrants: What is the evidence and where are the gaps? *Canadian Journal of Public Health* 95(3):14–18.

– 2007a. *Determinants of immigrant health*. Report to Public Health Agency of Canada. Ottawa: PHAC.

– 2007b. *Immigration and health: Reviewing evidence of the healthy immigrant effect in Canada. CERIS working paper no. 55.* Ed. M. Doucet. Toronto: Joint Centre of Excellence for Research on Immigration and Settlement.

Hyman I., and G. Dussault. 2000. Negative consequences of acculturation on health behaviour, social support and stress among pregnant Southeast Asian immigrant women in Montreal: An exploratory study. *Canadian Journal of Public Health* 91(5):357–61.

Hyman I., T. Forte, J. Du Mont, S. Romans, and M.M. Cohen. 2006. The association between length of stay in Canada and intimate partner violence among immigrant women. *American Journal of Public Health* 96(4):654–9.

Hyman I., R. Mason, and S. Guruge. (2008). The impact of post-migration change on marital relationships: A study of Ethiopian immigrant couples in Toronto. *Journal of Comparative Family Studies* 39(2):149-163.

Hynie, M. (2008). From conflict to compromise: Immigrant families and the processes of acculturation. From http://canada.metropolis.net/research-policy/litreviews/tylr_rev/tylr_rev-08.html#CONFLICT [accessed 1 May 2008].

Illich, I. 1999. *Deschooling society.* New York: Marion Boyars.

Interagency Coalition on AIDS and Development (ICAD). 2006a. Annotated bibliography, HIV/AIDS among persons from countries where HIV/AIDS is endemic, March 2006. Interagency Coalition on AIDS and Development. http://www.icad-cisd.com/pdf/publications/EndemicAnnot_Biblios_EN_FINAL.pdf [accessed 25 November 2007].

– 2006b. Fact sheet: HIV/AIDS and African and Caribbean communities in Canada. 30 June 2006. Interagency Coalition on AIDS and Development. http://www.icad-cisd.com/pdf/publications/HIV-AIDS_AfricanDiaspora_EN.pdf [accessed 25 November 2007].

Jaggar, A. 2002. A feminist critique of the alleged Southern debt. *Hypatia: A Journal of Feminist Philosophy* 17(2):119–42.

Jakubowski, L.M. 1997. *Immigration and the legalization of racism.* Halifax: Fernwood Publishing.

James, S.A., A.J. Schulz, and J. van Olphen. 2001. Social capital, poverty, and community health: An exploration of linkages. In *Social Capital and Poor Communities,* 165–88. Ed. S. Saegert, J.P. Thompson, and M.R. Warren. New York: Russell Sage Foundation.

Javed, N., and N. Gerrard. 2006. Bound, bonded and battered: Immigrant and visible minority women's struggle to cope with violence. In *Intimate partner violence: Reflections on experience, theory, and policy,* 33–46. Ed. M.R. Hampton and N. Gerrard. Toronto: Cormorant Books.

Jeffreys, M.R. 2005. Clinical nurse specialists as cultural brokers, change agents, and partners in meeting the needs of culturally diverse populations. *Journal of Multicultural Nursing and Health* 11 (2):40–9.

Jenkins, J., and M. Valiente. 1994. Bodily transactions of the passions: *El Calor* among Salvadorean women refugees. In *Embodiment and experience: The existential ground of culture and self*, 163–77. Ed. T. Csordas. Cambridge: Cambridge University Press:

Jezewski, M.A. 1990. Culture brokering in migrant farmworker health care. *Western Journal of Nursing Research* 12(4):497–513.

– 1993. Culture brokering as a model for advocacy. *Nursing and Health Care* 14(2):78–85.

Jezewski, M.A., and P. Sotnik. 2005. Culture and the Disability Services. In *Culture and Disability Services. Providing culturally competent services*, 15–27. Ed. J.H. Stone. Thousand Oaks, CA: Sage Publications.

Jiménez, M. 2008. Immigrants face growing economic mobility gap. *Globe and Mail*, 6 October, A1.

Joint United Nations Programme on HIV/AIDS (UNAIDS). 2006a. *Report on the global AIDS epidemic.* Geneva: UNAIDS.

– 2006b. *Operational guide on Gender and HIV/AIDS – A rights-based approach, 2005.* UNAIDS Inter-agency task team on gender and HIV/AIDS. Geneva: UNAIDS.

Joint United Nations Programme on HIV/AIDS (UNAIDS), and World Health Organization (WHO). 2007. *AIDS epidemic update, December 2007.* Geneva: UNAIDS and WHO.

Jones, S. 2004. Canada and the globalized immigrant. *American Behavioral Scientist* 47(1):1263–77.

Jordan, B., and F. Düvell. 2002. *Irregular migration: The dilemmas of transnational mobility.* Cheltenham, UK: Edward Elgar.

Judge, R. 2003. Social capital: Building a foundation for research and policy development. Policy Research Initiative. *Horizons* 6(3):7–12.

Justice Institute of British Colombia. 2007. *Empowerment of immigrant and refugee women who are victims of violence in their intimate relationships.* Report. Vancouver: Justice Institute of British Columbia.

Karlsen, S., and J. Nazroo. 2002. The relation between racial discrimination, social class, and health among ethnic minority groups. *American Journal of Public Health* 92(4):624-631.

Kawachi, I. 2001. Social capital for health and human development. *Development* 44(1):31–5.

Kawachi, I., and L.F. Berkman. 2001. Social ties and mental health. *Journal of Urban Health* 78(3):458–67.

Kawachi, I., B.P. Kennedy, K. Lochner, and D. Prothrow-Stith. 1997. Social capital, income inequality, and mortality. *American Journal of Public Health* 87:1491–8.

Kawachi, I., D. Kim, A. Coutts, and S.V. Subramanian. 2004. Commentary: Reconciling the three accounts of social capital. *International Journal of Epidemiology* 33(4):682–90.

Kawar, M. 2004. Gender and migration: Why are women more vulnerable? In *Femmes en movement: Genre, migrations et nouvelle divisions internationale du travail*. Ed. F. Reysoo and C. Verchuur. Commission suisse pour L`Unesco, Berne. www.iued.unige.ch [accessed 21 September 2007].

Kazemipur A., and S. Halli. 2000. The invisible barrier: Neighbourhood poverty and integration of immigrants in Canada, *Journal of International Migration and Integration* 1(1):85–100.

– 2001. The changing colour of poverty in Canada. *CRSA/RCSA* 38(2):217–38.

Kelly, J. 2006. *Advancing women in leadership*. Review of Race, gender, and leadership, by P.S. Parker. *Advancing Women* 21(summer):1.

Khan, B. 1997. Not so gay life in Pakistan in the 1980s and 1990s. *In Islamic homosexualities: Culture, history and literature*, 275–96. Ed. S.O. Murray and W. Roscoe, New York: NYU Press.

Kim, D., S.V. Subramanian, and I. Kawachi. 2006. Bonding versus bridging social capital and their associations with self rated health: A multilevel analysis of 40 US communities. *Journal of Epidemiology and Community Health* 60:116–22.

Kinitz, S.J. 2004. Social capital and health. *British Medical Bulletin* 69: 61–73.

Kinnon, D. 1999. *Canadian research on immigration and health*. Ottawa: Health Canada.

Kinsey, A.C., W.B. Pomeroy, and C.E. Martin. 1948. *Sexual behavior in the human male*. Philadelphia: W.B. Saunders.

Kinsey, A.C., W.B. Pomeroy, C.E. Martin, and P. Gebhard. 1955. Sexual behavior in the human female. Philadelphia: W.B. Saunders.

Kirrane, D.E. 1995. Valuing diversity: The role of minority associations. *Association Management* 47:49–55.

Kleinman, A., and J. Kleinman. 1997. The appeal of experience; the dismay of images: Cultural appropriation of suffering in our times. In *Social Suffering*, 1–24. Ed. V. Das, A. Kleinman, and M. Lock. Berkeley: University of California Press.

Kliewer, E.V., and R.H. Ward. 1988. Convergence of immigrant suicide rates to those in the destination country. *American Journal of Epidemiology* 127(3):640–53.

Knocke W., and R. Ng. 1999. Women's organizing and immigration: Comparing the Canadian and Swedish experiences. In *Women's organizing and public policy in Canada and Sweden*, 87–116. Ed. L. Briskin and M. Eliason. Montreal: McGill-Queen's University Press.

Kofman, E. 2004. Gendered global migrations: Diversity and stratification. *International Feminist Journal of Politics* 6(4):643–65.

Koser, K. 2000. Asylum policies, trafficking and vulnerability. *International Migration* 38(3):91–112.

Krieger, N. 2003. Genders, sexes, and health: What are the connections – and why does it matter? *International Journal of Epidemiology* 32:652–7.

Krieger, N., J. Chen, and J. Selby. 2001. Class inequalities in women's health: Combined impact of childhood and adult social class – A study of 630 US women. *Public Health* 115:175–85.

Krieger, N., D. Rowley, A. Herman, B. Avery, and M. Phillips. 1993. Racism, sexism, and social class: Implications for studies of health, disease and well-being. *American Journal of Preventative Medicine* 6 (suppl. 9):82–122.

Ku, L., and S. Matani. 2001. Left out: Immigrants' access to health care and insurance. *Health Affairs* 20:247–56.

Kunz, J. 2003. Social capital: A key dimension of immigrant integration. *Canadian Issues/Thèmes Canadiens*: April/avril.

– 2005. Orienting newcomers to Canadian society: Social capital and settlement. In *Social Capital in Action: Thematic Policy Studies*. Policy Research Initiative. http://policyresearch.gc.ca/page.asp?pagenm=pub%5Findex [accessed 8 March 2007].

Kunz-Ebrecht, S., C. Kirschbaum, and A. Steptoe. 2004. Work stress, socioeconomic status and neuroendocrine activation over the working day. *Social Science and Medicine* 58:1523–30.

Lai, D.W. 2004. Depression among elderly Chinese-Canadian immigrants from Mainland China. *Chinese Medical Journal* (Engl.) 117(5):677–83.

– 2005. Prevalence and correlates of depressive symptoms in older Taiwanese immigrants in Canada. *Journal of the Chinese Medical Association* 68(3):118–25.

Lamb, M.E. 2000. Research on father involvement: An overview. *Marriage and Family Review* 29(2/3):23–42.

Lammers, E. 1999. *Refugees, gender and human security: A theoretical introduction and annotated bibliography*. Utrecht: International Books.

Landenburger, K.M. 2007. Exploration of women's identity: Clinical approaches with abused women. In *Empowering survivors of abuse: Health care for battered women and their children*, 61–78. Ed. J.C. Campbell. Thousand Oaks, CA: Sage.

Langford, N., A. Fantino, and N. Waijaki. 1999. *Making the invisible visible: Relationship changes and stability of Edmonton immigrant couples*. Presentation to the Third Metropolis National Conference on Immigration. Vancouver, 14–16 January.

LaRossa, R. 1997. *The modernization of fatherhood: A social and political history.* Chicago: University of Chicago Press.

Lawson, E., F. Gardezi, L. Calzavara, W. Husbands, T. Myers, and W.E. Tharao. 2006. *HIV/AIDS stigma, denial, fear, and discrimination: Experiences and responses of people from African and Caribbean communities in Toronto.* Toronto: ACHO and University of Toronto HIV Social Behavioural, and Epidemiological Studies Unit.

Laurie, M., and R. Petchesky. 2008. Gender, health, and human rights in sites of political exclusion. *Global Public Health* 3 (suppl.1):25-41.

Lee, J.A. 2008. Homosexuality. In *The Canadian encyclopedia.* Ed. J.H. Marsh. http://thecanadianencyclopedia.com [accessed 1 May 2009].

Lewchuk, W., A. de Wolff, A. King, and M. Polyani. 2003. From job strain to employment strain: Health effects of precarious employment. *Just Labour* 3(fall):23–35.

Lewis, C., and M.E. Lamb. 2003. Fathers' influence on children's development: The evidence from two-parent families. *European Journal of Psychology of Education* 18(2):211–28.

Ley, D., and D. Hiebert. 2001. Immigration policy as population policy. *Canadian Geographer* 45(1):120–5.

Leyson, J.F.J. 2004. Philippines. In *Continuum complete international encyclopedia of sexuality.* Ed. R.T. Francour and R.J. Noonan. http://www.kinseyinstitute .org/ [accessed 1 May 2009].

Li, H.Z., and A.J. Browne. 2000. Defining mental illness and accessing mental health services: Perspectives of Asian Canadians. *Canadian Journal of Mental Health* 19(1):143–59.

Li, P. 2001. The racial subtext in Canada's immigration discourse. *Journal of International Migration and Integration* 2(1):77–97.

Lightman, E. 2008. *Poverty is making us sick: A comprehensive survey of income and health in Canada.* Toronto: Wellesley Institute.

Lin, N. 2000. Inequality in social capital. *Contemporary Sociology* 29(6):785–95.

Lincoln, Y.S., and E.G. Guba. 1985. *Naturalistic inquiry.* Beverly Hills, CA: Sage.

Lippel, K. 1998. Preventive reassignment of pregnant or breast-feeding workers: The Québec model. *New Solutions* 8(2):267–80.

Lister, R. 2005. Feminist citizenship theory: An alternative perspective on understanding women's social and political lives. In *Women and Social Capital,* 18–26. Ed. J. Franklin, Families and Social Capital ESRC Research Group.

Llácer, A., M.V. Zunzunegui, J. del Amo, L. Mazarrasa, and F. Bolumar.

2007. The contribution of a gender perspective to the understanding of migrants' health. *Journal of Epidemiology and Community Health* 61(suppl. II): ii4–ii10.

Lochner, K., I. Kawachi, and B.P. Kennedy. 1999. Social capital: A guide to its measurement. *Health and Place* 5(4):259–70.

Lock, M. 1993a. *Encounters with aging: Mythologies of menopause in Japan and North America.* Berkeley: University of California Press.

– 1993b. Cultivating the body: Anthropology and epistemologies of bodily practice and knowledge. *Annual Review of Anthropology* 22:133–55.

Lorber, J. 2005. *Breaking the bowls: Degendering and feminist change.* New York: W.W. Norton.

Lott, B. 2007. Introduction. *Women and leadership: Transforming visions and diverse voices*, 19–34. Ed. J.L. Chin, B. Lott, J.K. Rice, and J. Sanchez-Hucles. Malden, MA: Blackwell Publishing.

Low, S. 1994. Embodied metaphors: Nerves as lived experience. In *Embodiment and experience: The existential ground of culture and self*, 139–62. Ed. T. Csordas. Cambridge: Cambridge University Press.

Lundberg, U., and D. Parr. 2000. Neurohormonal factors, stress, health and gender. In *Handbook of gender, culture and health*, 21–41. Ed. R. Eisler and M. Hersen. Mahwah, NJ: Lawrence Erlbaum Associates Publishers.

Luther, R., and O. Prempeh. 2003. *Advocacy matters: Reviving? and sustaining community advocacy networks to support multiculturalism and anti-racism in the Ottawa region.* Report for the Community Advocacy Action Committee on Access and Equity and Canadian Heritage Multiculturalism Ottawa: Canadian Heritage Multiculturalism.

Lynam, M.J., and S. Cowley. 2007. Understanding marginalization as a social determinant of health. *Critical Public Health* 17(2):137–49.

Mackian, S. 2002. Complex cultures: Rereading the story about health and social capital. *Critical Social Policy* 22(2):203–25.

MacKinnon, M., and L. Howard. *Affirming immigrant women's health: Building inclusive healthy policy.* Maritime Centre of Excellence for Women's Health. http://www.acewh.dal.ca/eng/reports/ImmigrantHlthMack.pdf [accessed 23 May 2001].

MacPherson, D.W., and B. Gushulak. 2001. Human mobility and population health: New approaches in a globalizing world. *Perspectives in Biological Medicine* 44(3):390–401.

Mahler, S., and P. Pessar. 2001. Gendered geographies of power: Analyzing gender across transnational spaces. *Identities* 7(4):441–59.

Makinko, J., and B. Starfield. 2001. The utility of social capital in research on health determinants. *Milbank Quarterly* 79(3):387.

Malenfant, É.C. 2004. Suicide in Canada's immigrant population. *Health Reports* 15(2):9–17.

Marmot, M. 2007. Achieving health equity: From root causes to fair outcomes. *The Lancet* 370(9593):1153–63.

Marmot, M., and R. Wilkinson. 1999. Social determinants of health. In *Social organization, stress and health*. Ed. B. Marmot. Oxford: Oxford University Press.

Marsiglio, W., P. Amato, R. Day, and M. Lamb. 2000. Scholarship in fatherhood in the 1990s and beyond. *Journal of Marriage and the Family* 62:1173–91.

Martin, E. 1990. Toward an anthropology of immunology: The body as nation state. *Medical Anthropology Quarterly* 4(4):410–26.

– 1992. *The woman in the body: A cultural analysis of reproduction*. Boston: Beacon Press.

Matsuoka, A., and J. Sorenson. 1999. Engendering forced migration: Theory and practice. In *Engendering forced migration: Theory and practice*, 218–41. Ed. D. Indra. New York: Berghahn Books.

McDonald, J.T., and S. Kennedy. 2004. Insights into the 'healthy immigrant effect': Health status and health service use of immigrants to Canada. *Social Science and Medicine* 59(8):1613–27.

McDonough, P., V. Walters, and L. Strohschein. 2002. Chronic stress and the social patterning of women's health in Canada. *Social Science and Medicine* 54:767–82.

McIsaac, E. 2003. Immigrants in Canadian cities: Census 2001 – what do the data tell us? Ottawa: Institute for Research and Public Policy. http://www.triec.ca/docs/mcisaac.pdf [accessed 3 September 2007].

McKeown, I., S. Reid, and P. Orr. 2004. Experiences of sexual violence and relocation in the lives of HIV-infected Canadian women. *International Journal of Circumpolar Health* 63(2):399–404.

McLaren, A.T., and I. Dyck. 2004. Mothering, human capital, and the 'ideal immigrant.' *Women's Studies International Forum* 27:41–53.

Meadows, L.M., W.E. Thurston, and C. Melton. 2001. Immigrant women's health. *Social Science and Medicine* 52(9):1451–8.

Mehta, C., T. Nik, I. Mora, and J. Wade. 2002. *Chicago's undocumented immigrants: An analysis of wages, working conditions, and economic contributions*. Centre for Urban Economic Development. Chicago: University of Illinois.

Meintjes, S., A. Pillay, and M. Turshen. 2001. *The aftermath: Women in post-conflict transformation*. London and New York: Zed Books.

Messing, K., ed. 1999. *Integrating gender in ergonomic analysis*. Brussels, Belgium: Trade Union Technical Bureau.

Meyer, M., A. Estable, S. Torres, and N. Cermeño. 2009. *Addressing Health In-*

equities - A Model for Training Lay Health Promoters. Paper presented at the Canadian Public Health Association 2009 Annual Conference, Public Health in Canada: Strengthening Connections. Toronto, 7–10 June.

Meyer, M., S. Torres, N. Cermeño, L. MacLean, and R. Monson. 2003. Immigrant women implementing participatory research in health promotion. *Western Journal of Nursing Research* 25(7):815–34.

Michaud, J. 2005. *Conscience subalterne, conscience identitaire. La voix des femmes assistées au sein des organisations féministes et communautaires*. Ottawa: Presses de l'Université d'Ottawa.

Miron I., and J. Ouimette. 2007. *Les femmes aidantes naturelles dans les communautés francophones et acadiennes du Canada*. Alliance des femmes de la francophonie canadienne. Ottawa. http://www.affc.ca [accessed 3 March 2008].

Mohamoud, H. 2007. Material measures of exclusion among ethic groups in Ottawa: Employment access income inequality and poverty. Power Point presentation based on 2001 Census data. Ottawa: Social Planning Council.

Mohanty, C. 2003. *Feminism without borders: Decolonizing theory, practicing solidarity*. Durham, NC: Duke University Press.

Mohindra, K.S., and S. Haddad. 2005. Women's interlaced freedoms: A framework linking microcredit participation and health. *Journal of Human Development* 6(3):353–74.

Molyneux, M. 2002. Gender and the silences of social capital. *Development and Change* 33(2):167–88.

Moore, S., A. Shiell, P. Hawe, and V.A. Haines. 2005. The privileging of communitarian ideas: Citation practices and the translation of social capital into public health research. *American Journal of Public Health* 95(8):1330–7.

Moore Lappe, F., and P.M. Du Bois. 1997. Building social capital without looking backward. *National Civic Review* 86(2):119–28.

Morrow, M., O. Hankivsky, and C. Varcoe. 2004. Women and violence: The effects of dismantling the welfare state, *Critical Social Policy* 24(3):358–884.

Morrow, M., O. Hankivsky, and C. Varcoe, eds. 2007. *Women's health in Canada: Critical perspectives on theory and policy*. Toronto: University of Toronto Press.

Muennig, P., and M.C. Fahs. 2002. Health status and hospital utilization of recent immigrants to New York City. *Preventive Medicine* 35(3):225–31.

Muhonen, T., and E. Torkelson. 2004. Work locus of control and its relationship to health and job satisfaction from a gender perspective. *Stress and Health* 20:21–8.

Multicultural Health Broker's Co-op. 1998. Mission statement. Unpublished document.

Mulvihill, M., L. Mailloux, and W. Atkin. 2001. *Advancing policy and research responses to immigrant and refugee women's health in Canada.* Report for the Centres of Excellence in Women's Health. http://www.cwhn.ca [accessed 28 April 2006].

Munch, A., J.M. McPherson, and L. Smith-Lovin. 1997. Gender, children and social contact: The effects of childbearing for men and women. *American Sociological Review* 62:509–20.

Muntaner, C., and J.W. Lynch. 1999. Income inequality and social cohesion versus class relations: A critique of Wilkinson's neo-Durkheimian research program. *International Journal of Health Services* 29:59–81.

Murphy, T.F. 1997. *Gay science: The ethics of sexual orientation research.* New York: Columbia University Press.

Narayan, U. 1995. 'Male-order' brides: Immigrant women, domestic violence and immigration law. *Hypatia* 10(1):104–19.

Nath, J.K., and V.R. Nayar. 2004. India. In *Continuum complete international encyclopedia of sexuality.* Ed. R.T. Francour and R.J. Noonan. http://www .kinseyinstitute.org/ [accessed 1 May 2009].

National Center for Cultural Competence. 2004. *Bridging the cultural divide in health care settings: The essential role of cultural broker programs.* Georgetown University for Child and Human Development. http://nccc.georgetown. edu/documents/Cultural_Broker_Guide_English.pdf [accessed 5 April 2005].

National Council of Welfare. 2001. *The cost of poverty.* Ottawa: Minister of Public Works and Government Services.

National Forum on Health. 1997. *Canada health action: Building on the legacy.* Ottawa: Minister of Public Works and Government Services.

National Organization of Immigrant and Visible Minority Women of Canada (NOIVMWC). 2005. *Immigrant and visible minority women as full contributors to Canadian society: The livelihood project 15–16.* Report by Catalyst Research and Communications for the National Organization of Immigrant and Visible Minority Women of Canada. Ottawa: NOIVMWC.

Nazmabadi A. 1998. *The story of the daughters of Quchan: Gender and national memory in Iranian history.* Syracuse, NY: Syracuse University Press.

Nelson, G., and I. Prilleltensky, eds. 2005. *Community psychology: In pursuit of liberation and well-being.* New York: Palgrave Macmillan.

Neufeld, A., M. Harrison, K. Hughes, M. Stewart, and D.L. Spitzer. 2002. Immigrant women: Making connections to community resources for support in family caregiving. *Qualitative Health Research* 12(6):751-768.

Neville, S., and M. Henrickson. 2006. Perceptions of lesbian, gay and bisexual people of primary healthcare services. *Journal of Advanced Nursing* 55(4):407–15.

Newbold, K.B. 2005a. Health status and health care of immigrants in Canada: A longitudinal analysis. *Journal of Health Services Research and Policy* 10(2):77–83.

– 2005b. Self-rated health within the Canadian immigrant population: Risk and the healthy immigrant effect. *Social Science and Medicine* 60(6):1359–70.

Newbold, K.B., and J. Danforth. 2003. Health status and Canada's immigrant population. *Social Science and Medicine* 57(10):1981–95.

Ng, E., R. Wilkins, F. Gendron and J.-M. Berthelot. 2005. Dynamics of immigrants' health in Canada: Evidence from the National Population Health Survey. Ottawa, Statistics Canada: 11.

Ngo, H., and D. Este. 2006. Professional re-entry for foreign-trained immigrants. *Journal of International Migration and Integration*, 7(1):27–50.

Noh, S., V. Kaspar, and K.A.S. Wickrama. 2007. Overt and subtle racial discrimination and mental health: Preliminary findings for Korean immigrants. *American Journal of Public Health* 97(7):1269–74.

Noh, S., M. Speechley, V. Kaspar, and Z. Wu. 1992. Depression in Korean immigrants in Canada: Method of the study and prevalence of depression. *Journal of Nervous and Mental Disease* 180(9):573–7.

Nyers, P. 2006. *Access not fear: Non-status immigrants and city services, a preliminary report.* Unpublished manuscript.

Oakeshott, R. 1978. *The case for worker's co-ops.* London: Routledge and Kegan Paul.

O'Donnell, J., W. Johnson, L. D'Aunno, and H. Thornton. 2005. Fathers in child welfare: Caseworkers' perspectives. *Child Welfare League of America* 84(3):387–414.

Office des Affaires Francophones de l'Ontario. 2005. *Les minorités raciales Francophones en Ontario, Profil statistique.* Toronto.

Okeke, P., and D.L. Spitzer. 2005. In search of identity, longing for homelands: Intergenerational experiences of African youth in a Canadian Context. In *The African diaspora in Canada: Negotiating identity and belonging*, 205–24. Ed. W. Tettey and K. Puplampu. Calgary: University of Calgary Press.

Omidvar, R., and T. Richmond. 2005. Immigrant settlement and social inclusion in Canada. In *Social inclusion: Canadian perspectives*, 155–79. Ed. T. Richmond and A. Saloojee. Toronto: Fernwood Publications.

O'Neill, B.J. 2006. Toward inclusion of gay and lesbian people: Social policy changes in relation to sexual orientation. In *Canadian social policy: Issues and perspectives*, 331–48. 4th ed. Ed. A. Westhues. Waterloo, ON: Wilfrid Laurier University Press.

Ong, A. 1999. *Flexible citizenship: The cultural logics of transnationality.* Durham, NC: Duke University Press.

– 2003. *Buddha is hiding: Refugees, citizenship, the new America.* Berkeley: University of California Press.

Ontario Human Rights Commission. 2005. Racism and racial discrimination fact sheet. Ontario Human Rights Commission. http://www.ohrc.on.ca/english/publications/racism-and-racial-discrimination-fact2.shtml [accessed 7 August 2007].

Ontario Ministry of Health and Long-Term Care (OMHLTC). 2007a. Epidemiological fact sheet on HIV/AIDS in Ontario. Ontario Ministry of Health and Long-Term Care. http://www.health.gov.on.ca/english/public/pub/aids/pdf/hiv_epidemiological.pdf [accessed 1 October 2007].

– 2007b. Number (adjusted) and proportion of HIV diagnoses by year-quarter and sex, Ontario, 1996–2007. Ontario Ministry of Health and Long-Term Care. http://www.phs.utoronto.ca/ohemu/doc/Table1.pdf [accessed 1 October 2007].

Ontario Public Health Association (OPHA). June 2000. *Improving the access to and quality of public health services for lesbians and gay men: A position paper of the Ontario Public Health Association.* Toronto: OPHA. http://www.opha.on.ca [accessed 20 October 2008].

– 2002. *Equal access indicators for Ontario's mandatory core programming requirements.* Ontario Public Health Association (OPHA). http://www.opha.on.ca/resources [accessed 5 July 2007].

Ooka, E., and B. Wellman. 2003. Does social capital pay off more within or between ethnic groups? Analyzing job searches in five Toronto ethnic groups. In *Inside the Mosaic,* 199–226. Ed. E. Fong. Toronto: University of Toronto Press.

Ornstein, M. 2001. *Ethno-racial inequality in Toronto: Analysis of the 1996 Census.* Toronto: Institute for Social Research, York University.

Ornstein, M. 2006. *Ethno-racial groups in Toronto, 1971–2001: A demographic and socio economic profile.* Toronto: York University.

Ortiz, L.M. 2003. *Multicultural health brokering: Bridging cultures to achieve equity of access to health.* Diss. University of Alberta, Edmonton.

Ottawa Public Health (OPH). 2005. *HIV Epidemiology.* Ottawa: OPH Surveillance Unit.

– 2006. *Health status report: Measuring health in Ottawa to build a stronger and healthier community.* City of Ottawa. http://www.ottawa.ca/residents/health/publications/hsr/communicable_en.html [accessed 30 November 2007].

– 2007. *Summary of HIV/AIDS epidemiology.* OPH Surveillance Unit, Emerging Issues, Education, and Research Division. Ottawa: OPH.

Ottosson, D. 2008. *Sate-sponsored homophobia: A world survey of laws.* http://www.ilga.org [accessed 1 May 2009].

Oxman-Martinez, J., J. Hanley, L. Lach, N. Khanlou, S. Weerasinghe, and V. Agnew. 2005. Intersection of Canadian policy parameters affecting women with precarious immigration status: A baseline for understanding barriers to health. *Journal of Immigrant Health* 7(4):247–58.

Pachankis, J.E., and M.R. Goldfried. 2004. Clinical issues in working with lesbian, gay, and bisexual clients. *Psychotherapy, Theory, Practice, Training* 41(3):227–46.

Paisley, J.A., J. Haines, M. Greenberg, M.J. Makarchuk, S. Vogelzang, and K. Lewicki. 2002. An examination of cancer risk beliefs among adults from Toronto's Somali, Chinese, Russian and Spanish-speaking communities. *Canadian Journal of Public Health* 93(2):138–41.

Papademetriou, D. 2005. *The global struggle with illegal migration: No end in sight.* Migration Information Source, 1 September. Washington, DC: Migration Policy Institute.

Paradies, Y. 2006. A systematic review of empirical research on self-reported racism and health. *International Journal of Epidemiology* 35(4):888–901.

Parreñas, R. 2001. *Servants of globalization: Women, migration and domestic work.* Stanford, CA: Stanford University Press.

Parsons, R. 2001. Summer specific practice strategies for empowerment-based practice with women: A study of two groups. *Affilia* 2:159–79.

Patel, V., R. Araya, M. de Lima, A. Ludermir, and C. Todd. 1999. Women, poverty and common mental disorders in four restructuring societies. *Social Science and Medicine* 49:1461–71.

Patton, M.Q. 2002. *Qualitative research and evaluation methods.* Thousand Oaks, CA: Sage.

Pellicer, L.O. 2003. *Caring enough to lead: How reflective thought leads to moral leadership.* Thousand Oaks, CA: Corwin Press.

Perez, C.E. 2002. Health status and health behaviour among immigrants. *Health Reports* 13 (suppl.):1–13.

Perrin, B. 1998. *How does literacy affect the health of Canadians?* A profile paper presented to the Policy Development and Coordination Division.Health Promotion and Programs Branch, Health Canada http://www.hc-sc.gc.ca/hppb/healthpromotiondevelopment/pube/literacy-health/literacy.htm [accessed 10 October 2007].

Pevalin, D. 2002. *Intra-household differences in neighbourhood attachment and their associations with health. An analysis of the British Household Panel Survey.* Conference paper at Social Action for Health and Well-being, Health Development Agency. London, 21–2 June.

Pevalin, D.J., and D. Rose. 2002. *Social capital for health: Investigating the links between social capital and health using the British Household Panel Survey.* London: (NHS) Health Development Agency.

Picard, L., and G. Allaire. 2005. *Deuxième rapport sur la santé des Francophones de l'Ontario*. Sudbury, ON: Institut franco-ontarien.

Picot, G., and F. Hou. 2003. *The rise in low-income rates among immigrants in Canada*. Analytic studies research paper, series 11F0019MIE2003198. Analytic Studies Branch. Ottawa: Statistics Canada.

– 2009. *Immigrant characteristics, the IT bust and their effect on entry earnings of immigrants*. Ottawa: Statistics Canada.

Picot, G., F. Hou, and S. Coulombe. 2007. *Chronic low income and low-income dynamics among recent immigrants*. Ottawa: Statistics Canada.

Pilkington, P. 2002. Social capital and health: Measuring and understanding social capital at a local level could help to tackle health inequalities more effectively. *Journal of Public Health Medicine* 12(3):156–9.

Plaza, D. 2004. Disaggregating the Indo- and African-Caribbean migration and settlement experience in Canada. *Canadian Journal of Latin American and Caribbean Studies* 29(57/8):241–66.

Ploem, C. 2002. Studies document gender differences in HIV risk and impact. *Canadian HIV/AIDS policy and law review* 7(2–3):35.

Policy Research Initiative (PRI). 2005. *Social capital as a public policy tool: Measurement of social capital*. Reference document for public policy research, development, and evaluation. Ottawa: Sandra Franke.

Portes, A., and M. Mooney. 2002. Social capital and community development. In *The new economic sociology: Developments in an emerging field*, 303–29. Ed. M.F. Guillen, R. Collins, P. England, and M. Meyer. New York: Russell Sage Foundation.

Pottie, K., E. Ng, D. Spitzer, A. Mohammed, and R. Glazier. 2008. Language proficiency, gender and self-reported health: An analysis of the first two waves of the Longitudinal Survey of Immigrants to Canada. *Canadian Journal of Public Health* (November/December):505–10.

PRA Inc. 2004. *Évaluation de la capacité des communautés Francophones en situation minoritaire à accueillir de nouveaux arrivants*. Rapport fait pour le copte de la Fédération des communautés Francophones et acadienne du Canada, Ottawa. http://www.fcfa.ca [accessed 8 April 2007].

Premji, S., K. Messing, and K. Lippel. 2008. Broken English, broken bones? Mechanisms linking language proficiency and occupational health in a Montreal garment factory. *International Journal of Health Services* 38(1):1–19.

Press, I. 1969. Ambiguity and innovation: Implications for the genesis of the culture broker. *American Anthropologist* 71(2):205–17.

Public Health Agency of Canada (PHAC). 2001. Implementing the population health approach. www.phac-aspc.gc.ca/ph-sp/implement/index-eng.php [accessed 1 May 2009].

– 2006. *Canada communicable disease report: Estimates of HIV prevalence and incidence in Canada, 2005, 1 August.* Vol. 32, no. 15. Surveillance and Risk Assessment Division, Centre for Infectious Disease Prevention and Control, Public Health Agency of Canada. http://www.phac-aspc.gc.ca/publicat/ ccdr-rmtc/06vol32/dr3215ea.html [accessed 17 September 2007].

– 2007a. *HIV/AIDS epi updates, November 2007.* Surveillance and Risk Assessment Division, Centre for Infectious Disease Prevention and Control, Public Health Agency of Canada. http://www.phac-aspc.gc.ca/aids-sida/ publication/epi/pdf/epi2007_e.pdf [accessed 30 November 2007].

– 2007b. *HIV and AIDS in Canada. Selected surveillance tables to June 30, 2007.* Surveillance and Risk Assessment Division, Centre for Infectious Disease Prevention and Control, Public Health Agency of Canada. http://www .phac-aspc.gc.ca/aids-sida/publication/index.html#surveillance [accessed 9 December 2007].

– 2007c. *HIV and AIDS in Canada: Surveillance report to December 31, 2006.* Surveillance and Risk Assessment Division, Centre for Infectious Disease Prevention and Control, Public Health Agency of Canada. http://www .phac-aspc.gc.ca/aids-sida/publication/survreport/pdf/survrep1206.pdf [accessed 17 September 2007].

– 2007d. *What determines health? Determinants of health, key determinants, research and evidence base, health status indicators.* http://www.phac-aspc.gc.ca/ ph-sp/determinants/index-eng.php [accessed 2 May 2009].

Putnam, R. 1993. *Making democracy work: Civic traditions in modern Italy.* Princeton, NJ: Princeton University Press.

– 1995. Bowling alone: America's declining social capital. *Journal of Democracy* 6(1):64–78.

– 2001. Social capital: Measurement and consequences. *Canadian Journal of Policy Research* 2(1):41–51.

– 2007. *E Pluribus Unum*: Diversity and community in the twenty-first century. The 2006 Johan Skytte Prize Lecture. *Scandinavian Political Studies* 30(2):137– 74.

Quarter, J. 1992. *Canada's social economy: Co-operatives, non-profits and other community enterprises.* Toronto: James Lorimer.

Quell, C. 2002. *Official languages and immigration: Obstacles and opportunities for immigrants and communities.* Report for the Office of the commissioner of Official Languages. Ottawa: Minister of Public Works and Government Services Canada.

Raphael, D. 2000. Health inequalities in Canada. Current discourses and implications for public health action. *Critical Public Health* 10(2):193– 216.

– 2007. *Poverty and policy in Canada: Implications for health and quality of life.* Toronto: Canadian Scholars' Press.

– 2009. Escaping from the Phantom Zone: Social determinants of health, public health units and public policy in Canada. *Health Promotion International* 24(2):193–8.

Rappaport, J. 1987. Terms of empowerment/Exemplars of prevention: Toward a theory for community psychology. *American Journal of Community Psychology* 15(2):121–48. http://pao.chadwyc.com.proxy.bib.uottawa.ca [accessed 5 July 2007].

Raven, P., M. Rivard, Y. Samson, and M. VanderPlaat. 2003. Linking empowerment-based evaluation and social change. In *Making a difference: Research and families.* Ed. R. Munford and J. Sanders. St. Leonard's, Australia: Allen and Unwin.

Razack, S. 2000. From the clean snows of Petawawa: The violence of Canadian peacekeepers in Somalia. *Cultural Anthropology* 15(1):127–63.

Redwood-Campbell, L., N. Fowler, J. Kaczorowski, E. Molinaro, S. Robinson, M. Howard, and M. Jafarpour. 2003. How are new refugees doing in Canada? Comparison of the health and settlement of the Kosovars and Czech Roma. *Canadian Journal of Public Health* 94(5):381–5.

Reitmanova, S., and D.L. Gustafson. 2007. *Concepts and determinants of St. John's immigrants' mental health: Report for mental health decision makers, organizations and services providers in Newfoundland and Labrador. St. John's, NFLND.* http://www.nlcahr.mun.ca/research/reports_search/Immigrant_mental_health_reitmanova.pdf [accessed 16 July 2007].

Reitz, J.G. 2005. Tapping immigrants' skills: New directions for Canadian immigration policy in the knowledge economy. *Choices* 11(1):1–18.

Reijneveld, S., R. Verheij, L. van Herten, and D. de Bakker. 2001. Contacts of general practitioners with illegal immigrants. *Scandinavian Journal of Public Health* 29:308–13.

Remis, R.S., and M. Fikre-Merid. 2006. *Estimates and projections of HIV infection among persons from HIV-endemic countries in Ontario.* Presentation to the 1st African and Caribbean HIV/AIDS Research Summit, Toronto, 28 April. http://www.phs.utoronto.ca/ohemu/doc/Endemic%20plus.pdf [accessed 12 February 2008].

Remis, R.S., and M.F. Merid. 2004a. The epidemiologic characteristics of HIV infection and AIDS – Ottawa Public Health Unit, 1981–2003. Presentation to Community Planning Initiative, 12 October 2004. http://www.phs.utoronto.ca/ohemu/doc/2005/OttawaFinal.pdf [accessed 11 February 2007].

– 2004b. *The epidemiology of HIV infection among persons from HIV-endemic countries in Ontario: Update to December 2002, summary of findings.* Toronto: Ontario Ministry of Health and Long-Term Care, June 2004.

Remis, R.S., C. Swantee, L. Scheidel, M. Fikre, and J. Liu. 2007. *Report on HIV/ AIDS in Ontario 2005.* Toronto: Ontario Ministry of Health and Long-Term Care, March 2007.

Remis, R.S., C. Swantee, and J. Liu. 2010. *Report on HIV/AIDS in Ontario 2008, Ontario HIV Epidemiologic Monitoring Unit.* www.phs.utoronto.ca/ohemu [accessed 1 April 2011].

Remis, R.S., and E.P. Whittingham. 1999. *The HIV/AIDS epidemic among persons from HIV-endemic countries in Ontario, 1981–98: Situation report.* Department of Public Health Sciences, University of Toronto, November 1999.

Remennick, L. 1999. Women of the 'sandwich' generation and multiple roles: The case of Russian immigrants of the 1990s in Israel. *Sex Roles* 40(5/6):247–78.

Réseau francophone de santé du Nord de l'Ontario, Réseau de santé en français du Moyen Nord de l'Ontario, Réseau franco-santé du sud de l'Ontario, Réseau des services de santé en français de l'Est de l'Ontario. 2006. Préparer le terrain. Rapport provincial. http://santenordontario.ca/documents/ PLT_P_fr.pdf [accessed 10 October 2007].

Rice, J.J., and M.J. Prince. 2000. *Changing politics of Canadian social policy.* Toronto: University of Toronto Press.

Rigakos, G.S. 1995. Constructing the symbolic complainant: Police subculture and the nonenforcement of protection orders for battered women. *Violence and Victims* 10:227–47.

Rist, R.C. 1994. Influencing the policy process with qualitative research. In *Handbook of Qualitative Research,* 545–57. Ed. N.K. Denzin and Y.S. Lincoln. Thousand Oaks, CA: Sage.

Ritsner, M., I. Modai, and A. Ponizovsky. 2000. The stress-support patterns and psychological distress of immigrants. *Stress Medicine* 16:139–47.

Robinson, V., P. Tugwell, P. Walker, A.A. Ter Kuile, V. Neufeld, J. Hatcher-Roberts, C. Amaratunga, N. Andersson, M. Doull, R. Labonte, W. Muckle, F. Murangira, C. Nyamai, D. Ralph-Robinson, D. Simpson, C. Sitthi-Amorn, J. Turnbull, J. Walker, and C. Wood. 2007. Creating and testing the concept of an academic NGO for enhancing health equity: A new mode of knowledge production? *Education for Health* 7:53. http://www.educationforhealth .net/articles/subviewnew.asp?ArticleID=53 [accessed 30 November 2007].

Rollock, D., and Gordon, E. 2000. Racism and mental health into the 21st century: Perspectives and parameters. *American Journal of Orthopsychiatry* 70(11):5–13.

Roman, L.A., J.K. Lindsay, J.S. Moore, and A.L. Shoemaker. 1999. Community health workers: Examining the helper therapy principle. *Public Health Nursing* 16(2):87–95.

Rose, D., V. Preston, and I. Dyck. 2002. Gender and immigration. *horizons: Policy Research Initiatives* 5(2):12–13.

Rose, S., and S. Hatzenbuehler. 2009. Embodying social class: The link between poverty, income inequality and health. *International Social Work* 52(4):459–71.

Ross, F. 2001. Speech and silence: Women's testimony in the first five weeks of public hearings of the South African truth and reconciliation commission. In *Remaking a world*, 250–80. Ed. V. Das, A. Kleinman, M. Lock, M. Ramphele, and P. Reynolds. Berkeley: University of California Press.

Rousseau, C., and A. Drapeau. 2004. Premigration exposure to political violence among independent immigrants and its association with emotional distress. *Journal of Nervous and Mental Disease* 192(12):852–6.

Rousseau, C., A. Mekki-Berrada, and S. Moreau. 2001. Trauma and extended separation from family among Latin American and African refugees in Montreal. *Psychiatry* 64(1):40–59.

Rousseau, C., M.-C. Rufagari, D. Bagilishya, and T. Measham. 2004. Remaking family life: Strategies for re-establishing continuity among Congolese refugees during the family reunification process. *Social Science and Medicine* 59(5):1095–1108.

Rowe, W.S., J. Hanley, E.R. Moreno, and J. Mould. 2000. Voices of social work practice: International reflections on the effects of globalization. *Canadian Social Work Review* 2(1):65–87.

Ruan, F.F., and M.D. Lau. 2004. China. In *Continuum complete international encyclopedia of sexuality*. Ed. R.T. Francour and R.J. Noonan. http://www .kinseyinstitute.org/ [accessed 1 May 2009].

Rubin, H., and I. Rubin. 2001. *Community organizing and development*. 3d ed. Boston: Allyn and Bacon.

Rychetnik, L., and A. Todd. 2004. *Vic Health mental health promotion evidence review: A literature review focusing on the Vic Health 1999–2002 mental health promotion framework*. VicHealth: Victorian Health Promotion Foundation. http://www.vichealth.vic.gov.au [accessed 7 August 2007].

Safdar, S., and C.H. Lay. 2003. The relations of immigrant-specific and immigrant-nonspecific daily hassles to distress controlling for psychological adjustment and cultural competence. *Journal of Applied Social Psychology* 33(2):299–320.

Said, E. 1978. *Orientalism*. New York: Vintage Books.

Salaff, J., and A. Greve. 2004. Can women's social networks migrate? *Women's Studies International Forum* (27):149–62.

Salaff, J., A. Greve, and L. Ping. 2002. Paths into the economy: Structural barriers and the job hunt for skilled PRC migrants in Canada. *International Journal of Human Resource Management* 13(3):450–64.

Sales, R. 2002. The deserving and the undeserving? Refugees, asylum seekers and welfare in Britain. *Critical Social Policy* 22(3):456–78.

Sandelowski, M. 2000. What ever happened to qualitative description? *Research in Nursing and Health* 23:334–40.

Sassen, S. 2000. Women's burden: Counter-geographies of globalization and the feminization of survival. *Journal of International Affairs* 53(2):503–24.

Scasta, D. 1998. Historical perspectives on homosexuality. *Journal of Gay and Lesbian Psychotherapy* 2(4):3–17.

Schatzman, L., and A. Strauss. 1973. *Field research: Strategies for a natural sociology.* Englewood Cliffs: NJ: Prentice-Hall.

Scheder, J. 1988. A sickly-sweet harvest: Farmworker diabetes and social equality. *Medical Anthropology Quarterly* 2(3):251–77.

Schellenberg, G., and H. Maheux. 2007. Immigrants' perspectives on their first four years in Canada: Highlights from three waves of the Longitudinal Survey of Immigrants to Canada. *Canadian Social Trends* (April):2–34.

Scheper-Hughes, N. 1991. The subversive body: Illness and the micropolitics of resistance. *Anthropology UCLA* (spring):43–70.

– 1992. *Death without weeping: The violence of everyday life in Brazil.* Berkeley: University of California Press.

Scheper-Hughes, N., and M. Lock. 1987. The mindful body: A prolegomenon to future work in medical anthropology. *Medical Anthropology Quarterly* 1(1):6–41.

Schiebinger, L. 1999. Theories of gender and race. In *Feminist theory and the body: A reader*, 21–31. Ed. J. Price and M. Shildrick. New York: Routledge Press.

Schwanberg, S.L. 1996. Health care professionals' attitudes toward lesbian women and gay men. *Journal of Homosexuality* 31(3):71–83.

Sen, G., P. Östlin, and A. George. 2007. Unequal, unfair, ineffective and inefficient. Gender inequity in health: Why it exists and how we can change it. Final report to the WHO Commission on Social Determinants of Health. Geneva.

Sent, L., P. Ballem, E. Paluck, L. Yelland, and A.M. Vogel. 1998. The Asian women's health clinic: Addressing cultural barriers to preventive care. *Canadian Medical Association Journal* 159:350–4.

Sergiovanni, T. 2007. *Rethinking leadership.* 2d ed. Thousand Oaks, CA: Corwin Press.

Sharma, N. 2001. On being not Canadian: The social organization of 'migrant workers' in Canada. *CRSA/RCSA* 38(4):415–39.

Shimoni, R., D. Este, and D. Clark. 2003. Paternal engagement in immigrant and refugee families. *Journal of Comparative Family Studies* 34(4):555–68.

Siegmann, K.S., and S. Thieme, eds. 2007. *Coping on women's back: Social capital-vulnerability links through a gender lens.* International migration, multi-local livelihoods and human security: Perspectives from Europe, Asia and Africa, 30-31 August 2007. The Hague, Netherlands: Institute of Social Sciences.

Siegrist, J., and M. Marmot. 2004. Health inequalities and the psychosocial environment – Two Scientific Challenges. *Social Science and Medicine* 58:1463–73.

Silove, D., A. Steel, P. McGorry, and P. Mohan. 1998. Psychiatric symptoms and living difficulties in Tamil asylum seekers: Comparisons with refugees and immigrant. *Acta Psychiatrica Scandivavica* 97(3):175–81.

Silove, D., Z. Steel, and C. Watters. 2000. Policies of deterrence and the mental health of asylum seekers in Western countries. *Journal of the American Medical Association* 284:504–611.

Simich, L. 2006. Hidden meanings of health security: Migration experiences and systemic barriers to mental well-being among non-status migrants. *International Journal of Migration, Health and Social Care* 2(3/4):16–27.

Simich, L., M. Beiser, and F.N. Mawani. 2002. Paved with good intentions: Canada's refugee destining policy and paths of secondary migration. *Canadian Public Policy* 28(4):597–607.

– 2003. Social support and the significance of shared experience in refugee migration and resettlement. *Western Journal of Nursing Research* 25(7):872–91.

Simich, L., M. Beiser, M. Stewart, and E. Mwakarimba. 2005. Providing social support for immigrants and refugees in Canada: Challenges and directions. *Journal of Immigrant and Minority Health* 7(4):259–68.

Simich, L., H. Hamilton, and D. Este. 2005. Meeting the multilevel challenges of Sudanese well-being and social integration in Canada. Research proposal submitted to the Social Sciences and Humanities Research Council. Ottawa: University of Toronto and University of Calgary.

Simich, L., F. Mawani, F. Wu, and A. Noor. 2004. *Meanings of social support, coping and help-seeking strategies among immigrants and refugees in Toronto.* CERIS workshop paper, no. 31.

Simich, L., F. Wu, and S. Nerad. 2007. Status and Health Security: An exploratory study among irregular immigrants in Toronto. *Canadian Journal of Public Health* 98(5):369–73.

Smedley, A. 1993. *Race in North America: Origin and evolution of a worldview.* Boulder, CO: Westview Press.

Smith, D. 1984. The renaissance of women: Knowledge reconsidered: A feminist overview. Canadian Research Institute for the Advancement of Women. Ottawa: CRIAW Publications Committee.

Smith, D. 1987. *The everyday world as problematic: A feminist sociology*. Boston: Northeastern University Press.

Smith, K.L., F.I. Matheson, R. Moineddin, and R.H. Glazier. 2007. Gender, income and immigration differences in depression in Canadian urban centres. *Canadian Journal of Public Health* 98(2):149–53.

Social Planning Council of Ottawa. 2004. *Immigrants in Ottawa: Socio-cultural composition and socio-economic conditions*. Ottawa: Social Planning Council.

Speer, P.W., and J. Hughey. 1995. Community organizing: An ecological route to empowerment and power. *American Journal of Community Psychology* 23:729–48.

Spitzer, D.L. 2003. *Gender, stress and migration: Workshop synthesis report*. Presentation to the Eighth International Metropolis Conference. Vienna, Australia.

– 2004. In visible bodies: Minority women, nurses, time and the new economy of care. *Medical Anthropology Quarterly* 18(4):490–508.

– 2005. Engendering health disparities. *Canadian Journal of Public Health* 96(suppl. 2):S78–96.

– 2006. *Gender and sex-based analysis in health research: A guide for CIHR peer review committees*. Ottawa: Canadian Institutes for Health Research. http://www.cihr-irsc.gc.ca/e/32019.html [accessed 20 September 2007].

– 2007a. *Embodying inequalities: Globalization, health and foreign domestic workers*. Presentation to the Sixth Pan-European International Relations Conference, Torino, Italy.

– 2007b. Immigrant and refugee women: Re-Creating meaning in transnational context. *Anthropology in Action* 14(1/2):52–62.

– 2008. *Negotiating identities: The voices of African women in Alberta, Canada*. Institute for African Development, occasional paper. Ithaca, NY: Cornell University.

– 2009a. Policy (in) action: Policy-making, health and migrant women. In *Racialized Immigrant Women in Canada: Essays on Health, Violence and Equity*. Ed. V. Agnew. Toronto: University of Toronto Press.

– 2009b. Crossing cultural and bodily boundaries of migration and menopause. In *Crossing Cultural Boundaries*. Ed. S. Krajewski and L. Hernandez. Cambridge, UK: Cambridge Scholar's Publishing.

Spitzer, D.L., A. Neufeld, and S. Bitar. 2000. The impact of immigration policy on women's health and well-being: A synthesis of workshop findings. 5th International Metropolis Conference, Vancouver.

Spitzer, D.L., A. Neufeld, M. Harrison, K. Hughes, and M. Stewart. 2003. Caregiving in transnational perspective: My wings have been cut, where can I fly? *Gender and Society* 17(2):267–86.

Staeheli, L. 2003. Women and the work of community. *Environment and Planning* 35:815–31.

Statistics Canada. 1993. The violence against women survey. *The Daily,* 18 November 1993, 1-10.

Statistics Canada. 2003a. *Longitudinal survey of immigrants to Canada: Process, progress and prospects.* Ottawa: Ministry of Industry.

– 2003b. 2001 Census: Analysis series, Canada's ethnocultural portrait – the changing mosaic. Ottawa: Statistics Canada.

– 2003c. Census of population: Immigration, birthplace and birthplace of parents, citizenship, ethnic origin, visible minorities and aboriginal peoples. *The Daily,* 21 January.

– 2003d. Census of population: Earnings, levels of schooling, field of study and school attendance. *The Daily* 11 March, Statistics Canada. http://www .statcan.ca/Daily/English/030311/d030311a.htm [accessed 23 March 2007].

– 2003e. Longitudinal survey of immigrants to Canada. T*he Daily.* September. Statistics Canada. http://www.statcan.gc.ca/daily-quotidien/030904/ dq030904a-eng.htm [accessed 15 March 2011].

– 2005. Longitudinal survey of immigrants to Canada: A portrait of early settlement experiences. Ottawa: Statistics Canada.

– 2006. Portrait of the Canadian population in 2006: National portrait. Ottawa: Statistics Canada (2007). *Portrait of the Canadian Population in 2006: Highlights,* 2007. http://www12.statcan.ca/english/census06/analysis/ popdwell/highlights.efm [accessed 20 February 2007].

– 2007. Immigration in Canada: A portrait of the foreign-born Population, 2006 Census: Portraits of major metropolitan centres. Ottawa: Statistics Canada. http://www12.statcan.ca/census-recensement/2006/as-sa/97-557/ p28-eng.cfm [accessed 15 March 15 2011]

– 2008. Study: Health care use among gay, lesbian and bisexual Canadians. *The Daily* 19 March. www.statcan.gc.ca/daily-quotidien/080319/ dq080319b-eng.htm [accessed 30 October 2009].

Stearns, P.N. 1991. Fatherhood in historical perspective: The role of social change. In *Fatherhood and families in cultural context,* 28–52. Ed. F. Bozett and S. Hanson. New York: Springer.

Steele, L., C. Lemieux, J. Clark, and R. Glazier. 2002. The impact of policy changes on the health of recent immigrants and refugees in the inner city. *Canadian Journal of Public Health* 93(2):118–22.

Stein, C., V. Wemmerus, M. Ward, M. Gaines, A. Freeberg and T. Jewell. 1998. 'Because they're my parents': An intergenerational study of felt obligation and parental caregiving. *Journal of Marriage and the Family* 60 (August): 611–22.

Stephen, E., K. Foote, G. Hendershot, and C. Schoenborn. 1994. Health of the foreign-born population: United States, 1989–90. *Advance Data from Vital and Health Statistics* (241):1–12.

Stephens, C. 2008. Social capital in its place: Using social theory to understand social capital and inequalities in health. *Social Science and Medicine* 66:1174–84.

Stephens, T., and N. Joubert. 2001. The economic burden of mental health problems in Canada. *Chronic Diseases in Canada* 22(1):18–23.

Stephenson, P.H. 1995. Vietnamese refugees in Victoria, B.C.: An overview of immigrant and refugee health care in a medium sized urban centre. *Social Science and Medicine* 40(12):1631–42.

Stern, M.P., and M. Wei. 1999. Do Mexican Americans really have low rates of cardiovascular disease? *Preventive Medicine* 29(6): S90–5.

Stewart, M., J. Anderson, M. Beiser, E. Makwarimba, A. Neufeld, L. Simich, and D.L. Spitzer. 2008. Multicultural meanings of social support among immigrants and refugees. *International Migration* 46(3):123–59.

Stewart, M., J. Anderson, M. Beiser, A. Neufeld, D. Spitzer, and L. Simich. 2004. *Weaving together social support and health from a multicultural context.* Edmonton: Social Support Research Program. http://www.ssrp.ualberta .ca/pdf/multicultural_meanings_public_report.pdf [accessed 3 May 2007].

Stewart, M., J. Anderson, M. Beiser, A. Neufeld, D. Spitzer, E. Makwarimba, S. So, and Z. Jones. 2002. *Weaving together social support and health in a multicultural context.* Interim report submitted to SSHRC, September 2002.

Stone, R.A.T., B. Purkayastha, and T.A. Berdahl. 2006. Beyond Asian American: Examining conditions and mechanisms of earnings equality for Filipina and Asian Indian women. *Sociological Perspectives* 49(2):261–81.

Strier, R., and D. Roer-Strier. 2005. Fatherhood and immigration: Perceptions of Israeli immigrant fathers from Ethiopia and the former Soviet Union. *Families in Society* 86(1):121–33.

Sundquist, J. 1995. Ethnicity, social class and health: A population-based study on the influence of social factors on self-reported illness in 223 Latin American refugees, 333 Finnish and 126 South European labour migrants and 841 Swedish controls. *Social Science and Medicine* 40(6):777–87.

Suyemoto, K., and M. Ballou. 2007. Conducted monotones to coacted harmonies: A feminist (re)conceptualization of leadership addressing race, class, and gender. In *Women and leadership: Transforming visions and diverse voices*, 35–54. Ed. J. Lau Chin, B. Lott, J. Rice, and J. Sanchez-Hucles. Malden, MA: Blackwell Publishing.

Szasz, M. 1994. Introduction. In *Between Indian and white worlds: The cultural broker*, 4–19. Ed. M.C. Szasz. Norman, OK and London: University of Oklahoma Press

Takeda, Y., I. Kawachi, Z. Yamagata, S. Hashimoto, Y. Matsumura, S. Oguri, and A. Okayama. 2004. Multigenerational family structure in Japanese society: Impacts on stress and health Behaviours among women. *Social Science and Medicine* 59:69–81.

Tang, T.N., K. Oatley, and B.B. Toner. 2007. Impact of life events and difficulties on the mental health of Chinese immigrant women. *Journal of Immigrant and Minority Health* 9(4):281–90.

Tastsoglou, E., and A. Dobrowolsky. 2006. Crossing boundaries and making connections. In *Women, migration and citizenship: Making local, national and transnational connections*, 2–35. Ed. E. Tastsoglou and A. Dobrowolsky. Aldershot, UK: Ashgate Palgrave.

Tastsoglou, E., and V. Preston. 2005. Gender, immigration and labour market integration: Where we are and what we still need to know. *Atlantis* (30):46–59.

Teelucksingh, C., and Galabuzi, G.-E. 2005a. *Working precariously: The impact of race and immigrants' status on employment opportunities and outcomes in Canada.* Toronto: Canadian Race Relations Foundation.

– 2005b. Impact of race and immigrants status on employment opportunities and outcomes in the Canadian labour market. *CERIS Policy Matters* 22 (November).

Tharao, E., N. Massaquoi, and S. Teclom. 2006. *Silent voices of the HIV/AIDS epidemic: African and Caribbean women in Toronto, 2002–2004.* Toronto: Women's Health in Women's Hands.

Thomson, B., and S. Kinne. 1998. Social change theory: Applications to community health. In *Health Promotion at the Community Level: New Advances*, 29–45. 2d ed. Ed. N. Bracht, London: Sage.

Thomson, P. 1993. Developing and implementing culturally sensitive health promotion programs. In *Health and Cultures, Vol. 2*, 206–28. Ed. R. Masi, L. Mensah, and K.A. McLeod. London: Mosaic Press.

Thurston, W.E. 1998. Health promotion from a feminist perspective: A framework for an effective health system response to woman abuse. *Resources for Feminist Research* 26:175–202.

– 2007. Building healthy public policy. In *Canadian community as partner: Theory and multidisciplinary practice*, 138–47. 2d ed. Ed. A.R. Vollman, E.T. Anderson, and J. McFarlane, Philadelphia: Lippincott Williams and Wilkins.

Thurston, W.E., B. Clow, D. Este, T. Gordey, M. Haworth-Brockman, L. McCoy, R. Rapaport Beck, C. Saulnier, J. Smith, and L. Carruthers. 2006. *Immigrant women, family violence, and pathways Out of homelessness.* Calgary, AB: Department of Community Health Sciences, Faculty of Medicine, University of Calgary.

Thurston, W.E., J. Cory, and C.M. Scott. 1998. Building a feminist theoretical framework for screening of wife-battering: Key issues to be addressed. *Patient Education and Counselling* 33:299–304.

Thurston, W.E., and A. Eisener. 2002. *Sighting gender based analysis: Phase II of invisible women.* Winnipeg, MB: Prairie Women's Health Centre of Excellence.

– 2006. Successful integration and maintenance of screening for domestic violence in health settings: Moving beyond individual responsibility. *Trauma, Violence, and Abuse: A Review Journal* 7:83–92.

Thurston, W.E., G. MacKean, A. Vollman, A. Casebeer, M. Weber, B. Maloff, and J. Bader. 2005. Public participation in regional health policy: A theoretical framework. *Health Policy* 73:237–52.

Thurston, W.E., L.M. Meadows, C.M. Scott, A. Eisener, and D. Gavan. 2004a. *Participation of immigrant women in developing domestic violence health policy: The role of advocacy coalitions and policy networks.* Presented at RESOLVE Research Day Conference, Specialized Justice and Community Responses to Domestic Violence. Calgary, AB, 15–16 November.

– 2004b. *Immigrant women and domestic violence health policy: Preliminary analysis.* Presented at Diversity and Health: Connecting Research, Policy and Practice, Calgary, AB, 12 November.

Thurston, W.E., C.M. Scott, and A.R. Vollman. 2004. Public participation for healthy communities and public policy. In *Canadian community as partner: Theory and practice in nursing,* 124–56. Ed. A.R. Vollman, E.T. Anderson, and J. McFarlane. Philadelphia: Lippincott Williams and Wilkins.

Thurston, W.E. and B. Vissandjée. 2005. An ecological model for understanding culture as a determinant of women's health. *Critical Public Health* 15(3):229–42.

Todd, S. 2006. Social work and sexual and gender diversity. In *Social work in Canada,* 273–94. 2d ed. Ed. S. Hick. Toronto: Thompson Educational Publishing.

Todeschini, M. 2001. 'The Bomb's Womb? Women and the Atom Bomb.' In *Remaking A World: Violence, Social Suffering and Recovery,* 102–56. Ed. V. Das, A. Kleinman, M. Lock, M. Ramphele, and P. Reynolds. Berkeley: University of California Press.

Torres, A.M., and B. Sanz. 2000. Health care provision for illegal immigrants: Should public health be concerned? *Journal of Epidemiology and Community Health* 54:78–479.

Torres, S. 2009. *Addressing health inequities by incorporating lay health workers/ paraprofessionals in the public health workforce: Comparing Canada and the United States.* Paper presented at the Canadian Public Health Association 2009 Annual Conference, Public Health in Canada: Strengthening Connections, Winnipeg, 7-10 June.

Torres, S., N. Cermeño, and M. Smith. 2006. *Hispanic women's experiences in seeking and accessing health and social services in Ottawa.* Paper presented at the Second Mexico-Canada Health Week, Ottawa, 5 October.

Torres, S., A. Estable, L. MacLean, and M. Meyer. 2005. *Empowerment of lay health promoters: How women increased their own and their community's access to health and social services.* Paper presented to the Section on Women and Psychology, Canadian Psychological Association Conference, Montréal, 5 June.

Torres, S., M. Meyer, A. Estable, and N. Cermeño. 2009. *What do lay health workers do to facilitate access to health services? The example of Mujer Sana, Comunidad Sana (Healthy Women Healthy Communities).* Paper presented to the Canadian Association for Health Services and Policy Research (CAHSPR), Calgary, 11–14 May.

Tossutti, L. 2003. Does volunteerism increase the political engagement of young newcomers? Assessing the potential of individual and group-based forms of unpaid service. *Canadian Ethnic Studies* XXXV(3):70.

Triandis, H., R. Bentempo, M. Villareal, M. Asai, and N. Lucas. (1988). Individualism and collectivism: Cross-cultural perspectives on self-ingroup relationships. *Journal of Personality and Social Psychology* 54:323–338.

Triandis, H. 2001. Individualism-collectivism and personality. *Journal of Personality* 69(6):907–24.

Tripp-Reimer, T., and P. Brink. 1985. Cultural brokerage. In *Nursing interventions: Treatment for nursing diagnoses*, 352–64. Ed. G.M. Bulechek and J.C. McCloskey, Philadelphia: W.B. Saunders.

Tsigos, C., and G. Chrousos. 2002. Hypothalamic-pituitary-adrenal axis, neuroendocrine factors and stress. *Journal of Psychosomatic Research* 53:865–71.

Turner, V. 1967. Betwixt and between: The liminal period in rites de passage. In *The Forest of Symbols*. Ithaca, NY: Cornell University Press.

United Nations. 1994. Declaration on the elimination of violence against women. General Assembly resolution 48/104 of 20 December 1993. United Nations General Assembly. http://www.unhchr.ch/huridocda/huridoca .nsf/(Symbol)/A.RES.48.104.En [accessed 13 October 2007].

United Nations Children's Fund (UNICEF). HIV/AIDS and children: The big picture. http://www.unicef.org/aids/index_bigpicture.html [accessed 16 September 2007].

United Nations High Commission for Refugees. 2003. *Globe Appeal 2003 – Facts and figures*. http://www.unhcr.org/publ/PUBL/3ddcf8574.pdf [accessed 3 March 2008].

University of Victoria. *What is community-based research?* University of Victoria, Office of Community-based Research. http://www.uvic.ca/research/ocbr/whatis.html [accessed 20 November 2007].

University of Washington. *Community-based research principles*. University of Washington, School of Public Health and Community Medicine. http://sphcm.washington.edu/research/community.asp [accessed 20 November 2007].

Valkonen, T., A. Brancker, and M. Reijo. 1992. Mortality differentials between three populations – residents of Scandinavia, Scandinavian immigrants to Canada and Canadian-born residents of Canada, 1979–1985. *Health Reports* 4(2):137–59.

Valverde, M., and A. Pratt. 2002. From deserving victims to 'masters of confusion': Redefining refugees in the 1990s. *Canadian Journal of Sociology* 27(2):135–61.

VanderPlaat, M. 1998. Empowerment, emancipation and health promotion policy. *Canadian Journal of Sociology* 23(1):71–90.

– 2007. *Integration outcomes for immigrant women in Canada: A review of the literature 2000–2007*. AMC working paper, no. 7. Halifax: Atlantic Metropolis Centre.

VanderPlaat, M., and G. Barrett. 2006. Building community capacity in governance and decision making. *Community Development Journal* 41:25–36.

VanderPlaat, M., Y. Samson, and P. Raven. 2001. The politics and practice of empowerment evaluation and social interventions: Lessons from the Atlantic community action program for children regional evaluation. *Canadian Journal of Program Evaluation* 16(1):79–98.

Van Kemenade S., J.F. Roy, and L. Bouchard. 2006. Social networks and vulnerable populations: Findings from the GSS. Social capital and health: Maximizing the benefits, Health Policy Research, Health Canada. http://hc-sc.gc.ca/sr-sr/pubs/hpr-rpms/bull/2006-capital-social-capital/2006-capital-social-capital-4_e.html [accessed 7 August 2007].

Viruell-Fuentes, E.A. 2007. Beyond acculturation: Immigration discrimination, and health research among Mexicans in the United States. *Social Science and Medicine* 65(7):1524–35.

Varcoe, C. 2001. Abuse obscured: An ethnographic account of emergency nursing in relation to violence against women. *Canadian Journal of Nursing Research* 32:95–115.

Varcoe, C., O. Hankivsky, and M. Morrow. 2007. Introduction: Beyond gender matters. In *Women's health in Canada: Critical perspectives on theory and policy*, 3–30. Ed. M. Morrow, O. Hankivsky, and C. Varcoe. Toronto: University of Toronto Press.

Veronis, L. 2006. *Rethinking transnationalism: Citizenship and immigrant participation in neoliberal Toronto*. PhD diss. University of Toronto.

Vissandjée, B., M. DesMeules, and A. Apale. 2006. Putting migration and ethnicity on the women's health map. *Canadian Women Health Network* 8(3/4):16–17.

Vissandjée, B., M. Desmeules, Z. Cao, S. Abdool, and A. Kazanjian. 2004. Integrating ethnicity and immigration as determinants of Canadian women's health. In *Women's health surveillance report: Supplementary chapters*, 5–7. Ottawa: Canadian Institute for Health Information.

Vissandjée, B., and I. Hyman. 2011. Preventing and managing diabetes at the intersections of gender, ethnicity and migration. In *Health inequities in Canada: Intersectional frameworks and practices*. Vancouver: UBC Press.

Vissandjée, B., I. Hyman, I., D.L. Spitzer, N. Kamrun, and A. Apale. 2007. Integration, clarification, substantiation: Sex, gender, ethnicity and migration as determinants of women's health. *Journal of International Women's Studies* 8(4):32–48.

Vissandjée, B., and L. Maillet. 2007. L'empowerment et l'expérience de l'immigration au Canada: Multiples déterminants dans une réalité complexe (chapitre 6). In *Problèmes sociaux-Tome IV*, 139–58. Ed. Henri Dorvil. Québec: Presse de l'Université du Quebec.

Vissandjée, B., W. Thurston, A. Apale, and N. Kamrun. 2007. Women's health: At the intersection of gender and the experience of migration. In *Women's health in Canada: Critical perspectives on theory and policy*. Ed. M. Morrow, O. Hankivsky, and C. Varcoe. Toronto: University of Toronto Press.

Vissandjée, B., W. Thurston, A. Apale, and K. Nahar. 2007. Women's health at the intersection of gender and the experience of international migration. In *Women's health in Canada: Critical perspectives on theory and policy*, 221–43. Ed. M. Morrow, O. Hankivsky, and C. Varcoe. Toronto: University of Toronto Press.

Vissandjée, B., M. Weinfeld, S. Dupéré, and S. Abdool. 2001. Sex, gender, ethnicity, and access to health care services: Research and policy challenges for immigrant women in Canada. *Journal of International Migration and Integration* 2(1):55–75.

Vissandjée, B., S. Wieringa, and A. Apale. 2009. Exploring social capital among women in the context of migration: Gender sensitive pathway to a healthier life. In *Racialized immigrant women in Canada: Essays on health, violence and equity*. Ed. V. Agnew. Toronto: Centre for Feminist Research.

Voyer, J.-P. 2004. Foreward. *Journal of International Migration and Integration* 5(2):159–64.

Wakefield, S., and B. Poland. 2005. Family, friend or foes? Critical reflections on the relevance and role of social capital in health promotion and community development. *Social Science and Medicine* 60(12):2819–32.

Wales, J. 1995. Does stress cause diabetes? *Diabetic Medicine* 12(2):109–12.

Walls, N.E. 2008. Toward a multidimensional understanding of heterosexism: The changing nature of prejudice. *Journal of Homosexuality* 55(1):20–70.

Wang, Z., S. Ramcharan, and E. Love. 1989. Cancer mortality of Chinese in Canada. *International Journal of Epidemiology* 18(1):17–21.

Warner, T. 2002. *Never going back: A history of queer activism in Canada.* Toronto: University of Toronto Press.

Watters, C., and D. Ingleby. 2004. Locations of care: Meeting the mental health and social care needs of refugees in Europe. *International Journal of Law and Psychiatry* 27:549–70

Wayland, S. 2006. *Unsettled: Legal and policy barriers for newcomers in Canada.* Ottawa: Community Foundations of Canada and Law Commission of Canada.

Weber, L., and D. Parra-Medina. 2003. Intersectionality and women's health: Charting a path to eliminating health disparities. *Advances in Gender Research* 7:181–230.

Weekes, N., J. MacLean, and D. Berger. 2005. Sex, stress and health: Does stress predict health symptoms differently for the two sexes? *Stress and Health* 21:147–56.

Weeks, J. 2004. Sexual orientation: Historical and social construction. In *International encyclopedia of the social and behavioral sciences*, 13998–14002. Ed. N.J. Ameiser and P.B. Baltes. http://www.sciencedirect.com/science/referenceworks/ [accessed 1 May 2009].

Weerasinghe, S., and L. Williams. 2002. *Health and the intersections of diversity: A challenge paper on selected program, policy and research issues.* http://canada.metropolis.net/events/Diversity/Challeng_papers/Health_e.doc [accessed 1 May 2009].

Weidman, H.H. 1982. Research strategies, structural alterations and clinically applied anthopology. In *Clinically applied anthropology: Anthropologists in health science settings*, 201–41. Ed. N.J. Chrisman and T.W. Maretski. Amsterdam: D. Reidel Publishing.

Weinstock, M. 1996. Does prenatal stress impair coping and regulation of hypothalamic-pituitary-adrenal axis. *Neuroscience and Biobehavioral Review* 21(1):1–10.

Weir, E. 2002. Caring for refugees. *Canadian Medical Association Journal* 166(11):1441.

Weisman, C. 2000. Review of empowerment and women's health: Theory, methods, and practice by Jane Stain. (London: Zed, 1997.) *Health Politics and Law* 25(3):607–11.

Weitz, T., and C. Estes. 2001. Adding aging and gender to the women's health agenda. *Journal of Women and Aging* 13(2):3–20.

West, C. 1998. Lifting the 'political gag order': Breaking the silence around partner violence in ethnic minority families. In *Partner violence: A comprehensive review of 20 years of research*, 184–209. Ed. J.L. Jasinski and L.M. Williams. Thousand Oaks, CA: Sage.

Whittle, K.L., and M. Inhorn. 2001. Rethinking difference: A feminist reframing of gender/race/class for the improvement of women's health research. *International Journal of Health Services* 31(1):147–65.

Wickberg, E. 1982. *From China to Canada: A history of Chinese communities in Canada*. Toronto: McClelland and Stewart.

Wlkinson, R. 2001. *Mind the gap: Hierarchies, health and human evolution*. New Haven: Yale University Press.

Wilkinson, R., and M. Marmot, eds. 2003. *Social determinants of health: The solid facts*. 2d ed. Copenhagen: World Health Organization Europe.

Williams, D.R. 1999. Race, socioeconomic status, and health: The added effects of racism and discrimination. *Annals of the New York Academy of Sciences* 896(1):173–88.

– 2005. The health of U.S. racial and ethnic populations. *Journals of Gerontology Series B-Psychological Sciences and Social Sciences* 60 (Special Issue 2):53–62.

Williams, L. 2004. Culture and community development: Towards new conceptualizations and practice. *Community Development Journal* 39(4):345–59.

Willms, M. 2005. Canadian immigration law and same-sex partners. *Canadian Issues* (spring):17–20.

Wilson, D. 1995. *The Canadian health care system*. Edmonton: author.

Wilson, D., and S. Neville. 2009. Culturally safe research with vulnerable populations. *Contemporary Nurse* 33(1):69–79.

Women's Health Bureau (WHB). 2003. *Exploring concepts of gender and health*. Ottawa: Women's Health Bureau.

Wong, Y.L.R., and A.K.T. Tsang. 2004. When Asian immigrant women speak: From mental health to strategies of being. *American Journal of Orthopsychiatry* 74(4):456–66.

World Health Organisation (WHO). 1998. *Health promotion glossary*. Geneva: D. Nutbeam.

– 2002. *World report on violence and health*. Ed. E. Krug, L. Dahlberg, J. Mercy, A. Zwi, and R. Lozano. Geneva: WHO.

– 2003. *Health promotion glossary*. Division of Health Promotion Education and Communication, Health Education and Health Promotion Unit. http://www.who.int/hpr/support.material.shtml [accessed 5 July 2007].

– 2006a. *Engaging for health: 11th general programme of work 2006–2015: A global health agenda*. Geneva: WHO.

– 2006b (October). *The constitution of the World Health Organization*. http://www.who.int [accessed 1 May 2009].

– 2007. *Gender, women, and health: Women and HIV/AIDS*. Geneva: WHO.

World Health Organization Commission on the Social Determinants of Health. 2009. Closing the gap in a generation: Health equity through action on the social determinants of health, 1–246. Geneva: WHO.

Wright, C. 2000. Nowhere at home: Gender, race and the making of anti-immigrant discourse in Canada. *Atlantis* 24(2):38–48.

Young, D., D.L. Spitzer, and F. Pang. (1998). *Understanding the Health Needs of Canadian Immigrants*. Edmonton, AB: Prairie Metropolis Centre.

Young, I.M. 2005. *On female body experience: 'Throwing like a girl' and other essays*. Oxford: Oxford University Press.

Young, L. 2002. *Women's electoral participation in bringing worlds together: The study of political participation of women in Canada and lessons for research on newcomers and minority political participation*. Ottawa: Citizenship and Immigration Canada.

Yuval-Davis, N. 1997a. Ethnicity, gender relations and multiculturalism. In *Debating cultural hybridity*, 193–208. Ed. P. Werbner and T. Modood. London, Zed Press.

– 1997b. *Gender and nation*. London: Sage.

Zelkowitz, P., J. Schinazi, L. Katofsky, J.F. Saucier, M. Valenzuela, R. Westreich, and J. Dayan. 2004. Factors associated with depression in pregnant immigrant women. *Transcultural Psychiatry* 41(4):445–64.

Zietsma, D. 2007. *Canadian immigrant labour market in 2006: First results from Canada's Labour Force Survey*. Ottawa: Statistics Canada.

Zimmer, J.C., and W.E. Thurston. 1998. Attitudes, beliefs, and practices of nursing students concerning HIV/AIDS: Implications for prevention in women. *Health Care for Women International* 19:327–42.

Zoller, H. 2005. Women caught in the multi-causal web: A gendered analysis of healthy people 2010. *Communication Studies* 56(2):175–92.

Contributors

Stephanie Ann Claire Alexander holds an honours BA in psychology from Concordia University in Montréal and an MSc in community health from Université de Montréal. She began a PhD in health promotion in the fall of 2008 in order to examine the way the intersection of gender, socio-economic position, and elements of the social context shape the smoking behaviour of youth. Stephanie has five years' experience conducting research in public health and has worked on various health promotion projects, gaining experience in qualitative health research, interview methods, and both qualitative and quantitative data analysis. Her main research interests involve seeking a better understanding of the ways in which health behaviours are gendered and differentially influence men's and women's health outcomes.

Carol Amaratunga is a research associate emerita with the Justice Institute of British Columbia. In 2008 she retired from the position of dean of applied research. She previously held the Ontario Women's Health Council chair in Women's Health Research, Faculty of Medicine, Institute of Population Health, University of Ottawa. She established a Women's Health Research Unit (WHRU) at the University of Ottawa with a special focus on gender and women's health, including gender and disaster management. Prior to joining the University of Ottawa in 2003, Carol was the principal investigator and executive director of the Atlantic Centre of Excellence for Women's Health, Dalhousie University, Halifax. Her research interests centre on the social determinants of health and health interventions with a focus on the health and well-being of disadvantaged populations and 'forgotten' communities in pandemic, disaster, and post-conflict situations. In addition to a doctorate in educational theory/adult education from the University of Toronto, Dr Amaratunga holds an MSc in agricultural economics and extension education and a BA in sociology and anthropology from the University of Guelph.

Alisha Nicole Apale is an MSc student in the TropEd Erasmus Mundus Program for International Health. She also holds a degree in health care management and is a fellow with CARTHA, a non-profit organization of young and experienced professionals working in global health partnerships. She has worked as a research assistant and project co-coordinator with Professor Bilkis Vissandjée at the University of Montreal for three years, in collaboration with the Shastri Institute and Aga Khan Health Services, India. She has also worked on a number of community development and health research projects in Thailand, India, Kenya, and England. She is currently conducting research on private-public partnerships for health in urban slum settlements in Nairobi, Kenya.

Laura Bisaillon is a PhD student at the Institute of Population Health, University of Ottawa, where she worked as a research assistant for the GOAL project as part of the Women's Health Research Unit. Laura earned degrees in urban planning (McGill), political studies (Bishop's), and international relations (Strasbourg). Her research is focused on immigrant women's health and the health of racialized communities in relation to HIV/AIDS. Qualitative methods, including visual art and narrative, are Laura's methods of choice. In addition to her work in HIV/AIDS advocacy at regional and international levels, she is currently involved in a children's HIV/AIDS book project and the organization of a 'Body Mapping' workshop and art exhibition. She is committed to promoting the involvement of HIV+ women in policy and planning. Laura's work has taken her to Africa, Asia, and the Caribbean to work in maternal health, HIV/AIDS policy development, teaching, refugee health and camp planning, social housing, organizational development, and post-emergency housing reconstruction.

Nubia Cermeño completed the Lay Health Promotion Program given by Mujer Sana, Comunidad Sanaworks in 2003. She then completed a diploma in social service work from Algonquin College. Nubia is currently employed as a settlement worker for the Catholic Immigration Centre/Newcomer Centre in Ottawa, and she volunteers her time to improve the lives of the Hispanic and other ethnocultural communities in the region. Lastly, she is the best-known – if not only – Latin American woman singer in the Ottawa area.

Parin Dossa is professor of anthropology at Simon Fraser University. Her teaching and research interests include diaspora and migration, gender and health, aging culture and ethnicity, ethnographic methods, and structural violence in war and peace. Her ethnographic work has focused on Muslim women in Canada and on the coast of Kenya. She is the author of *Politics and Poetics of Migration: Narratives of Iranian Women from the Diaspora* (Canadian Scholars Press 2004) and *Racialized Bodies and Disabling Worlds: Storied Lives of Immigrant Muslim Women* (University of Toronto Press 2009), and co-producer of two video documentaries. Her work has resulted in several interrelated projects such as differently-abled women, policy implications of storytelling, testimonial narratives and social marginality, and social suffering and everyday life. Currently she is working on a project entitled 'Writing Trauma: Testimonial Narratives of Afghan Women – Homeland to Diaspora.'

Alma Estable, BA, MSW (social administration and policy), is a principal in Gentium Consulting. Alma has successfully managed many projects at the national, provincial, and municipal levels. She has 20 years of experience in community-based social research, program planning, evaluation, writing, and policy development, with a focus on human rights, equity, and global issues. This experience includes the development and implementation of policies to ensure racialized and ethnocultural equity in public institutions, gender analysis, and minority access to health and social services. Alma is a member of the Canadian Evaluation Society and the Ontario Association of Consultants, Counsellors, Psychotherapists and Psychometrists (OACCPP). Alma's long history of involvement with immigrant women's organizations and active community participation complements, grounds, and enriches much of her research on social issues. She is a member of the Latin American Women's Support Organization (LAZO).

David C. Este is a professor within the Faculty of Social Work at the University of Calgary. His major teaching interests include social work practice with immigrants/refugees and racialized minorities, mental health, the management of human service organizations, and qualitative research methodologies. His research focuses on different aspects of the immigrant/refugee experience in Canada, the mental health service delivery system, colouration in the non-profit sector, and the health and well-being of people of African descent residing in Canada. David has also worked as an evaluation consultant for the Calgary Health Region, Immigrant Services Calgary, and the Canadian Mental Health Association. In addition to a master's degree in history from the University of Waterloo, Dr Este obtained his MSW from the University of Toronto in 1982 and a PhD from the Faculty of Social Work, Wilfrid Laurier University, in 1994.

Allison Farber is pursuing a master's degree in epidemiology and is a research assistant at the Women's Health Research Unit, University of Ottawa. Allison completed a BSc in life sciences at Queen's University, where she volunteered with the Queen's AIDS Awareness Committee educating university students about HIV/AIDS prevention. Furthermore, Ms Farber has volunteered for several years with the Canadian Working Group on HIV and Rehabilitation.

Ana Mercedes Guerra, BSW, has been working as a social worker for the South East Ottawa Centre for a Healthy Community since 1993. She has been providing counselling to clients from all walks of life and from various ethnocultural backgrounds. In the past three years, in coordination with the Canadian Mental Health Association, Ana Mercedes Guerra has specialized in working with clients who are survivors of war trauma and torture. Fluent in Spanish and English, Ana Mercedes Guerra is a member of the Latin American Women's Support Organization (LAZO).

Ilene Hyman is an assistant professor in the Dalla Lana School of Public Health at the University of Toronto. She has over 20 years of experience in public health and public health research in Canada and overseas. Dr Hyman's expertise is in the areas of health, women's health, and access to health care for immigrant and racialized populations. She has most recently been involved in conducting research examining intimate partner violence in newcomer communities, including studies of prevalence, risk factors, and help-seeking behaviour. She is also the author of several policy reports related to women's health and immigration and health.

Lucie Kalinda is the past coordinator for the International Twinning Partnership HIV/AIDS, a partnership between the Women's Health Research Unit at the University of Ottawa and the National University of Rwanda. Lucie holds a doctorate in medicine from the University of Kinshasa (Democratic Republic of Congo) and has postgraduate training in ophthalmology. For the past five years, Lucie has served as senior health policy advisor at the Inuit Tapiriit Kanatami in Ottawa, a non-profit advocacy organization representing Inuit peoples across Canada. Her work centres on advocacy, policy development, and strategic planning. Dr Kalinda actively volunteers in activities related to sustainable development, poverty, and hunger and disease reduction, with a focus on the well-being of people in developing countries. Dr. Kalinda is currently residing and practicing medicine in South Africa.

Michèle Kérisit, a professor at the School of Social Work at the University of Ottawa, held a master's degree in Anthropology (Carleton University) and a doctorate in sociolinguistics (Université de Rennes, France). Her most recent research focused on the practices of municipal governments regarding the inclusion of ethnic and racialized diversity within their policies and services, and on family reunification and how it affects French-speaking immigrant and refugee women in Ontario. Dr Kérisit has also conducted research on issues of health for aging francophone women in Ontario, and has published, with Sylvie Frigon, *Du corps des femmes: Contrôles, surveillances et résistances* (Les presses de l'Université d'Ottawa 2000); with Andrée Côté and Marie-Louise Côté, *Sponsorship ... For Better or For Worse: The Impact of Sponsorship on the Equality Rights of Immigrant Women* (Status of Women Canada 2001), and, with a collective of researchers, *L'impact du conflit armé sur l'intégration des femmes immigrantes et des réfugiées Francophones en Ontario* (Rapport présenté au Mouvement ontarien des femmes immigrantes Francophones, MOFIF, 2004).

Sujatha Liyanage is a recent postdoctoral fellow with the Women's Health Research Unit (WHRU) of the Institute of Population Health at the University of Ottawa. Dr Liyanage holds a doctorate in medicine from the Belarus State Medical Institute in Minsk, and an MSc and MD in community medicine from the University of Colombo, Sri Lanka. For 16 years, she served as a medical doctor in curative and preventive sectors under the Ministry of Health in Sri Lanka. In the field of Public Health in Sri Lanka, Sujatha was employed as a medical officer of health where she was also actively involved in maternal mortality surveillance programs. Dr Liyanage's research interests include maternal and child health, women's health, and special-needs children. Dr Liyanage currently resides in Toronto.

Félicité Murangira is the past coordinator, Global Ottawa AIDS Link project, Women's Health Research Unit, University of Ottawa. She was responsible for linking the community to academia for knowledge exchange and innovative best practices in HIV prevention, care, treatment, and support. She has a bachelor of law degree from the University of Burundi, and has been an advocate for newcomers in Ottawa for the last 17 years. Ms Murangira has worked at the Ottawa Carleton Catholic School Board for 10 years as a board community liaison officer and for five years at the Somerset West Community Health Centre in Ottawa as the ethnocultural HIV/AIDS community coordinator. Félicité is co-founder and co-chair of the African and Caribbean Health Network of Ottawa. In 2006, Ms Murangira was awarded both the YMCA-YWCA Women of Distinction Award and the Planet Africa Volunteer of the Year Award. In 2007, she co-led a team visit to the National University of Rwanda as part of the twinning linkage initiative on gender and HIV/AIDS. She remains an untiring advocate for women's health, gender and race equality.

Brian O'Neill is an associate professor at the University of British Columbia's School of Social Work. He received a bachelor of arts in psychology from the University of Windsor, a master of social work from Carleton University, and a doctorate in social work from Wilfrid Laurier University. Dr O'Neill is interested in discovering how social relations related to gender, ethnicity, and sexuality that run through social institutions such as social services reproduce inequity and disadvantage. His research focuses on professional education as well as health and social services, particularly from the standpoint of gay and lesbian people, with the goal of contributing to the development of more inclusive organizational policies and practices.

Lucenia Ortiz has been co-executive director of the Multicultural Health Brokers Co-op in Edmonton, Alberta, since 2002. In addition to a background in public health and urban and regional planning from the University of the Philippines, Dr Ortiz completed her doctorate in human ecology at the University of Alberta in 2003. Lucenia has extensive experience working with immigrant and refugee communities since she came to Canada in 1994. She has coordinated various initiatives aimed at addressing barriers to access and participation of ethnic minorities in health and social service sectors. Dr Ortiz's research interests focus on issues of social exclusion and equity. She is also involved in developing and delivering cultural competency workshops for various service providers in the health and social development sectors.

Melissa Rowe is the coordinator of the African and Caribbean Health Network of Ottawa and an independent consultant with 30 years of professional experience. Ms Rowe holds master of social work and bachelor of social work honours degrees from Carleton University, Ottawa. Through community mobilization partnerships, Melissa advocates for culturally appropriate care, treatment, and support for members of the African and Caribbean communities affected by HIV/AIDS. A registered social worker, Melissa is also a cultural competency consultant, diversity trainer, and health educator. She has developed cross-cultural and anti-racist training-of-trainers programs. Melissa has an ongoing interest in issues related to ethnocultural communities' access to health and social support services. In addition, Ms Rowe is a certified anger solution specialist who has expertise in critical incident stress management.

Laura Simich is an anthropologist and research director at the Center for Immigration and Justice at the Vera Institute of Justice in New York City. She is also an assistant professor in the Culture, Community and Health Studies Program, Department of Psychiatry, University of Toronto, and an affiliate scientist at the Centre for Addiction and Mental Health, Toronto. Dr Simich specializes in qualitative community-based and policy-oriented research. In Canada, her research focused on socio-cultural determinants of mental well-being among immigrants, particularly social support and resilience during refugee resettlement. She developed the popular self-help guide for mental health promotion, *Alone in Canada: 21 Ways to Make It Better, a Guide for Single Newcomers to Canada,* available from www.camh.net/About_Addiction_Mental_Health/Mental_Health_Information/alone_in_canada.html. Her current applied research interests include criminal justice and immigrant mental health in the United States.

Denise Spitzer is the Canada Research Chair in gender, migration, and health at the University of Ottawa, where she is an associate professor affiliated with the Institute of Women's Studies and a principal scientist in the Institute of Population Health. She holds a master's degree and doctorate in anthropology and undergraduate degrees in biology and

Chinese language and literature. Dr Spitzer is interested in examining how global processes – intersecting with gender, ethnicity, migration status, and other social identifiers – are implicated in health and well-being. Her work focuses primarily on immigrant and refugee women, and engages with critical perspectives of the body; transnationalism and constructions of identity; the impact of policy on health; agency and social support; community-based research; and intersectional analysis. She is currently involved in a series of linked research projects with migrants who came to Canada under the auspices of the Live-In Caregiver Program, and in a program of research examining the impact of upheavals in the global economy on various communities of migrant workers and their families.

Kamala Sproule is a community-based social researcher and program evaluator. She received her master of social work from the University of British Columbia in 2002. For 10 years prior to receiving her MSW, Kamala was an English as a second language instructor in non-profit multicultural agencies where she witnessed the systemic and cultural ways in which queer content and identity are excluded or silenced. For the past five years, her community-based research has focused on issues pertaining to marginalized groups, in particular women and people of colour, immigrants and refugees, queer people, and survival sex trade workers. Her research process stresses capacity and relationship building by including the marginalized groups in the research process. The goals of her research have been to raise mainstream community awareness around issues of disenfranchisement, facilitate community development, and increase capacity within marginalized groups via a participatory research process.

Admasu A. Tachble obtained his PhD in social work from the University of Calgary. He also holds a masters degree in development studies (ISS, The Hague) and bachelor's degree in political science and international relations (Ethiopia), Dr Tachble has extensive international development experience in Ethiopia and has worked primarily with multicultural families in Canada. Currently, he is a research associate at the Department of Psychosocial Resources with Alberta Health Services – Cancer Care in Calgary. His research interests include immigrant resettlement, immigrant/refugee fathers, ethnicity, and health outcomes that encompass patient-centred care in a multicultural setting.

Wilfreda (Billie) Thurston has a BA in psychology and a master's and doctorate in health research and social epidemiology. She worked in family and children's services and addictions, and was director of a shelter for women escaping abusive relationships. Dr Thurston is a professor in the Department of Community Health Sciences and director of the University of Calgary Institute for Gender Research. Her program of research and training includes development and evaluation of health promotion programs and health services; prevention of violence against women; public participation in health policy development; and the interplay of the social determinants of health, particularly gender and culture, among marginalized populations. She recently conducted a national study on homelessness among immigrant women who have left abusive relationships, and piloted an international project on health policy and prevention of domestic violence that has resulted in the development of collaborative relationships across Canada and around the world.

Sara Torres holds a bachelor's degree in social work and a master's in social administration and policy. Since 1987, Sara has been working with both the Latin American and Canadian women's communities in Ottawa, as well as with other international communities, most specifically El Salvador. Sara is a member of the Latin American Women's Support Organization (LAZO). Fluent in Spanish, English, and French, Ms Torres has experience in developing and delivering adult training programs in academe and the community on various issues, including participatory action research, multicultural health promotion, and anti-oppression workshops. She has experience in implementing and supervising research projects, including conducting qualitative data analysis and program evaluations. Sara is completing a PhD in population health at the University of Ottawa.

Madine VanderPlaat is a sociologist at Saint Mary's University in Halifax, specializing in community well-being with a focus on citizen participation and marginalized populations, evaluation research, gender analysis, and participatory research strategies. She has worked extensively with the Public Health Agency of Canada and Citizenship and Immigration Canada. From 2004 to 2007 she worked with partners in Cuba, Chile, and Brazil exploring resiliency in coastal communities. She also collaborated with faculty at the Human Rights and Health Research Unit at the National School for Public Health, Oswaldo Cruz

Foundation, in Rio de Janeiro. She currently works with faculty at Shaanxi Normal University in Xi'an, China, developing multidisciplinary, inter-sectoral approaches to ecosystems and human well-being. She is a director of the Atlantic Metropolis Centre, one of five Centres of Excellence committed to comparative research and public policy development on migration and diversity in Canada and around the world.

Bilkis Vissandjée, a professor in the School of Nursing at the University of Montreal, holds a doctorate in population planning and international health. Her work focuses on the relationship between sex, gender, ethnicity, and migration as social determinants of health. Specifically, her research addresses the need for gender and migration sensitive indicators that value and reflect women's lives, work, productivity, and social, cultural, and economic security over the lifespan. Dr Vissandjée is a member of a Québec advisory board at the Ministry of Health in Québec, whose mandate is to contribute to equitable access to quality care for the diversity of women, men, families, and groups, especially newcomers. She also sits on the advisory board of the CIHR Institute of Gender and Health and has long-standing collaborations with institutions such as the International Development Research Council, the Shastri Indo-Canadian Institute, The Aga Khan Foundation, and the United Nations Development Program, among others.

Index